Neurological Differential Diagnosis

D1355613

Neurological Differential Diagnosis

A Prioritized Approach

Roongroj Bhidayasiri, MD, MRCP(UK), MRCPI

Department of Neurology
David Geffen School of Medicine at UCLA and
Parkinson Disease Research, Education and Clinical Center (PADRECC) of West Los Angeles
Veterans Affairs Medical Center
Los Angeles, CA

Michael F. Waters, MD, PhD

Department of Neurology
David Geffen School of Medicine at UCLA
Los Angeles, CA

Christopher C. Giza, MD

UCLA Brain Injury Research Center
Divisions of Neurosurgery and Pediatric Neurology
David Geffen School of Medicine at UCLA
Los Angeles, CA

Blackwell
Publishing

First published 2005

Library of Congress Cataloging-in-Publication Data

Bhidayasiri, Roongroj.
    Neurological differential diagnosis : a prioritized approach / by Roongroj Bhidayasiri, Michael F.
Waters, Christopher C. Giza.
    p. ; cm.
    Includes index.
    ISBN-13: 978-1-4051-2039-5 (alk. paper)
    ISBN-10: 1-4051-2039-8 (alk. paper)
1. Nervous system--Diseases--Diagnosis--Handbooks, manuals, etc. 2. Diagnosis, Differential--Hand-
books, manuals, etc.
[DNLM: 1. Nervous System Diseases--diagnosis--Handbooks. 2. Diagnostic Techniques, Neurological-
-Handbooks.] I. Waters, Michael F. II. Giza, Christopher C., 1965- III. Title.

    RC348.B485 2005
    616.8'0475--dc22

                                                                                    2005001189

ISBN 13: 978-1-4051-2039-5
ISBN 10: 1-4051-2039-8

A catalogue record for this title is available from the British Library

Set in 10/13 pt Minion by Sparks, Oxford – www.sparks.co.uk
Printed and bound in India by Gopsons Papers Limited, New Delhi

Commissioning Editor: Stuart Taylor
Development Editor: Kate Bailey and Katrina Chandler
Production Controller: Kate Charman

For further information on Blackwell Publishing, visit our website:
http://www.blackwellpublishing.com

The publisher's policy is to use permanent paper from mills that operate a sustainable forestry policy,
and which has been manufactured from pulp processed using acid-free and elementary chlorine-free
practices. Furthermore, the publisher ensures that the text paper and cover board used have met acceptable environmental accreditation standards.

Although every effort has been made to ensure that drug doses and other information are presented
accurately in this publication, the ultimate responsibility rests with the treating physician. Neither the
publishers nor the authors can be held responsible for any consequences arising from the use of information contained herein. Any product mentioned in this publication should be used in accordance
with the prescribing information prepared by the manufacturers.

Dedication

To my loving grandmother, Pranom Chivakiat, my parents, Mitr & Nisaratana Bhidayasiri, all my teachers of neurology, and lastly all my patients who have taught me much about neurology.

RB

I would like to dedicate this work to my family, friends, and colleagues, especially Alejandra, for helping to keep my tank full.

MFW

To my wonderful wife, Rosanne, who gave me our son and greatest joy, Vincent, and my parents, Chester & Yueh-hua who started me on my journey.

CCG

Contents

Foreword

Every time a physician encounters a patient for the purpose of diagnosis and treatment, a complicated process occurs. It is obvious that this process must be successful if a physician is to choose an optimal therapy in a timely fashion. Such reasoning requires the physician to identify important facts in the history from the patient, family members, and, in some cases, witnesses. The appearance of the patient and the physical examination confirm suspicions identified from the history. The importance of signs and symptoms must be ranked in terms of their relative importance to the diagnosis at hand, eliminating artifactual information as well as true findings that are irrelevant to the current diagnosis, such as those related to prior diagnoses. The resulting set of facts must then be applied to a large store of possible disorders weighted by the patient's demographic features such as gender, age, ethnicity, habits, and geographical factors as well as the time-intensity relationship (e.g. acute, subacute, chronic) and temporal pattern (e.g. progressive, episodic, relapsing) of the onset of the medical problem at hand.

The nervous system provides a unique set of deductive reasoning opportunities in that its architecture is not homogeneous but compartmentalized by functional systems composed of groups of cell bodies and the fiber tracts that connect them. This information can then be applied to possible diagnoses constrained by anatomical localization, temporal features, and demographics. What emerges is a short, prioritized list by likelihood, and, most importantly, concern for possibilities that could be life threatening or produce irreparable damage to the nervous system. This working diagnosis is then confirmed, first during the physical examination itself, and later by laboratory methods including electrophysiological tests, imaging, and analysis of body fluids or biopsy material. Once confirmed, treatment may begin.

Thus, a large body of information is sifted down to the salient facts and converging in overlapping indicators that allow the selection of this short differential diagnostic list. In many ways, this is an exercise in probability. In fact, numerous attempts have been made to reduce the diagnostic decision-making process to a mathematical one. Computers are especially well suited to help in collecting and processing clinical information. They can be used to retain large lists with the capability of convergence on the most likely answer, with special attention to those diagnoses that may be life threatening. The applications of symbolic logic, probability theory, value theory, and Boolean algebra have all been employed in these automated strategies. Such approaches have taught us what we see and know from the clinic on an everyday basis. Medical diagnostics should emphasize the fundamental importance of considering combinations of symptoms or symptom complexes. This is important because all too often an evaluation is made of a sign or symptom by itself, without respect to the other features of the disorder, often leading to errors. The consideration of a combination of signs and symptoms that a patient does and does not have, in relation to possible combinations of disease, is a most effective and efficient approach to the diagnostic process.

This text is a marvelous example of providing the practical and probabilistic approach to patients with disorders of the nervous system. It emphasizes probability because a neurological diagnosis can rarely be made with absolute certainty at the bedside, but rather a short list of the 'most likely' diagnoses is made and then one is later confirmed. At the same time, the authors have made the important contribution of also identifying those potential diagnoses that would acutely be life threatening or result in irreparable damage to the brain, spinal cord, or peripheral nerves. The importance of this strategy is self-evident. By clustering their approach in accordance with the usual categories of neurological disorders, the process of identifying a complex of patient symptoms, signs, demographic factors, and temporal relationships leading to the appropriate diagnosis is simplified for the reader.

The authors have done a superb job in producing a text that is efficient, easy to use, practical, and accurate. Their motivation comes from practical experience. The clinician, particularly the clinician in training, needs to be able to find and quickly assess information about the patient with whom they are concerned at that moment. It is their job to sift through the facts and artifacts, as noted above, and bring the salient information to be merged with the compendium of lists and diseases provided in this text.

Great diagnosticians, from experience and through their ability to generate an instant rapport with the patient, arrive at accurate diagnoses in a remarkably efficient fashion. Great diagnosticians also have an excellent memory for the facts of their field. Good memory alone and the ability to efficiently prioritize data provided by the patient are not enough, however. It is the ability to rapidly converge those data sets to a short list or a final diagnosis that makes a good physician a great diagnostician. This text provides a vehicle to help the reader think in that fashion and move toward that role model. The authors have done a masterful job in facilitating the process. I am certain they can be persuaded to apply these strategies to future projects and to expand this approach within the fields of neurology and neurosurgery.

A final comment: diagnoses, diseases, signs, and symptoms, along with their probabilities, life threatening potentials, and other quantifiable variables are all part of the practice of medicine. These issues are the factors that allow us to determine what is wrong with a patient and provide treatments for their benefit. The patient with an illness is also a human being in trouble who seeks the help of another person with special knowledge and training. That distinction and the compassion required to help both the person and the patient is as important as any drug or procedure that we as physicians can provide.

John C. Mazziotta, MD, PhD
Los Angeles, California
March 30, 2004

Preface

This book has its roots in our perceived need for a concise text to assist the practitioner in prioritizing likely diagnoses when encountering a patient complaining of neurological problems or deficits. Though many references exist on neurological disease and differential diagnoses, few offer easily referable likely diagnoses based on common complaints and presentation. When one approaches differential diagnosis in neurology, there is frequently a feeling of overwhelming information. It is often one's first appreciation of the complexities of neurological disease and the elegance of the neurological system when realizing that seemingly 'anything can cause anything'. When constructing a neurological differential diagnosis, it is often inevitable that a page-long laundry list is quickly compiled. And, although it is true that one cannot make a diagnosis that one doesn't think of, it is also true that the overwhelming majority of diagnoses can be made by considering the top five or so possibilities. Common things are commonly seen. Moreover, it is also true that one practices today in an environment of limited time and limited resources. Therefore, shouldn't one be considering the most likely diagnoses first, working up those possibilities, and moving forward if that approach fails to yield the answer? The caveat, of course, is that dangerous or disabling diagnoses must be considered early on to limit death and disability. These principles have directed the construction of this book. While many of the differentials are somewhat lengthy, they are arranged to direct the reader to consider the most likely and most dangerous possibilities first, saving the lesser possibilities for those instances when a comprehensive differential is required for an accurate diagnosis. This book is not, nor is it intended to be, an exhaustive reference. It is, however, an attempt to rationally focus one's attention in a 'high-yield' manner. In writing this text, we are seeking to strike a balance between being comprehensive and being practical. It is our hope that you will find this book a valuable resource when confronted with the task of formulating a neurological differential diagnosis. Collectively, we all wish we had had it during our training, particularly on those late nights in the emergency department.

Roongroj Bhidayasiri, Michael F. Waters, Christopher C. Giza

Acknowledgments

We wish to thank the following reviewers for their thoughtful comments and suggestions that have been of immense help to us in the development of this book.

Robert Baloh *(Neuro-ophthalmology and Neuro-otology)*
Jeff Bronstein *(Movement Disorders)*
Dennis Chute *(Neuroanatomy and Neuropathology)*
Timothy Cloughsey *(Neuro-oncology)*
Robert Collins *(Diagnostic Tests)*
George Ellison *(Clinical Syndromes)*
Stanley Fahn *(Movement Disorders)*
Michael Graves *(Peripheral Neurology)*
Leif Havton *(Spinal Cord Disorders)*
Joanna Jen *(Neurogenetics)*
Mario Mendez *(Neuropsychiatry and Dementias)*
Noriko Salamon *(Neuroradiology)*
Raman Sankar *(Pediatric Neurology)*
Jeffrey Saver *(Vascular Neurology)*
Nancy Sicotte *(Infectious, Inflammatory and Demyelinating Disorders)*
John Stern *(Paroxysmal Disorders)*

How to Use this Book

The purpose of this book is to clarify the possible diagnoses for a given neurological presentation, but in a fashion that prioritizes the differential diagnosis (DDx), based on the frequency of a particular disorder or on the potential for death/disability if the diagnosis is missed acutely.

This book is divided into chapters covering major points of neurological differential diagnosis. Some chapters will include more descriptive listings, such as Chapter 2: Clinical Syndromes. However, most chapters will adhere to a format of covering a particular set of related neurological problems. At the beginning of each chapter there will be an outline listing the disorders covered therein. Following this may be some general discussion of approach or work-up. The majority of each chapter will be devoted to lists of diagnoses related to a common primary sign or symptom that will be the title of a given differential diagnosis.

Each topic will have a gray box that covers the general approach to this particular clinical complex. These include descriptions of commonly confused entities, assistance in organizing the diagnostic work-up, and even clinical 'pearls' that are relevant to the entities being considered.

The individual diagnoses will generally be arranged in decreasing order of frequency or decreasing order of acute mortality/morbidity. Very common or very threatening diagnoses will be listed first, often with a few descriptive points to allow the reader to quickly discern salient clinical distinctions between these 'top contenders'. Correspondingly, less emphasis is placed on the specific order of low frequency or low morbidity disorders, and less detail is provided for these diagnoses.

Bold indicates the most likely diagnoses for a particular sign/symptom/differential, as determined by epidemiology and clinical experience. Sometimes the most common diagnoses may be diagnoses of exclusion. Often the most common diagnoses will not be the most dangerous.

Italics indicate diagnoses that are less likely, but are life threatening or disabling in the acute or subacute period, and thus should be considered and ruled out. Diagnoses likely to result in late death or disability (tumors, motor neuron disease, etc.) may not be listed thus. (Note that this use of italics has meant that we have ignored the usual convention of using italics for the binomial nomenclature of organisms. Thus, *E. coli*, for example, appears in italics only if it is part of a life-threatening diagnosis.)

Bold italics indicate diagnoses that are both common for the given differential and potentially immediately life threatening or disabling.

A diagnosis that is not in **bold** or *italics* does not imply that this diagnosis is unimportant. These diagnoses are either less common or not acutely dangerous or debilitating. However, they may still result in progressive problems or even death, particularly if they remain undiagnosed for a longer duration of time.

It is appropriate to initially consider a differential diagnosis (DDx) by focusing on **very common** or *very dangerous* entities. However, during the course of evaluation and work-up, and as these possibilities are ruled out, the less common or less acutely threatening diagnoses must be considered until the definitive diagnosis is made. *Furthermore, if a diagnosis is made but the clinical symptomatology is atypical or changing, or the response to intervention is different from what is normally anticipated, the clinician must revisit the original differential diagnosis to ensure that the correct etiology is not missed.*

Approaching neurological differential diagnosis

Many generalists and neurological trainees may initially approach neurological diagnosis as a 'black box'. However, even with only a basic understanding of neurology, it is possible to generate and follow comprehensive differentials to arrive at a correct diagnosis.

First, *one should consider if there is an obvious or very likely diagnosis* for a given patient. Nonetheless, it is important, even in apparently simple cases, to **avoid becoming fixated on a particular diagnosis too early**, as this may lead one to ignore contradictory data that might actually lead to the correct diagnosis.

Secondly, *consider what are the patient's main signs/symptoms*. A prioritized DDx may be generated for each major symptom. Diagnoses that overlap between these lists should then be primary considerations for the work-up and treatment of that particular patient. It is important to use prioritized DDx lists, to properly weight commonly occurring conditions. This does not preclude returning to the original DDx if an initial diagnostic assumption should prove to be incorrect or inconsistent with new data or symptoms.

When generating a neurological DDx without a handbook, there are several approaches. One of the simplest is to consider the patient's primary problem, and to list potential disorders that affect each level of the neuraxis. Thus, when approaching a patient with leg weakness, one may generate a comprehensive (although not prioritized) DDx by starting at the muscle and moving cranially.

1 Myopathy
2 Neuromuscular junction disorder
3 Neuropathy
4 Plexopathy/radiculopathy

5 Spinal cord disorder
6 Cerebral disorder

Another method of generating a comprehensive DDx is to think about categories of disease/etiologies and consider diagnostic possibilities for each potential etiology. Using the same example of leg weakness, the following DDx might be made:

1 Metabolic: peripheral neuropathy (uremia, nutritional deficiency)
2 Endocrine: thyroid disease, diabetes
3 Drugs/medicines: corticosteroids, aminoglycosides
4 Infectious: polio, viral myositis
5 Congenital: tethered cord, spina bifida occulta, syrinx
6 Immunologic/inflammatory: myositis, neuritis, myelitis
7 Neoplastic: paraneoplastic syndrome, tumor
8 Ischemic: cerebral infarction, spinal cord infarction
9 Degenerative: motor neuron disease
10 Demyelinating: MS, Guillain-Barré
11 Compressive: radiculopathy, compression neuropathy
12 Toxic/occupational: toxin exposure

Either of these methods is a good starting place, but then the diagnoses need to be prioritized. Patient demographics, other symptoms, exam findings, and results from diagnostic tests all serve to fine tune this comprehensive DDx into a 'working DDx'.

Probability is of great importance for a good diagnostician. At least three points of probability should be considered with each differential.

1 How common is the disease being considered?
2 How common is this disease in the particular demographic to which the patient belongs?
3 How common are the patient's particular signs/symptoms as a presentation of the disease being considered?

For example, a young woman presents with an acute headache, in association with blurred vision and nausea. She is concerned about the possibility of a brain tumor. While it is possible for a brain tumor to present in this manner, it is very unlikely. Furthermore, young women are not a particular demographic at risk for rapidly progressive brain tumors. Migraine headaches could also cause these symptoms, and happen to be more common in young females. In fact, all of the patient's symptoms would fit with such a diagnosis. It would then be important to obtain information regarding particular aspects of the patient's problem that would help distinguish between these possibilities and settle on a most likely diagnosis.

Let us presume that examination shows no focality and no papilledema, and her family history is positive for migraines. Her headache came on over 10–15 minutes, and this is the second headache of this sort she has experienced over the last month. In this clinical setting, progressive increased intracranial pressure becomes less likely, and migraine moves to the top of the differential.

What if her headache was actually progressively worsening over the last 3 weeks? The possibility of raised intracranial pressure is more likely. What if her neurological exam showed a sixth nerve palsy and papilledema? This could be evidence of a focal intracranial mass, or even signs of nonfocal, generalized increased intracranial pressure. The working differential diagnosis now includes mass lesion, hydrocephalus, and pseudotumor cerebri, all ranked higher than migraine headache. This hypothetical illustrates how one might use prioritization to arrive at the correct diagnosis.

This text is designed to assist in prioritizing the DDx from the start, without overlooking rare but potentially serious diagnoses. Primary topics may be searched by chapter outline or through the index at the end of the book.

Other general notes regarding format

Any lists of characteristic signs/symptoms for a specific diagnosis are to be considered in addition to the primary sign/symptom listed in the differential's title. In other words, in the ataxia DDx, the clinical signs and symptoms listed for, say, SCA1, are *in addition to* the primary symptom of ataxia.

In general, major diagnoses or diagnostic categories will be numbered (1, 2, 1.1, 1.2, 1.1.1, etc.). Clinical characteristics and information about a diagnosis or category will be bulleted (•, ♦, ▪, etc.).

When an inheritance pattern is known and is relevant, it will generally be noted. The following abbreviations will be used: AD = autosomal dominant; AR = autosomal recessive; XL = X-linked.

Chapter 1

Neuroanatomy and Neuropathology

Neuroanatomy and normal functions

General

Blood-brain barrier

- The blood-brain barrier (BBB) isolates the CNS from the molecular and cellular constituents of the blood.
- It has characteristic features of vascular structures, including a vascular basement membrane, vascular endothelial cells, and perivascular macrophages.
- In addition, it has characteristic features unique to the CNS, including:
  - tight junctions between vascular endothelial cells,

- the coating of blood vessels and pial surface of the brain by astrocytic foot processes,
- a complete absence of fluid-phase endocytosis, and
- highly restricted receptor mediated endocytosis.
- The BBB can be broken down by viral, bacteria, or fungal infections.
- The BBB is also incomplete in the vicinity of many brain tumors.
- This fact is used to advantage in neuroimaging studies, where contrast agents such as gadolinium and iodine-containing compounds may pass across areas of faulty BBB and result in increased signals on MRI and CT scans, respectively.

The BBB is absent in the following regions. This arrangement allows relatively free passage of large protein molecules into and out of these regions.

1 Basal hypothalamus
2 Pineal gland
3 Area postrema of the fourth ventricle
4 Small areas near the third ventricle

Major brain structures and functions

- We provide this table as a quick guide to major intracranial structures and their functions. Some structures may have more than one function, although only the main function is included.

Structure	Main function
Amygdala	Emotions/autonomic functions
Basal ganglia • Caudate • Putamen • Globus pallidus • Subthalamic nucleus	Frontal lobe connected • Motor functions • Output structure of basal ganglia • Output structure of indirect pathway of basal ganglia circuitry
Central canal	Continuation of ventricular system in the spinal cord
Cerebellar peduncles • Superior cerebellar peduncles • Middle cerebellar peduncles	Outflow pathway from cerebellum • Inflow pathway from cerebrum to cerebellum
Cerebellum	Coordinates movement of the body
Cerebral peduncles	Carry motor information from brainstem to spinal cord
Circular sulcus	CSF space between insula and overlying opercular cortex

Continued

Structure	Main function
Corpus callosum	Interconnects cerebral hemispheres
Foramen of Monro	Connecting lateral and third ventricles
Hippocampus	Memory
Hypothalamus	Regulating appetite, thirst, sexual drive, neuroendocrine and autonomic functions
Inferior colliculus	Auditory system
Insula	Emotions/autonomic functions
Internal capsule	Connections of motor pathway between cerebral cortex and cerebral peduncles
Periaqueductal gray	Pain experience/modulation
Pyramids	Carrying motor information from brainstem to spinal cord
Septum pellucidum	Separate lateral ventricles
Superior colliculus	Visual system
Sylvian aqueduct	Connecting third and fourth ventricles
Thalamus	Relay information center from brainstem to cortex and between cortical regions

Common neurotransmitters

- A large number of molecules act as neurotransmitters at chemical synapses. These neurotransmitters are present in the synaptic terminal and their action may be blocked by pharmacologic agents.
- The major steps in neurotransmitter processing are:
  1 synthesis,
  2 storage,
  3 release,
  4 reception, and
  5 inactivation.
- Abnormal activities of these neurotransmitters have been implicated in various neurological disorders.

Neuro-transmitters	Precursor, enzymes	Receptors	Areas of concentration	Related disorders
Acetylcholine (Ach)	Choline, Choline-O-acetyltransferase	Nicotinic Muscarinic	Basal nucleus of Meynert, Limbic system, NM junctions, Parasympathetic neurons, Autonomic ganglia	Alzheimer disease, Myasthenia gravis, Botulism

Neuro-transmitters	Precursor, enzymes	Receptors	Areas of concentration	Related disorders
Dopamine	Phenylalanine, Tyrosine hydroxylase DOPA decarboxylase	D1 D2 (main receptors) D3, D4, D5	Nigrostriatal pathway, Hypothalamus	Parkinson disease, Prolactinoma, Schizophrenia
Norepinephrine (NE)	Phenylalanine, Tyrosine hydroxylase Dopamine-β-hydroxylase	α-receptor β-receptor	Locus coeruleus, Lateral tegmental nuclei, Sympathetic ganglia	Sleep-wake cycle
Glutamate	α-Ketoglutarate, Glutamate dehydrogenase	NMDA, Kainate, AMPA	Cerebral cortex, Brainstem, Spinal cord, Hippocampus	Epilepsy, Migraine, Stroke
Gamma-aminobutyric acid (GABA)	Glutamate, Glutamic acid decarboxylase (GAD)	$GABA_A$ $GABA_B$	Striatonigral system, Cerebellum, Hippocampus, Cerebral cortex	Sleep, Epilepsy Anxiety
Glycine	Serine		Spinal cord, Brainstem	Tetanus, Strychnine poisoning
Serotonin	Tryptophan, Tryptophan hydroxylase		Raphe nuclei	Levels of arousal, Pain modulation, Migraine, Depression

Reflexes

- The afferent nerve emanating from the receptor endings project on alpha motor neurons in the spinal cord, which in turn supply the extrafusal fibers. Thus, when a muscle is stretched by tapping its tendon, the stimulated receptor endings initiate an impulse in the afferent nerves, which stimulates the alpha motor neurons and results in a reflex muscle contraction. As soon as the muscle contracts, the tension in the intrafusal muscle fibers decreases, the receptor response diminishes, and the muscle relaxes. This is the concept of all monosynaptic stretch reflexes.

Reflexes	Center	Afferent nerve	Efferent nerve
Deep reflexes			
Jaw	Pons	Trigeminal nerve	Trigeminal nerve
Biceps	C5, 6	Musculocutaneous nerve	Musculocutaneous nerve

Continued

Reflexes	Center	Afferent nerve	Efferent nerve
Deep reflexes			
Triceps	C6, 7	Radial nerve	Radial nerve
Periosteoradial	C6, 7, 8	Radial nerve	Radial nerve
Wrist flexion	C6, 7, 8	Median nerve	Median nerve
Wrist extension	C7, 8	Radial nerve	Radial nerve
Patellar (knee jerk)	L2, 3, 4	Femoral nerve	Femoral nerve
Achilles (ankle jerk)	S1, 2	Tibial nerve	Tibial nerve
Superficial reflexes			
Corneal	Pons	Trigeminal nerve	Facial nerve
Nasal (sneeze)	Brainstem and upper cervical cord	Trigeminal nerve	Combinations of trigeminal, facial, glossopharyngeal, vagus, and spinal nerve of expiration
Pharyngeal and uvula	Medulla	Glossopharyngeal nerve	Vagus nerve
Upper abdominal	T7, 8, 9, 10	T7, 8, 9, 10	T7, 8, 9, 10
Lower abdominal	T10, 11, 12	T10, 11, 12	T10, 11, 12
Cremasteric	L1	Femoral nerve	Genitofemoral nerve
Plantar	S1, 2	Tibial nerve	Tibial nerve
Anal	S4, 5	Pudendal nerve	Pudendal nerve
Visceral reflexes			
Light	Midbrain	Optic nerve	Oculomotor nerve
Accommodation	Occipital cortex	Optic nerve	Oculomotor nerve
Ciliospinal	T1, 2	A sensory nerve	Cervical sympathetics
Oculocardiac	Medulla	Trigeminal nerve	Vagus nerve
Carotid sinus	Medulla	Glossopharyngeal nerve	Vagus nerve
Bulbocavernosus	S2, 3, 4	Pudendal nerve	Pelvic autonomic fibers
Bladder and rectal	S2, 3, 4	Pudendal nerve	Pudendal nerve and autonomic fibers

Cranial floor/foramina

- The internal, or superior, surface of the skull base forms the floor of the cranial cavity. It is divided into three fossae: anterior, middle, and posterior.
- A number of openings (termed foramens) provide entrance and exit routes through the floor of the cranial cavity, for vascular structures, cranial nerves, and the medulla.

Foramina	Structures
ANTERIOR CRANIAL FOSSA	
Cribiform plate of ethmoid	Olfactory nerves
MIDDLE CRANIAL FOSSA	
Optic foramen	Optic nerve Ophthalmic artery Meninges
Superior orbital fissure	Oculomotor nerve Trochlear nerve Abducens nerve Ophthalmic division of the trigeminal nerve (V1) Superior ophthalmic vein
Foramen rotundum	Maxillary division of the trigeminal nerve (V2)
Foramen ovale	Mandibular division of the trigeminal nerve (V3)
Foramen lacerum	Internal carotid artery Sympathetic plexus
Foramen spinosum	Middle meningeal artery and vein
Foramen of Vesalius	Emissary veins and clusters of venules
POSTERIOR CRANIAL FOSSA	
Internal acoustic meatus	Facial nerve Vestibulocochlear nerve Internal auditory artery
Jugular foramen	Glossopharyngeal nerve Vagus nerve Spinal accessory nerve Sigmoid sinus
Hypoglossal canal	Hypoglossal nerve
Foramen magnum	Medulla Meninges Spinal accessory nerve Vertebral arteries Anterior and posterior spinal arteries

Cranial nerves

Ganglia related to cranial nerves

- Two types of ganglia are related to cranial nerves.
  - The first type contains cell bodies of afferent somatic or visceral axons within the cranial nerves. These ganglia are somewhat similar to the dorsal root ganglia.
  - The second type contains the synaptic terminals of visceral efferent axons, together with postsynaptic parasympathetic neurons that project peripherally.

Ganglia	Cranial nerve	Functional type
Ciliary	III, Oculomotor	Visceral efferent (parasympathetic)
Semilunar	V, Trigeminal	Sensory afferent
Pterygopalatine	VII, Facial	Visceral efferent (parasympathetic)
Submandibular	VII, Facial	Visceral efferent (parasympathetic)
Geniculate	VII, Facial	Visceral afferent (taste)
Spiral	VIII, Vestibulocochlear	Sensory
Vestibular	VIII, Vestibulocochlear	Sensory
Otic	IX, Glossopharyngeal	Visceral efferent (parasympathetic)
Inferior and superior	IX, Glossopharyngeal	Somatic afferent, visceral afferent (taste)
Intramural	X, Vagus	Visceral efferent (parasympathetic)
Inferior and superior	X, Vagus	Somatic afferent, visceral afferent (taste)

Cranial nerves: exits and functions

- The 12 pairs of cranial nerves exit from the forebrain (the first two) and brainstem. They provide sensory and motor function for the head and convey special senses (sight, smell, hearing, balance, and taste) and participate in the control of viscera.
- Cranial nerves can be purely sensory, motor or mixed and can contain efferent or afferent autonomic fibers.
- All but one of the cranial nerves exit the brain from the ventral or lateral surface and are visible on ventral view. The olfactory and optic nerves are found on the forebrain, while the rest are located in the brainstem.

Cranial nerves	Type, nuclei	Brain region entry/exit	Foramina	Functions
I, Olfactory	Sensory	Uncus and posterior inferior frontal lobes	Cribiform plate of ethmoid	Sense of smell
II, Optic	Sensory	Thalamus (lateral geniculate body)	Optic foramen	Vision
III, Oculomotor	Motor and parasympathetic Oculomotor and Edinger-Westphal nuclei	Midbrain	Superior orbital fissure	Eye movement Pupillary constriction
IV, Trochlear	Motor Trochlear nucleus	Midbrain	Superior orbital fissure	Control of superior oblique muscle
V, Trigeminal	Sensory, motor Main sensory, spinal, mesencephalic, motor nuclei	Pons	V1: Superior orbital fissure V2: Foramen rotundum V3: Foramen ovale	Control of muscles of mastication Sensation on the face, mouth and anterior/ mid-cranial fossa
VI, Abducens	Motor Abducens nucleus	Pontomedullary junction	Superior orbital fissure	Control of lateral rectus muscle
VII, Facial	Motor, sensory, parasympathetic Facial, superior salivatory, solitary nuclei	Pontomedullary junction	Internal acoustic meatus	Control of muscles of facial expression Sense of taste in anterior 2/3 of the tongue, control of lacrimation
VIII, Vestibulo-cochlear	Sensory Cochlear (2) and vestibular (4) nuclei	Pontomedullary junction	Internal acoustic meatus	Hearing and balance
IX, Glosso-pharyngeal	Motor, sensory, parasympathetic Ambiguus, inferior salivatory, solitary nuclei	Medulla	Jugular foramen	Control of stylopharyngeus muscle, parotid gland Sense of taste in posterior 1/3 of the tongue
X, Vagus	Motor, sensory, parasympathetic Dorsal motor, ambiguus, solitary nuclei	Medulla	Jugular foramen	Control of pharyngeal muscles Visceral autonomic sensation and control

Continued

Cranial nerves	Type, nuclei	Brain region entry/exit	Foramina	Functions
XI, Accessory	Motor Spinal accessory, ambiguus nuclei	Cervicomedullary junction	Jugular foramen	Control of sternocleidomastoid and trapezius muscles
XII, Hypoglossal	Motor, Hypoglossal nucleus	Medulla	Hypoglossal canal	Control of the tongue

Cranial nerve I (olfactory nerve)

- Although the olfactory system is not of major importance in neurological diagnosis, certain clinical information useful in neuroanatomical localization can be attained by investigating the sense of smell.
- Olfactory pathway:
  - Olfactory epithelium → olfactory bulb → olfactory tract → lateral (primary), medial, and intermediate olfactory areas → medial forebrain bundle, striae medullaris, and striae terminalis → reticular formation and cranial nerve nuclei responsible for visceral responses.
- Lateral or primary olfactory area includes cortex of the uncus, entorhinal area, limen insula, and part of amygdaloid body.
- Because olfactory loss is usually unilateral, each nostril must be tested separately.

Causes of olfactory impairment:

1 **Head injury**
  - Can cause tearing of the olfactory fibers that traverse the cribiform plate, thereby resulting in ipsilateral loss of olfaction (anosmia).
  - Closed head injury can also produce impairment of olfactory recognition despite preserved olfactory detection.
2 Tumors
  - Frontal lobe masses in the floor of anterior cranial fossa can cause ipsilateral anosmia, ipsilateral optic atrophy, and contralateral papilledema, called Foster-Kennedy syndrome.
  - Temporal lobe mass involving primary olfactory area can result in olfactory hallucinations with phantom smell (usually unpleasant).
3 Rare causes of anosmia:
  - Congenital anosmia or hyposmia: can occur secondary to cleft palate in males
  - Familial dysautonomia
  - Turner syndrome
  - Kallmann syndrome: permanent anosmia, hypogonadotropic hypogonadism

Cranial nerve II (optic nerve)

- Functions: special sensory. Provides light perception and visual information from the retinas.
- Retinal ganglion cells are actually extensions of the CNS and not strictly speaking nerves. However, by convention, pre-chiasm pathways are referred to as the optic nerves, and post-chiasm pathways are referred to as the optic tracts.
- Because the image projected on the retina is inverted and reversed, images from the lower visual field project to the primary visual cortex superior to the calcarine fissure and images in the right visual field project to the left primary visual cortex. The inverse is also true.
- Complete evaluation of the visual system should include visual acuity, visual fields by confrontation, color vision, pupillary response (both direct and consensual), and ophthalmoscopic exam (evaluating the optic disk for pallor, swelling, and margins). Symptoms should be characterized as positive (flashing lights, fortification spectra) or negative (blind spots).
- The afferent papillary light reflex bypasses both the lateral geniculate body as well as the cortex.

Clinical spectrum	Lesion localization
Monocular visual deficits	Anterior to the optic chiasm including eye, retina, or optic nerve
Bitemporal visual field deficits	At the optic chiasm
Monocular blindness and contralateral field deficit	Ipsilateral optic nerve with contralateral nasal retinal fibers in the chiasm
Bitemporal hemianopia	Optic chiasm
Homonymous hemianopia with preservation of central vision	Lateral geniculate body
Binocular homonymous visual field deficits	Optic tract, lateral geniculate nucleus, optic radiations, or visual cortex
Contralateral homonymous hemianopia	Primary visual cortex superior and inferior to the calcarine fissure or entire optic radiation
Contralateral superior quadrantanopsia (pie in the sky)	Optic radiations in the temporal lobes or primary visual cortex inferior to the calcarine fissure
Contralateral inferior quadrantanopsia (pie on the floor)	Optic radiations in the parietal lobes or primary visual cortex superior to the calcarine fissure
Variable homonymous hemianopia with macular sparing	Occipital lobe

MONOCULAR VISUAL LOSS: ACUTE OR TRANSIENT

1 **Vascular**
  - Typically a central or branch retinal artery occlusion of the ophthalmic artery.
    1.1 *Embolism*: cardiac origin or commonly artery-to-artery emboli from ipsilateral internal carotid disease.
    1.2 Atherosclerosis: resulting in critical stenoses, associated with hypertension and diabetes.
    1.3 Migraine with scotoma
    1.4 *Vasculitis: temporal arteritis*
    1.5 Vasospasm: migraine or *hypertensive crisis*
    1.6 *Hypotension* with critical arterial stenosis
2 Ocular
    2.1 Structural
        2.1.1 *Retinal detachment*
        2.1.2 Retinitis pigmentosa
    2.2 Infectious: frequently associated with HIV infection
        2.2.1 Cytomegalovirus
        2.2.2 Histoplasmosis
        2.2.3 Toxoplasmosis

CHRONIC, PROGRESSIVE MONOCULAR VISUAL LOSS

1 **Optic neuritis**
  - Accompanied by pain and color desaturation.
  - May be presenting symptom of multiple sclerosis.
2 Anterior ischemic optic neuropathy: stepwise, painless visual loss
3 Optic nerve compression
  - Associated with proptosis, restricted eye movement, retro-orbital pain, headache.
    3.1 Neoplastic process
    3.2 Vascular malformation
4 Leber optic neuropathy
  - Typically males 10–30 years old.
  - Painless monocular vision loss over days.
  - Mitochrondrial disorder. Progresses to bilateral involvement.

BINOCULAR VISION LOSS

May be complete, central sparing, or a field cut.

1 *Cerebral infarction*
  - May involve optic tracts or primary visual cortex (typically central sparing or field cut).
2 Ocular etiologies
    2.1 *Bilateral papilledema*

Cranial nerve III (oculomotor nerve)

- The oculomotor nerve supplies four extraocular muscles (medial, superior, inferior recti, and inferior oblique) as well as the levator of the lid, and contains parasympathetic fibers that supply the sphincter of the pupil and ciliary body.
- The complete peripheral third nerve palsy causes ptosis, a fixed and dilated pupil, and a 'down and out' resting eye position.
- Partial third nerve palsy may cause variable ptosis, variable paresis of eye adduction, elevation, depression, and variable pupillary involvement.
- Patients with non-isolated third nerve palsy should undergo neuroimaging with attention to areas suggested by associated signs and symptoms.
- Compression of the third nerve by aneurysm characteristically causes pupillary dilatation and unresponsiveness. Occasionally, it can spare the pupil and the pupillary involvement may occur later. Therefore, a pupillary sparing third nerve palsy does not always rule out compressive lesions.

Structure involved	Physical signs	Etiology
Oculomotor nucleus	Ipsilateral complete third nerve palsy, contralateral ptosis and superior rectus paresis	*Stroke (brainstem)* Tumor Demyelination
Oculomotor fasciculus		*Stroke (brainstem)* Tumor Demyelination
• Fascicle, red nucleus, superior cerebellar peduncle	Isolated third nerve palsy with contralateral ataxia and tremor or *Claude syndrome*	
• Fascicle, cerebral peduncle	Ipsilateral third nerve palsy with contralateral hemiparesis or *Weber syndrome*	
• Fascicle, red nucleus, substantia nigra	Ipsilateral third nerve palsy and choreiform movement or *Benedikt syndrome*	
Oculomotor nerve in the subarachnoid space	Complete third nerve palsy with or without other cranial nerve involvement	Ischemia *Aneurysm* *Trauma (herniation)* *Meningitis* Metastasis
Oculomotor nerve in the cavernous sinus	Painful or painless third nerve palsy with or without paresis of CN IV, V1, VI	*Sinus thrombosis* *Hemorrhage* Tumor *Meningitis* *Aneurysm* Granulomatous disease
Oculomotor nerve in the superior orbital fissure	Third nerve palsy with or without paresis of CN IV, V1, VI, often with proptosis	Tumor, *Aneurysm* Trauma Local infection, *meningitis*
Oculomotor nerve in the orbit	Third nerve palsy, may be selected superior or inferior third nerve palsy, proptosis may present	Tumor *Aneurysm* Trauma

Cranial nerve IV (trochlear nerve)

- Functions: somatic motor. Supplies efferent innervation to the superior oblique muscle of the eye. This muscle effects inward rotation (intorsion) as well as downward and lateral movement of the eye.
- Anatomy: Nucleus: near midline midbrain tegmentum → decussates in superior medullary velum → exits brainstem caudal to inferior colliculus → wraps around cerebral peduncle, between superior cerebellar and posterior cerebral arteries, lateral to CNIII → anteriorly into cavernous sinus → along lateral wall of cavernous sinus → superior orbital fissure → medially along orbital roof.

- The smallest cranial nerve (approximately 2,400 axons).
- The cranial nerve with the longest intracranial course.
- The only cranial nerve with complete decussation.
- The only cranial nerve to exit the brainstem dorsally.

Common clinical pathologies
1 Vascular
   - *Aneurysms* of the posterior cerebral or superior cerebellar artery may compress the trochlear nerve.
2 Inflammation
   - Inflammatory processes may affect the trochlear nerve.
3 Cavernous sinus pathology
   - Multiple pathologies of the cavernous sinus, including:
     - Mass lesions: tumors, granulomatous disease
     - *Local infection, meningitis*
     - Venous thrombosis

Clinical correlates
- Lower motor neuron lesions of the trochlear nerve may cause vertical diplopia which is most pronounced on contralateral downward gaze.
- Patients may present with a head tilt towards the non-paretic nerve to compensate for the action of the paralyzed superior oblique.

Cranial nerve V (trigeminal nerve)

- The trigeminal nerve is a mixed nerve that provides sensory innervation to the face and mucous membranes of the oral and nasal cavities as well as motor innervation to the muscles of mastication.
- The motor portion leaves the skull via the foramen ovale, forming the mandibular nerve, which supplies the muscles of mastication (masseter, temporalis, medial and lateral pterygoid muscles). In addition, motor fibers are given off to the tensor tympani, tensor veli palatini, mylohyoid, and the anterior belly of the digastric muscles.
- The sensory portion involves three major nuclear complexes within the brainstem:
  1 The spinal nucleus of the trigeminal nerve: conveys the sensations of pain, temperature, and light touch from the face and mucous membranes.
  2 The main sensory nucleus of the trigeminal nerve: conveys tactile and proprioceptive sensation.

3 The mesencephalic nucleus: receives proprioceptive impulses from the masticatory muscles and from muscles supplied by other motor cranial nerves.
* The sensory root leaves the pons to form the Gasserian ganglion, which further gives rise to three nerve trunks, the ophthalmic, maxillary, and mandibular divisions.

Structure involved	Physical signs	Etiology
Supranuclear lesions: technically not CN V neuropathies, but can mimic symptoms with hemifacial anesthesia		
Unilateral supranuclear lesions • Corticobulbar fibers (mild paresis due to bilateral innervation) • Thalamic lesions • Parietal lesions	Deviation of the jaw 'away from' the lesion Anesthesia of the contralateral face Depressed contralateral corneal reflex	**Stroke** Demyelination Tumor
Bilateral supranuclear lesions	Pseudobulbar palsy Exaggerated jaw jerk	
Nuclear lesions: usually involve other brainstem structures. Therefore, the localization is based on 'the company they keep' of other cranial nerve involvement		
Dorsal midpons: involving the motor nucleus	Ipsilateral paresis, atrophy, fasciculations of muscles of mastication	***Stroke (brainstem)*** **Demyelination** Tumor *AVM* *Syringobulbia*
Caudal pons to C4 level: involving the spinal nucleus, e.g. lateral medullary syndrome	Ipsilateral facial analgesia, hypesthesia, and thermoanesthesia Onion-skin sensory loss (lower medulla/upper cervical lesions)	
Lesions affecting mesencephalic nucleus	No neurological signs, except depressed ipsilateral jaw jerk	
Preganglionic trigeminal nerve roots: usually associated with involvement of the CN VI, VII, and VIII		
Preganglionic lesions	Ipsilateral facial pain, paresthesia, numbness, and sensory loss Depressed corneal reflex Trigeminal motor paresis +/- Ipsilateral tinnitus/deafness (CN VIII), facial nerve paresis (CN VII), ipsilateral abducens nerve palsy +/- Cerebellar signs	**Tumors** (meningioma, schwannoma, metastasis, nasopharyngeal) *Herpes zoster infection* *Meningitis: TB, fungal, bacterial* Carcinomatous meningitis Trauma Sarcoidosis

Structure involved	Physical signs	Etiology
Preganglionic trigeminal nerve roots: usually associated with involvement of the CN VI, VII, and VIII		
Trigeminal neuralgia	Sudden, excruciating unilateral pains, usually in the V2, V3 distribution	**Idiopathic** **Demyelination** CP angle tumors Aberrant blood vessels
Lesions in the Gasserian ganglion or near temporal apex		
Gasserian ganglion lesions	Unilateral paroxysmal pain Ipsilateral facial numbness Unilateral pterygoid or masseter paresis +/- Ipsilateral abducens nerve palsy	**Herpes zoster infection** **Tumors (meningioma,** **schwannoma,** **metastasis,** **nasopharyngeal)** *Meningitis, Abscess* Carcinomatous meningitis Trauma Granulomatous lesions Syphilis
Gradenigo syndrome (temporal apex)	Pain and sensory disturbances in ophthalmic distribution Ipsilateral abducens palsy Oculosympathetic paresis	**Osteitis/petrositis,** **mastoiditis, otitis** Trauma Tumors *Meningitis*
Raeder paratrigeminal syndrome	Unilateral oculosympathetic paresis, consisting of miosis and ptosis, without facial anhidrosis Unilateral head, retro-orbital pain	**Tumors** Granulomatous lesions
Lesions in the cavernous sinus		
Cavernous sinus lesions (only V1, V2, not V3)	Damage the ophthalmic and maxillary divisions Ophthalmoparesis from involvement of abducens or oculomotor nerves Oculosympathetic paresis No masticatory involvement	**Tumors** *Carotid aneurysm* *Carotico-cavernous fistula* *Meningitis* Trauma Granulomatous (sarcoid, Tolosa-Hunt)
Lesions in the superior orbital fissure		
Superior orbital fissure lesions (only V1, not V2 or V3)	Ipsilateral pain, paresthesia, and sensory loss in the ophthalmic (V1) distribution +/- Abducens, trochlear, and oculomotor nerves palsy	**Tumors** *Aneurysms* Trauma *Meningitis,* local infection

Continued

Structure involved	Physical signs	Etiology
Peripheral branches: often damaged in isolation		
Ophthalmic division (V1) – distally in the face	Paresthesia, pain, and sensory loss confined to the cutaneous supply of its branches (e.g. nasociliary, frontal or lacrimal)	**Trauma – facial fractures** **Herpes zoster infection** Tumors
Maxillary division (V2) – foramen rotundum, pterygopalatine fossa, orbital floor, infraorbital foramen, in the face	Numbness or discomfort in a maxillary distribution	**Trauma – facial fractures** **Herpes zoster infection** Tumors, especially nasopharyngeal (Numb cheek-limp lower lid syndrome)
Mandibular division (V3) – foramen ovale, zygomatic arch, in the face	Numbness or discomfort in the mandibular division Masticatory paralysis Pain, swelling, and numbness in the jaw (isolated mental neuropathy, numb chin syndrome, Roger sign)	Trauma – facial fractures Herpes zoster infection Tumors Systemic cancer (numb chin syndrome)

Cranial nerve VI (abducens nerve)

- The sixth nerve nucleus is located in lower pons. The nucleus contains motor neurons for the lateral rectus and interneurons traveling via the medial longitudinal fasciculus (MLF) to the contralateral medial rectus subnucleus of the third nerve. The sixth nerve nucleus contains all the neurons responsible for horizontal conjugate gaze. The fascicle leaves the nucleus and travels within the substance of the pontine tegmentum, adjacent to the medial lemniscus and the corticospinal tract. It enters the subarachnoid space (prepontine cistern), courses nearly vertically along the clivus, travels over the petrous apex of the temporal bone where it is tethered in Dorello canal. It then enters the cavernous sinus lateral to the internal carotid artery and medial to the ophthalmic division of the trigeminal nerve to enter the orbit via the superior orbital fissure.
- Patients with nonisolated sixth nerve palsy should undergo neuroimaging for further evaluation, with attention to areas suggested by physical signs or symptoms. Vasculopathic sixth nerve palsies can be observed for 4–12 weeks without neuroimaging. The recovery rate is 70% in patients with DM, HTN, and atherosclerosis.
- Aneurysm is a rare cause of acquired sixth nerve palsy (3.3%). Sixth nerve palsy can result after lumbar puncture, spinal anesthesia or occurs in pseudotumor cerebri.

Structure involved	Physical signs (in addition to sixth nerve palsy)	Etiology
Lower pontine lesions		
Nuclear lesions	Horizontal gaze palsy rather than abduction deficits, other brainstem signs, e.g. ipsilateral facial palsy	*Stroke (brainstem)* **Demyelination** Tumor
Fascicular lesions	Other brainstem signs, e.g. CN V, VII, VIII, ataxia, Horner syndrome	Trauma Congenital
Lesions in subarachnoid space	Unilateral or bilateral sixth nerve palsy Nonlocalizing finding as it can be due to increased intracranial pressure	Following procedures, LP *Nonlocalizing sign of increased ICP* Metastasis Inflammation *Infection: meningitis*
Lesions in the petrous apex	Involvement of other cranial nerves including V, VII, VIII or facial pain	Nasopharyngeal tumor Mastoiditis (Gradenigo syndrome) Trauma Inflammation
Lesions in the cavernous sinus	Involvement of other cranial nerves including III, IV, V1 or Horner syndrome	*Cavernous sinus thrombosis* *Cavernous carotid fistula* Tumors from pituitary, skull base, sphenoid sinus Inflammation, e.g. Tolosa-Hunt syndrome
Lesions in the orbit	Proptosis Chemosis	Tumors Inflammation Infection Trauma

Cranial nerve VII (facial nerve)

- Functions
  - Branchial motor: efferent supply of the stapedius, stylohyoid, posterior belly of the digastric, buccinator, platysma, occipitalis, orbicularis oculi, and orbicularis oris muscles.
  - Visceral motor: efferent supply to lacrimal, submandibular, and sublingual glands, and mucus membranes of the nose, hard, and soft palate.
  - Somatic sensory: afferent supply from the concha of the auricle, postauricular skin, and external tympanic membrane.
  - Special sensory: taste from the anterior two-thirds of the tongue, hard and soft palate.

- The differentiation between upper and lower motor neuron pathology of CN VII is an important one and usually easy to do clinically. Because of bilateral cortical innervation to the branchial motor nuclei subserving the frontalis muscles, upper motor neuron lesions spare the forehead, whereas lower motor neuron lesions involve the forehead.
- Deficits referable to the brainstem are nearly always accompanied by multiple CN pathologies, especially CN VI and to a lesser extent CN VIII

Structure involved	Physical signs	Etiology
Lower motor neuronopathy	Upper and lower facial paralysis	**Bell palsy, idiopathic**: often in the setting of an antecedent illness
Lesion of the lingual nerve distal to its junction with the chorda tympani	Loss of general sensation, taste, and secretion	**Infection: herpes,** meningitis (bacterial, mycobacterium, Lyme, fungal), middle ear, syphilis, parotitis
Lesion in the facial canal	Loss of taste and secretion, muscle paralysis, preservation of general sensation	**Guillain-Barré syndrome**: weakness and areflexia, uni- or bilateral facial palsy Vasculitis: rarely affects VII in isolation Autoimmune: often with other CN palsies; sarcoidosis, amyloidosis, Behcet, polyarteritis nodosum
Lesion within the internal acoustic meatus	CN VII and CN VIII deficits in combination*	Tumor: parotid gland, middle ear, (especially schwannoma), temporal bone, meningeal carcinomatosis
Lower motor nerve lesion proximal to its exit from the stylomastoid foramen where a branch serving the stapedius muscle is given off	Hyperacusis in combination with lower motor neuron symptoms	Trauma: intracranial carotid artery dissection, facial laceration, temporal bone fracture
Upper motor neuronopathy	Lower facial paralysis	**Stroke**: ~85% ischemic, ~15% hemorrhagic, may occur in the brainstem, thalamus, internal capsule, or cortex, typically acute onset, often additional deficits
Brainstem lesion	CN VII and VI deficits in combination	Tumor: metastatic or primary CNS, gradual onset Abscess: often in the setting of systemic illness, frequently accompanied by additional deficits

* Etiology excludes Bell palsy and Guillain-Barré.

FACIAL PALSY, BILATERAL

1 Miller-Fisher variant of Guillain-Barré syndrome

2 Infectious:

- **Lyme disease,** usually associated with aseptic meningitis (a combination called Bannwarth syndrome) or with a slightly erythematous indurated face resembling painless cellulitis.

- HIV disease
- Others include TB, syphilis, cryptococcosis

3 Systemic:
- **Sarcoidosis:** most common.
- Systemic lupus erythematosis
- Diabetes mellitus

4 Neuromuscular:
- Myotonic dystrophy; myotonia, frontal balding, diabetes mellitus, cardiomyopathy
- Oculopharyngeal muscular dystrophy; severe ptosis, ophthalmoplegia, dysphagia

5 Neoplastic:
- Carcinomatous meningitis
- Pontine glioma

Cranial nerve VIII (vestibulocochlear nerve)

- Functions: special sensory. Auditory information from the cochlea and balance information from the semicircular canals.
- The nuclei of the vestibular complex all contribute to fibers of the medial longitudinal fasciculus which coordinates the stimulation of extraocular muscles to allow the eyes to fixate on an object when the head is moving.
- Because of extensive bilateral projections, unilateral lesions above the level of the cochlear nucleus do not cause deafness.

Otologic vertigo

Syndrome	Frequency of otologic vertigo	Duration of vertigo	Additional features	Etiology
Benign paroxysmal positional vertigo (BPPV)	~50%	Seconds to minutes	Nausea, emesis, nystagmus	Otolith malpositioning in posterior semicircular canal
Ménière disease	~15%	Minutes to days	Progressive hearing loss, thyroid disease	Presumed dilatation and rupture of endolymph
Vestibular neuronitis	~15% (with labyrinthitis	Weeks and longer	Nausea, nystagmus, ataxia	Presumed viral infection of vestibular nerve
Labyrinthitis	As vestibular neuronitis	As vestibular neuronitis	As vestibular neuronitis plus tinnitus, hearing loss or both	As vestibular neuronitis

Hearing loss

Classification	Rinne test	Weber test	Common etiologies
Conductive	Bone greater than air (negative)	Lateralized to ear with greatest loss	**Otitis media** **Cerumen impaction** **Oteosclerosis** Perforation of tympanic membrane
Sensorineural	Air greater than bone (positive)	Lateralized to ear with preserved hearing	**Congenital** **Presbyacusis** **Noise-induced** Ménière disease Ototoxicity
Neural	Air greater than bone (positive)	Lateralized to ear with preserved hearing	Schwannoma Vascular infarct

Cranial nerve IX (glossopharyngeal nerve)

- The glossopharyngeal nerve contains motor, sensory, and parasympathetic fibers. It is in close anatomical relationship with cranial nerves X and XI.
  1. Motor fibers: originate from nucleus ambiguus and supply the stylopharyngeus and the constrictor muscles of the pharynx.
  2. Sensory fibers: include taste afferents and supply the posterior third of the tongue, and pharynx and general visceral afferents from the same regions.
  3. Parasympathetic fibers: carry secretory and vasodilatory fibers to the parotid gland.
- The nerve travels through the jugular foramen, and passes between the internal carotid artery and the internal jugular vein.
- Lesions affecting the glossopharyngeal nerve usually involve the vagus nerve. Therefore, syndromes affecting both nerves are much more common than nerve lesions occurring in relative isolation.

Structure involved	Physical signs	Etiology
Supranuclear lesions		
Unilateral lesions	No neurological deficits because of bilateral corticobulbar inputs	
Bilateral lesions	Pseudobulbar palsy, including severe dysphagia, emotional lability, spastic tongue, dysarthria	**Stroke** Tumors Trauma Neurodegenerative process

Structure involved	Physical signs	Etiology
Nuclear and intramedullary lesions		
Brainstem lesions, e.g. lateral medullary lesions	Usually involves other cranial nerves Dysarthria, dysphagia	*Stroke (brainstem)* Demyelination Tumors
Extramedullary lesions		
Cerebellopontine angle lesions	Can also involve CN IX, in addition to CN VII, VIII Tinnitus, vertigo, deafness, ataxia Cerebellar signs	**Acoustic neuroma** Meningioma Metastasis
Jugular foramen lesions (Vernet syndrome)	Ipsilateral trapezius and sternocleidomastoid paresis Dysphonia, dysphagia Ipsilateral palatal droop and vocal cord paralysis Ipsilateral loss of taste in the posterior third of the tongue Dull, unilateral, aching pain behind the ear	**Glomus jugulare tumors** *Aneurysms* *Jugular thrombosis* Basal skull fractures *Meningitis* Trauma
Lesions within retroparotid and retropharyngeal space		
Collett-Sicard syndrome	Cranial nerve IX, X, XI, XII signs	**Tumors** (parotid, carotid body, lymph nodes)
Villaret syndrome	Cranial nerve IX, X, XI, XII and Horner syndrome	Granulomatous lesions/ lymph nodes (TB, sarcoid, fungi) *Aneurysm* *Carotid dissection* Trauma to nerve
Distal lesions		
Glossopharyngeal neuralgia	Unilateral sudden stabbing pain in the distribution of CN IX and X, precipitated by cough, talking, swallowing	**Idiopathic** Lesions (tumors, nodes, inflammation) in the peripheral distribution

Cranial nerve X (vagus nerve)

- The vagus nerve contains motor, sensory, and parasympathetic nerve fibers.
  1 Motor fibers: originate from dorsal motor nucleus and nucleus ambiguus, supplying all striated muscles of the soft palate, pharynx, and larynx, except the tensor veli palatini and stylopharyngeus muscles.

2 Sensory fibers: carry taste sensation from epiglottis, hard and soft palates, pharynx, general visceral sensations, and exteroceptive sensations.
3 Parasympathetic fibers: innervating cardiac and abdominal viscera.
- It leaves the skull via jugular foramen, along with the accessory nerve (CN XI). In the neck, the vagus nerve proper descends within a sheath common to the internal carotid artery and the internal jugular vein, giving off the cardiac rami. At the root of the neck, it gives off recurrent laryngeal nerves on both sides, supplying all muscles of the larynx except the cricothyroid muscle.
- Myopathies (polymyositis) may involve laryngeal/pharyngeal muscles and mimic vagal nerve involvement.

Structure involved	Physical signs	Etiology
Supranuclear lesions		
Unilateral lesions	No neurological deficits because of bilateral inputs	
Bilateral lesions	Pseudobulbar palsy, including severe dysphagia, emotional lability, spastic tongue, dysarthria	**Stroke** Tumors Trauma Neurodegenerative

Nuclear lesions within the brainstem
Bilateral nuclear lesions with complete paralysis are fatal.

Nuclear lesions	Ipsilateral palatal, pharyngeal, and laryngeal paralysis, dysarthria, dysphagia; associated with cerebellar/other cranial nerve involvement	*Stroke (brainstem)* **Neurodegenerative** (ALS): may be bilateral **Tumors** **Syringobulbia** Demyelination Polio: may be bilateral Trauma
Jackson syndrome	Cranial nerve X, XI, XII signs	*Stroke (brainstem)*
Schmidt syndrome	Cranial nerve X, XI signs	**Tumors** Idiopathic

Extramedullary lesions		
Jugular foramen syndrome (Vernet)	Cranial IX, X, and XI signs	See under Cranial nerve IX (**glomus tumors**, etc.)
Tapia syndrome	Cranial nerve X, XII, +/- XI	**Tumors** (neurofibroma, parotid) Trauma

Structure involved	Physical signs	Etiology
Lesions within retroparotid and retropharyngeal space		
Collett-Sicard syndrome	Cranial nerve IX, X, XI, XII signs	**Tumors** (parotid, carotid body, lymph nodes)
Villaret syndrome	Cranial nerve IX, X, XI, XII and Horner syndrome	Granulomatous lesions/ lymph nodes (TB, sarcoid, fungi)
		Aneurysm
		Carotid dissection
		Trauma to nerve

Lesions in the vagus nerve proper
Unilateral lesions of the nerve itself do not cause prominent autonomic symptoms.

Lesions of the vagus nerve proper	Ipsilateral vocal cord paralysis	Tumors
	Unilateral laryngeal anesthesia	Guillain-Barré syndrome
		Diphtheric neuropathy
		Aneurysm
		Trauma
		Adenopathy

Lesions in the recurrent laryngeal nerve (left side is more common)
No palatal weakness, no dysphagia, no pharyngeal sensory loss, as these fibers have already separated.

Unilateral lesion	Transient hoarseness (paralyzed vocal cord lies near the midline.)	*Aortic aneurysm*
		Tumors (lung, mediastinal, thoracic lymph nodes)
Bilateral lesion (after thyroidectomy)	Inspiratory stridor	**Idiopathic** (up to 1/3)
	Dyspnea on exertion	Enlarged left atrium
	Aphonia	Trauma
		Post-thyroidectomy

Cranial nerve XI (the spinal accessory nerve)

- The spinal accessory nerve is a purely motor nerve. It originates from the medulla and upper spinal cord. The column of cells are somatotopically arranged with C1, C2 innervating ipsilateral sternocleidomastoid muscle (SCM) and C3, C4 innervating ipsilateral trapezius muscle.
- The cranial and spinal roots exit from the skull through the jugular foramen. The cranial roots join the vagus nerve to supply the pharynx and larynx, the spinal portion enters the neck between the internal carotid artery and the internal jugular vein.

- Weakness of the unilateral SCM results in weakness in turning the head to the **opposite** side. Weakness of the unilateral trapezius causes the shoulder to be lower on the affected side with the scapula displaced downward and laterally. Scapular winging due to trapezius weakness is *present at rest* and *worsens with shoulder abduction*; if due to serratus weakness, winging is *absent at rest* and *worsens with shoulder flexion*.
- The most common cause of isolated spinal accessory nerve palsy is related to surgical procedures within the posterior triangle of the neck.
- Isolated lesions of the spinal accessory nerve do not cause any sensory deficits.
- Myopathies (polymyositis, muscular dystrophy) may mimic bilateral CN XI palsies.

Structure involved	Physical signs	Etiology
Supranuclear/nuclear lesions		
Hemispheric lesions	Contralateral hemiplegia Head is turned away from the hemiplegic side	**Stroke** Tumors *Trauma*
Nuclear lesions	Weakness of trapezius & SCM	Syringobulbia Neurodegenerative (ALS) *Stroke (brainstem)* Tumors Poliomyelitis
Infranuclear lesions		
Lesions within the skull and foramen magnum (Involving cranial nerves IX, X, XII)	Weakness of trapezius & SCM Dysphonia, dysphagia, loss of taste on the posterior third of the tongue, ipsilateral tongue paresis and atrophy	**Extramedullary tumors** (meningioma, neurinoma) *Meningitis* Occipital bone disease Trauma
Jugular foramen syndrome (Vernet syndrome)	See under cranial nerve IX	See under cranial nerve IX (**tumors**)
Lesions of the spinal accessory nerve within the neck		
Within the posterior triangle of the neck	Ipsilateral weakness of the SCM and trapezius without affecting other cranial nerves	Complications of surgical procedures, including node biopsy, carotid endarterectomy, venous cannulation

Cranial nerve XII (hypoglossal nerve)

- The hypoglossal nerve supplies all of the intrinsic and all but one of the extrinsic muscles of the tongue. The exception is the palatoglossus muscle, which is supplied by cranial nerve X.
- The hypoglossal nucleus is located in the tegmentum of the medulla, between the dorsal vagal nucleus and the midline.
- The hypoglossal nerve exits the cranium through the hypoglossal foramen. At one point, it lies between the internal carotid artery and the internal jugular vein.
- Lesions of this nerve result in ipsilateral tongue weakness deviating to the weak side.
- Most common associated cranial neuropathies include vagus nerve and facial nerve palsies.
- It is affected in the medial medullary syndrome. **This is a key feature used to differentiate medial from lateral medullary syndrome.**

1 **Tumors**
  - Most common cause, accounting for 49%.
  - Usually malignant, consisting of metastases (to medulla or meninges) and nasopharyngeal carcinoma.
2 *Trauma*
  - Second most common cause (12%), usually due to a penetrating wound rather than blunt trauma.
  - Injury to the 10th, 11th cranial nerves, oculosympathetic trunk, and the carotid artery often coexists.
3 *Stroke (brainstem)*
  - Accounts for 6%, most common being infarction.
  - An important finding in medial medullary syndrome. Others include contralateral weakness, contralateral loss of discriminative touch, and kinesthesia.
4 Others
  - Hysterical tongue deviation (6%)
  - Surgery, especially carotid endarterectomy (5%)
  - Multiple sclerosis
  - Infections, presumably viral (4%), Guillain-Barré syndrome (4%)

(Ref: Keane J.R. Twelfth-nerve palsy. Analysis of 100 cases. *Arch Neurol* 1996; 53: 561–566.)

Cortical and subcortical structures

Aphasia and anatomical localization

> • Benson and Geschwind popularized a bedside language examination into six parts, providing useful localizing information and is well worth a few minutes to take.
> • The six parts are as follows:
>   • spontaneous speech,
>   • naming,
>   • repetition,
>   • comprehension,
>   • reading, and
>   • writing.
> • Apraxia can sometimes be difficult to differentiate from ability to comprehend. Therefore, it is recommended to test comprehension by tasks that do not require a motor act, for example, yes or no questions or by pointing response.

Aphasia	Features	Localization (dominant hemisphere)
Global aphasia	Impairment of all six parts with **nonfluent or mute speech**	Large lesion involving both inferior frontal and superior temporal regions
Broca aphasia	**Nonfluent speech** with impaired naming, repetition, and others, but **intact comprehension**	Posterior part of the inferior frontal gyrus
Wernicke aphasia	**Fluent speech** with **impaired** naming, repetition as well as **comprehension**	Posterior part of the superior temporal gyrus +/- inferior parietal lobule
Conduction aphasia (disconnection syndrome)	Fluent speech with **impaired repetition**, naming, but **intact comprehension**	Arcuate fasciculus, superior temporal gyrus or inferior parietal lobule
Anomic aphasia	Fluent speech with intact comprehension, naming, repetition, and others, but **impaired naming**	Less specific in localization, suggest left hemispheric pathology
Transcortical (T) aphasia	Intact repetition Nonfluent in T. mixed and motor aphasia Fluent in T. sensory aphasia	Lesions sparing the perisylvian cortex

Brodmann areas

- Division and classification of the cerebral cortex have been attempted by many investigators. However, the most commonly used classification system is **Brodmann**, which is based on cytoarchitectonics and uses numbers to label individual areas of the cortex.
- These anatomically defined areas have been used as a reference base for localization of physiologic and pathologic processes. More recently, particular cortical areas have been localized with the use of functional neuroimaging.

Brodmann area	Name	Function	Connections
Frontal lobe			
Area 4	Primary motor cortex	Voluntary simple movement	Origin of corticospinal tract
Area 6	Premotor cortex	Combine with area 4 for complex movements	Contribute to part of corticospinal tract, project to area 4
Area 8	Frontal eye field	Eye movements	Paramedian pontine reticular formation (PPRF)
Area 44, 45	Broca area	Language (dominant hemisphere)	Wernicke area via arcuate fasciculus
Parietal lobe			
Area 3, 1, 2	Primary sensory cortex (postcentral gyrus)	Somatosensory	Input from VPL, VPM
Area 5, 7	Parietal convexity posterior to postcentral gyrus	Visual and somatosensory association area	Occipital cortex
Temporal lobe			
Area 41, 42	Primary auditory cortex (Heschl gyri)	Processing of auditory stimuli	Input from medial geniculate
Area 22	Wernicke area (Planum temporale and posterior superior temporal gyrus)	Language comprehension (dominant hemisphere)	Different inputs from auditory association cortex, visual association cortex and Broca area

Continued

Brodmann area	Name	Function	Connections
Occipital lobe			
Area 17	Primary visual cortex (striate or calcarine cortex)	Processing of visual stimuli	Input from lateral geniculate, projects to area 18, 19
Area 18, 19	Visual association cortex (extrastriate cortex)	Processing of visual stimuli	Input from area 17

Frontal lobe lesions

Lesion location	Clinical features
Orbitofrontal cortex	Social disinhibition Witzelsucht
Dorsolateral prefrontal cortex	Depression Apathy Loss of task set Primitive reflexes Frontal ataxia
Medial frontal cortex	Akinetic mutism (bilateral lesions)
Precentral gyrus	Monoplegia or hemiplegia
Broca area (inferior part of dominant frontal lobe)	Non-fluent aphasia
Supplementary motor area	Paralysis of head and eye movement to opposite side Head turns toward 'disease' hemisphere and eyes look in the same direction
Paracentral lobule (posterior part of the superior frontal gyrus)	Loss of cortical inhibition results in incontinence of urine and feces. **Likely to occur with ventricular dilatation in normal pressure hydrocephalus**

Hydrocephalus

- Hydrocephalus is characterized by an increased amount of CSF in the ventricles.
- Hydrocephalus is classified as communicating or noncommunicating hydrocephalus.

- In adults, hydrocephalus is associated with a significant increase in intracranial pressure. Patients usually manifest with headache, vomiting, altered consciousness, and edema of optic disks. MR imagings may reveal rounded lateral margins of the lateral ventricles, associated with transependymal flow.
- On the contrary, if hydrocephalus develops in early childhood (before the closure of sutures), the skull yields to the increased pressure by widening of the sutures and a progressive increase in head circumference. Nonetheless, rapid increases in intracranial pressure can still result in headache, vomiting, altered consciousness, and irritability. A 'sunset sign' may be evident in neonates, where the upper eyelids are retracted and the globes are directed downwards.

Features	Communicating hydrocephalus	Noncommunicating or obstructive hydrocephalus
Definition	There is a free communication between the ventricles and subarachnoid spaces	CSF in the ventricles cannot reach the subarachnoid spaces because of obstruction at different levels
Site of lesions	Usually distal to the ventricular system, e.g. in the subarachnoid spaces over the convexities or obstruction at the perimesenchalic cistern	Foramen of Monro Aqueduct of Sylvius Foramina of Magendie & Luschka
Causes	Previous infections resulting in fibrosis, abnormalities of arachnoid granulations	Ventricular hemorrhage, intracranial tumors with compression to the foramens or intraventricular tumors with obstruction of the foramens, congenital atresia
Neuroradiological findings	Enlargement of all the ventricular cavities as well as subarachnoid spaces	At foramen of Monro: enlargement of lateral ventricle on the side of obstruction or both At aqueduct of Sylvius: enlargement of the third and both lateral ventricles At foramina of Magendie & Luschka: enlargement of the third, fourth, and both lateral ventricles

Papez circuit

- Papez circuit is a route in which the limbic system communicates between the hippocampus, thalamus, hypothalamus, and cortex.
- Limbic system is **not a true lobe of the brain** but rather a functional collection of structures that regulate higher activities such as memory and emotion. It commonly includes parahippocampal gyrus, hippocampus, congulate gyrus, and uncus.
- Bilateral lesions of any structures of Papez circuit have been reported to cause amnesia.

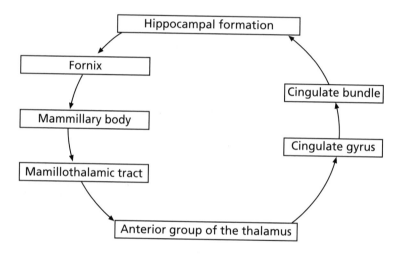

Substantia nigra

- The substantia nigra is a pigmented mass of neurons between the cerebral peduncles and tegmentum.
- It is composed of two zones: a dorsal zona compacta containing melanin pigment and a ventral zona reticulata containing iron compounds.
- The neuronal populations of the substantia nigra consist of pigmented and nonpigmented neurons. Pigmented neurons outnumber nonpigmented neurons two to one.
- The neurotransmitter in pigmented neurons is dopamine, while it is either cholinergic or GABAergic for nonpigmented neurons.
- There is a characteristic pattern of neuronal loss in the substantia nigra in various neurological conditions as listed below.

Pattern of cell loss:

Disorders	Pigmented neurons	Nonpigmented neurons	Distribution
Idiopathic Parkinson disease	Yes	No	Central loss
Postencephalitic Parkinsonism	Yes	No	Uniform loss
Parkinson dementia complex	Yes	Yes	Uniform loss
Multiple system atrophy	Yes	No	Medial and lateral loss with sparing of the central part
Huntington disease	Yes	Yes	No specific pattern

Peripheral nerves (see Chapter 8: Peripheral Neurology)

Spinal cord

Ascending fiber systems in the spinal cord

- All afferent axons in the dorsal roots have their cell bodies in the dorsal root ganglia. Further, different ascending systems decussate at different levels. In general, ascending axons synapse within the spinal cord before decussating.

Tract	Origin	Ending	Function	Location in the cord
Dorsal column	Skin, joint, tendons	Dorsal column nuclei, second-order neurons projecting to contralateral thalamus	Proprioception, two-point discrimination, fine touch	Dorsal column (cross in medulla at lemniscal decussation)
Spinothalamic tracts	Skin	Dorsal horn, second-order neurons projecting to contralateral thalamus	Temperature, sharp pain, crude touch	Ventrolateral column (cross in the cord 1–2 levels above entry)
Dorsal spinocerebellar tract	Muscle spindles, Golgi tendon organs, touch and pressure receptors	Cerebellar paleocortex	Movement and positioning mechanisms	Lateral column (via ipsilateral inferior cerebellar peduncle)
Ventral spinocerebellar tract	Muscle spindles, Golgi tendon organs, touch and pressure receptors	Cerebellar paleocortex	Movement and positioning mechanism	Lateral column (via contralateral and ipsilateral superior cerebellar peduncle)

Continued

Tract	Origin	Ending	Function	Location in the cord
Spinoreticular tract	Deep somatic structures	Reticular formation of brainstem	Deep and chronic pain	Ventrolateral column (diffuse and polysynaptic)

Ref: Waxman S.G. *Clinical Neuroanatomy*, 25th edn, 2003, New York, Lange Medical Books/McGraw-Hill.

Descending fiber systems in the spinal cord

- Examination of a cross-section of the spinal cord reveals major descending tracts, including corticospinal tract, vestibulospinal tract, rubrospinal tract, reticulospinal tract, descending autonomic tract, tectospinal tract, and medial longitudinal fasiculus.
- The corticospinal fibers originate in the contralateral cerebral cortex, and 90% of its fibers cross in the decussation of the medullary pyramids, with the remaining 10% traveling ipsilaterally as anterior corticospinal tract. Finally, a small fraction (0–3%) of the corticospinal axons descend, without decussating, as uncrossed fibers within the lateral corticospinal tract.

Tract	Origin	Ending	Function	Location in the cord
Lateral corticospinal tract	Motor and premotor cortex	Anterior horn cells (interneurons and LMNs)	Fine motor function	Lateral column (crosses in medulla at pyramidal decussation)
Anterior corticospinal tract	Motor and premotor cortex	Anterior horn cells (interneurons and LMNs)	Gross and postural motor function (proximal and axial structure)	Anterior column (uncrossed)
Vestibulospinal tract	Lateral and medial vestibular nucleus	Anterior horn interneurons and motor neurons for extensors	Postural reflexes	Ventral column
Rubrospinal tract	Red nucleus	Ventral horn interneurons	Motor function	Lateral column
Reticulospinal tract	Brainstem reticular formation	Dorsal and ventral horn	Modulation of sensory transmission, esp. pain and spinal reflexes	Anterior column

Tract	Origin	Ending	Function	Location in the cord
Descending autonomic	Hypothalamus, brainstem nuclei	Preganglionic autonomic neurons	Modulation of autonomic functions	Lateral columns
Tectospinal	Midbrain, superior colliculus	Ventral horn interneurons	Reflex head turning	Ventral column
Medial longitudinal fasiculus (MLF)	Vestibular nuclei	Cervical gray	Coordination of head and eye movements	Ventral column (intermingled with tectospinal tract)

Ref: Waxman S.G. *Clinical Neuroanatomy*, 25th edn, 2003, New York, Lange Medical Books/McGraw-Hill.

Neuropathology

Central nervous system

Brain biopsy: indications and techniques

- Brain biopsy is an invasive and expensive diagnostic procedure, associated with a small but definite risk of morbidity and mortality.
- It is usually regarded as the last resort in a diagnostic evaluation, although it is commonly used to confirm a definite diagnosis, particularly in patients with mass lesions.
- It cannot be overemphasized that the neurologist, neurosurgeon, neuroradiologist, and neuropathologist should fully discuss the case. Careful arrangements must be made in advance for optimal specimen handling and interpretation.

Indications	Techniques
Mass lesions • The most common indication • Common differential diagnosis usually includes neoplasm, infection, or demyelination.	Stereotactic brain biopsy • Good for deep and small lesions. • Can be done under local anesthesia with CT or MRI-guidance. • Sensitivity is 90–95%, but very much depends on techniques, tissue handling, and experience of the neuropathologist. • Intraoperative neuropathological consultation is often essential to ensure that a good specimen is obtained. • A specimen size is usually 2 mm thick cores with a length of 8–10 mm. • Complications include 0.04%–5% risk of hemorrhage and 0.2% risk of death. Unexpected diagnosis occurs in 12% of cases.

Continued

Indications	Techniques
Multifocal atypical lesions • Biopsy is usually performed as a last resort to obtain the diagnosis.	Stereotactic brain biopsy or open biopsy

Diffuse lesions	Open biopsy
	  • More tissue can be acquired.
	  • Usually performed under general anesthesia.
	  • Dural and arachnoid biopsies can be obtained.
	  • A specimen is usually of 1 cm in size of cortex and underlying white matter.
	  • Right frontal lobe is commonly chosen for biopsy unless a focal area of more intense involvement is identified.

Arteriovenous malformation versus cavernous malformation

- Four types of vascular malformations are recognized:
  - Arteriovenous malformation (AVM)
  - Cavernous malformation (CM)
  - Venous malformation (VM)
  - Capillary telangiectasia (CaT)
- AVMs and CMs are commonly seen surgically, while VMs and CaTs are often seen incidentally at autopsy.
- The most common vascular malformation seen in surgical neuropathology is the AVM. This consists of a complex mass of blood vessels and gliotic neural parenchyma. Patients usually present with hemorrhages or seizures as young adults.
- The other vascular malformations, CMs, are classically angiographically occult vascular malformations, which may present with hemorrhage, seizures, or a mass lesion in adolescents and young adults. CMs are distinguishable from other types of malformations on the basis of a central nidus, where the cavernous vascular spaces are separated only by collagenous tissue, without intervening neural parenchyma.

Features	Arteriovenous malformation	Cavernous malformation
Angiographic appearance	Usually obvious (although occult findings can be seen)	Usually occult
Abnormal arteries	Yes Vascular media is replaced by a collagenous scar, or markedly thinned with aneurismal dilatation.	No

Features	Arteriovenous malformation	Cavernous malformation
Nidus	No	Yes
Intervening parenchyma	Yes	Peripherally
Gliosis	Yes (adjacent to abnormal vessels)	May be present
Calcifications	May be present	May be present
Hemosiderin	Rare	Common
Multiple	Rare	Common
Familial	Rare	Common

Modified from: Prayson R.A., Cohen M.L. *Practical Differential Diagnosis in Surgical Neuropathology.* 2000, Totowa, Humana Press.

Granulomatous inflammation of the CNS

- The majority of cases of CNS granulomatous diseases are infectious in etiology, especially tuberculosis, or represent sarcoidosis.
- The distinction of tuberculous infection and sarcoidosis is of particular importance, especially from a therapeutic standpoint. However, the diagnosis of neurosarcoidosis is often difficult because of varied and nonspecific neurological manifestations. The leptomeninges are the most frequent site of CNS involvement by sarcoidosis, although it has a similar affinity to involve the base of brain as does tuberculous meningitis.
- In general, granulomata are preferentially perivascular in location and are often associated with a chronic inflammatory cell infiltrate consisting of primarily T lymphocytes, B lymphocytes, and monocytes. Granulomatous inflammatory disorders are characterized by the presence of multinucleated giant cells (epitheloid syncytial macrophages).
- Common clinical manifestations of granulomatous disease include cranial neuropathies and/or obstructive hydrocephalus.

1 **Mycobacterial infection**
- Mycobacterium tuberculosis is the most common cause.
- There are two major pathological manifestations in CNS tuberculosis: infection involving the leptomeninges (with or without secondary ventriculitis) and inflammation confined to the parenchyma corresponding to a tuberculoma (caseating granuloma).
- Posterior fossa tuberculoma may mimic a tumor.
- M. leprae causes leprosy. M. avium-intracellulare may cause meningitis in immunocompromised individuals.

2 **Neurosarcoidosis**
   - Histologically, sarcoidosis is characterized by non-caseating granulomas with large epithelioid cells and minimal necrosis. This is an important distinction from tuberculosis.
   - Involvement of the central and peripheral nervous system in sarcoidosis occur in approximately 5% of patients with this disease.
   - Of patients with nervous system involvement facial nerve palsy is the most common presenting cranial neuropathy. Cranial neuropathies are the most common neurological signs/symptoms (53%), followed by parenchymal involvement (48%), aseptic meningitis (22%), peripheral neuropathy (17%), myopathy (15%), and hydrocephalus (7%).

3 Neurosyphilis
   - Can produce meningovascular and parenchymatous involvement.
   - Chronic leptomeningeal inflammation with spinal arachnoiditis and meningeal thickening is not uncommon.

4 Fungal infections
   - For example, cryptococcosis, aspergillosis, coccidioidomycosis, and histoplasmosis.
   - Can produce meningitis as well as numerous cortical and subcortical micro-abscesses.

5 Foreign body giant cell reaction
   - For example, suture materials, dermoid cyst rupture, history of traumatic brain injury, history of intravenous drug abuse.
   - Histologically characterized by multinucleated giant cells containing polymorphonuclear inclusion bodies within their cytoplasm.

6 Germinoma
   - The presence of small granulomas and giant cells in the setting of a pineal gland tumor should raise the suspicious of germinoma.

7 Wegener granulomatosis
   - Histologically characterized by necrotizing granulomas and vasculitis affecting predominantly medium and small vessels.
   - Neurological involvement occurs in 30% of patients and includes aseptic chronic meningitis. Mononeuritis multiplex is also common, seen in 15% of patients.
   - Typical systemic pathological features include granulomatous lesions of the upper and lower respiratory tracts, focal segmental glomerulopathy, and necrotizing vasculitis, associated with symptoms related to upper and lower airways.

8 Lymphomatoid granulomatosis
   - Although the lungs are primarily involved, the upper respiratory tract is usually spared, unlike in Wegener granulomatosis.

- Neurological features can occur in 30% of patients, with the most common CNS findings being necrotizing inflammatory masses in the parenchyma.
- 13% of patients progress to lymphoma.

9 Tolosa-Hunt syndrome
- Idiopathic granulomatous inflammation of the cavernous sinus is characterized by painful ophthalmoplegia and rapid response to corticosteroids.

10 Others: uncommon
- Rheumatoid arthritis
- Langerhan cell histiocytosis

Heterotopias

- A cortical heterotopia is characterized by islands of gray matter along the route of neuroblast migration. The islands consist of a collection of normal neurons in abnormal locations secondary to arrest of the radial migration of neuroblasts, no later than the fifth month of gestation.
- The cause of incomplete migration is unknown.
- They are associated with a wide variety of genetic, vascular, and environmental causes.

Three types are recognized:

1 **Nodular (subependymal) heterotopia**
- Subependymal masses of gray matter that form clusters of round nodules.
- Usually localized at the corner of lateral ventricles.
- Normal development and mild symptoms with onset of seizures in the first two decades of life.

2 Laminar (focal subcortical) heterotopia
- Variable symptoms and signs depending on the extent of the heterotopia.
- The larger the heterotopia, the more severe the developmental delay.

3 Band heterotopia (double cortex)
- Moderate to severe developmental delay and intractable seizures.

Neurofibrillary tangles

- Neurofibrillary tangles are non-membrane bound masses of filaments, which are stained positive with silver stain.
- The structures are composed of 10–20 nm filaments in paired helix configuration, crossover every 80 nm.
- They are associated with phosphorylated tau protein (i.e. A68). Tau is a microtubule protein that promotes tubule stability and assembly.

Tangles are seen in a variety of pathologies including:

1 **Alzheimer disease**
   - Other pathologies include neuronal loss, neuritic plaques, and granulovacuolar degeneration. Hirano bodies and amyloid angiopathy can also be seen.
   - Tangles are also seen in Down syndrome: by the age of 40 years, almost 100% of patients develop a pathology of Alzheimer disease but they can be asymptomatic.
2 Normal aging
   - Exists in small numbers.
3 Progressive supranuclear palsy
   - Salient features include predominant axial Parkinsonism and vertical ophthalmoparesis.
4 Subacute sclerosing panencephalitis
   - Progressive fatal condition secondary to measles infection, characterized by dementia, myoclonus, seizures, ataxia, and dystonia
5 Others
   - Dementia pugilistica
   - Myotonic dystrophy
   - Kuf disease
   - Cockayne syndrome
   - Niemann-Pick disease

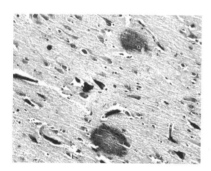

Plaques and tangles (Bielschowsky silver stain)

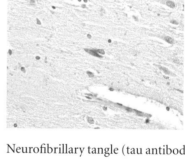

Neurofibrillary tangle (tau antibody)

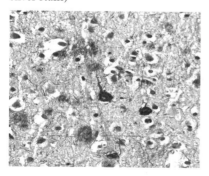

Neurofibrillary tangle (Bielschowsky silver stain)

Pathological neuronal inclusions

- In addition to normally occurring nonpathologic substances such as lipofuscin, neuromelanin, and Marinesco bodies, a wide variety of abnormal intranuclear and intracytoplasmic inclusions may be seen in neurons.

Intranuclear

Inclusion	Disease
Cowdry type A	HSV
	VZV
	CMV
	SSPE
	JCV (PML)
Cowdry type B	Acute polio
Intranuclear inclusions	Huntington disease

HSV – herpes simplex virus, VZV – varicella zoster virus, CMV – cytomegalovirus, SSPE – subacute sclerosing panencephalitis, JCV – JC virus, PML – progressive multifocal leukoencephalopathy.

Intracytoplasmic

Inclusion	Disease
Neurofibrillary tangles	Alzheimer disease
Pick bodies	Pick disease
Lewy bodies	Parkinson disease
	Diffuse Lewy body disease
Negri bodies	Rabies
Polyglucosan bodies	Polyglucosan disease (PGB)
Lafora bodies	Myoclonic epilepsy
Bunina bodies	Amyotrophic lateral sclerosis

Ref: Fuller G.N., Goodman J.C. *Practical Review of Neuropathology.* 2001, Philadelphia, Lippincott Williams & Wilkins.

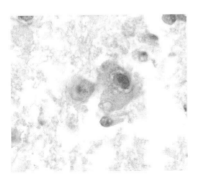

Cowdry type A inclusion, cytomegalovirus infection (H&E stain)

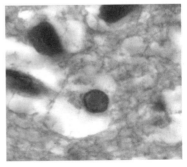

Cowdry type A inclusion, herpes simplex type I infection (H&E stain)

Pigmented lesions in the CNS

- Among all the pigmented lesions in the CNS, metastatic malignant melanoma is the most common.
- Other differential diagnoses in this group represent rare entities. However, distinguishing these lesions from malignant melanoma is critically important, since some of the lesions are benign and therefore the treatment is vastly different.

1 **Metastatic malignant melanoma**
   - Most common pigmented lesion in the CNS.
2 Melanocytoma
   - The proliferating cells are melanocytes with the predilection for the leptomeninges.
   - Most of the lesions are benign, pigmented, meningeal-based tumors, so called meningeal melanocytoma.
   - Half of lesions are located intracranially, especially in the posterior fossa. The rest occur in the spinal canal as intradural extramedullary masses in the cervical and thoracic regions.
   - While most meningeal melanocytomas occur without cutaneous stigmata, some patients have pigmented skin lesions, raising the possibility of metastatic malignant melanoma or a neurocutaneous syndrome.
3 Melanocytic schwannoma
   - Distinctive psammomatous melanocytic schwannoma is easily recognized and can be associated with Carney complex (myxomas, spotty pigmentation, endocrine overactivity, and multiple psammomatous melanotic schwannoma).
4 Meningeal melanocytosis
   - Refers to a set of lesions characterized by a diffuse proliferation of melanocytic cells within leptomeninges without a dominant mass lesion.
   - Presentation is usually in childhood and can manifest with increased intracranial pressure with hydrocephalus. Neuroimaging often reveals diffuse meningeal enhancement. CSF cytology is usually positive.
   - The main differential diagnosis in this rare disorder is superficial siderosis due to chronic leakage of blood into the CSF, which may accompany meningeal melanocytomas.
   - Although the proliferating cells may appear cytologically benign, meningeal melanocytosis is a lethal disorder, with death often occurring within a year of diagnosis.

Positive CSF cytology without a history of malignancy

- CSF samples that show malignant cells in the absence of any history of malignancy represent a special dilemma.
- This accounts for approximately 11% of patients with positive CSF malignant cytology. Most occult carcinomas with leptomeningeal manifestations are in the lung or the stomach. However, the primary sites are unknown in the majority of cases. Breast carcinoma commonly involves the leptomeninges, but is usually clinically apparent prior to meningeal spread.
- The diagnosis and classification of malignancy that presents initially in the CSF should proceed in a stepwise fashion. The first distinction is whether the cells are hematopoietic or nonhematopoietic. Then, the carcinomas can be further divided into adenocarcinoma, squamous cell carcinoma, small cell carcinoma, or undifferentiated carcinoma. In the next step, clinical and radiographic investigation will provide further clues to the diagnosis. As a general rule, most small cell carcinoma originates from the lung, whereas most squamous cell carcinoma comes from the head and neck.

Type of malignancy	Percentage of cases first diagnosed by positive CSF cytology
Unknown primary	70
Gastric adenocarcinoma	67
Bronchogenic carcinoma	18
Malignant melanoma	8
Primary CNS tumor (e.g. medulloblastoma, glioblastoma, etc.)	5
Malignant lymphoma	2

Ref: Bigner S.H., Johnston W.W. The diagnostic challenge of tumors manifested initially by the shedding of cells into cerebrospinal fluid. *Acta Cytol* 1984; 28: 29–36.

Rosenthal fibers

- Rosenthal fibers are opaque, homogeneous, brightly eosinophilic intracytoplasmic structures, which exhibit elongated, anfractuous (corkscrew or lumpy-bumpy) profiles.

Rosenthal fibers are observed in:
1 Reactive states
   - Most often those associated with significant chronicity, such as syringomyelia and around the margins of nonglial, slow-growing tumors, such as craniopharyngioma and hemangioblastoma.

2 Metabolic/genetic disorders
- Rosenthal fibers are morphological hallmarks of **Alexander disease** (of which some forms are now known to arise from mutations of the gene encoding glial fibrillary acidic protein, GFAP).
3 Neoplasia
- Most characteristic of pilocytic astrocytoma.
- It can also be found in a wide variety of gliomas.

The importance of recognizing Rosenthal fibers in an astrocytic neoplasm cannot be overemphasized. The nuclear polymorphism of most pilocytic astrocytomas is more than sufficient to suggest anaplastic astrocytoma; the identification of Rosenthal fibers significantly mitigates the risk of this potential overdiagnosis.

4 Others
- Axonal neuropathy

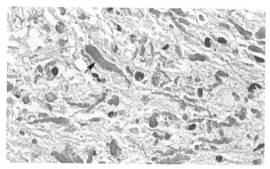

Rosenthal fibers

Senile plaques

- Plaques are extracellular 20–150 μm structures consisting of a central pink amyloid core surrounded by blunt swollen neuritic processes.
- The amyloid is composed of Aβ peptide, derived by proteolytic breakdown from a normal neuronal membrane protein called amyloid precursor protein (APP). Like tangles, they stain well with silver stains.
- There are four main types of plaques; diffuse, primitive, classic, and burnt-out. It is believed that there is progression from diffuse through finally burnt-out plaques. However, there is no definitive evidence for this.

1 Elderly individuals
- Plaques occur in the cortex with increased frequency in aging. In normal aging, the plaques are mainly diffuse.
- There may be small numbers of neuritic plaques, most associated with ubiquitin- and chromogranin-immunoreactive neuritis that do not contain tau protein.

2 Alzheimer disease (AD)
- ◆ Plaques are widely distributed in the brain of patients with AD. The neocortex and hippocampus are always involved. Most neuritic plaques include tau-immunoreactive dystrophic neurites.
3 Amyloid angiopathy
4 Down syndrome

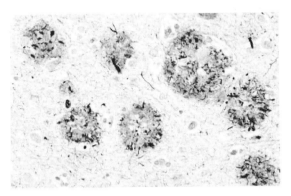

Senile plaques

Synucleinopathies

- The synucleinopathies are a subset of neurodegenerative disorders that have in common a pathological lesion composed of fibrillary aggregates of insoluble α-synuclein protein in selective populations of neurons and glia.
- Synuclein belongs to a family of brain proteins. It consists of three members: α-, β-, and γ-synuclein. The α-synuclein gene is located on chromosome 4, and only α-synuclein is associated with the filamentous inclusions. In diseases where it aggregates, α-synuclein changes conformation and aggregates with fibrils of β-sheet structure similar to other amyloid proteins.
- Abnormal filamentous aggregates of misfolded α-synuclein protein are the major components of Lewy bodies, dystrophic (Lewy) neuritis, and the Papp-Lantos filaments in oligodendroglial and neurons in multiple system atrophy linked to degeneration of affected brain regions.

1 **Lewy body disorders**
- ◆ Lewy bodies are intracytoplasmic inclusions composed of several proteins, including ubiquitin and α-synuclein. α-synuclein immunohistochemistry is now widely used to recognize this pathological marker in both brainstem and cortical lesions.

- The presence and distribution of Lewy bodies has led to a clinicopathological classification of Lewy body disorder spectrum.
  - 1.1 **Parkinson disease** (PD): brainstem type of Lewy bodies
    - Sporadic form: most common
    - Familial form: 10% of cases
      - Autosomal dominant with α-synuclein mutations
      - Autosomal recessive with parkin gene or DJ-1 mutations
  - 1.2 Dementia with Lewy bodies (DLB): both cortical and classic Lewy bodies
    - DLB is now recognized as the most frequent cause of degenerative dementia after AD.
  - 1.3 Normal aging
    - Lewy bodies occur in the substantia nigra and brainstem in up to 10% of normal individuals.
  - 1.4 Pure autonomic failure
2 Non-Lewy body disorders
  - 2.1 Multiple system atrophy (MSA)
    - The histological hallmark is the presence of α-synuclein-positive cytoplasmic inclusions in oligodendroglia, which is required for diagnosis.
    - Different clinical subtypes are recognized, including MSA-P, MSA-C and MSA-A.
  - 2.2 Neurodegeneration with brain iron accumulation type 1 (NBIA I)
    - Previously referred to as Hallervorden-Spatz disease.
    - Represents a pantothenate-kinase associated neurodegeneration caused by the PANK2 gene, linked to chromosome 20p12.3–13.
    - Axonal spheroids, the hallmark of this condition, contain immunoreactive neurofilament proteins, ubiquitin, superoxide dismustase, amyloid precursor protein, and α-synuclein.

Tauopathies

- A heterogeneous group of dementing illnesses and movement disorders, neuropathologically characterized by the presence of neuronal or neuronal and glial filamentous inclusions composed of tau, are collectively known as tauopathies.
- The phosphorylated tau, encoded by a single gene localized on the long arm of chromosome 17, is a microtubule-associated protein involved in microtubule assembly and stabilization. Tau is primarily expressed by neurons.
- Through alternative mRNA splicing, six tau isoforms are expressed in adult human brain, which differ from one another by the presence of three or four 31 or 32-amino-acid-long tandem repeats in the C-terminal microtubule binding region together with 0, 29, or 58 amino acid inserts in the N-terminal region.

1 Primary tauopathies
  - In this group of diseases, the characteristic neuropathological feature is the presence of abundant filamentous tau pathological findings in the absence of extracellular protein deposits.
  - The majority of such conditions are sporadic, with the exception of fronto-temporal dementia with parkinsonism, linked to chromosome 17, which is the major familial form of primary tauopathy.
    - Progressive supranuclear palsy (PSP)
    - Corticobasal ganglionic degeneration (CBGD)
    - Pick disease
    - Frontotemporal dementia (FTD) with Parkinsonism, linked to chromosome 17
2 Secondary tauopathies
  - In this group of diseases, the pathological changes include not only filamentous tau inclusions, but also extracellular, aggregated deposits of a secondary protein.
    - **Alzheimer disease**: most common
    - Gerstmann-Sträussler-Scheinker syndrome (GSS)
    - BRI2 gene related dementias
    - Familial British dementia (FBD)
    - Familial Danish dementia (FDD)

Tumors: demyelination vs. glioma

- A significant number of neuroimaging studies in patients with demyelination may show lesions with a tumor-like appearance. This probably represents the acuteness and severity of the demyelinating lesion(s).
- When this problem arises, clinical and radiological differentiation from glioma is often difficult, necessitating biopsy of the lesion(s).
- Even with biopsy, there is considerable difficulty in differentiating between the two. This is because tumor-like demyelinating lesions can also demonstrate hypercellularity, pleomorphism, necrosis, astrocytic mitosis as well as microcystic changes.
- The following histopathologic features suggest that a clinically diagnosed 'tumor' is not a true neoplasm.
  - Abundant lipid-laden macrophages
  - Evenly spaced astrocytes with well-developed processes
  - Sharp demarcation
  - Perivascular chronic inflammation

Features	Tumor-like demyelinating lesions	Glioma
Pleomorphism	Present	Present
Microcystic changes	Present	Present
Mitotic figures	May be present	Present
Lipidized astrocytes	May be present	May be present
Lipidized macrophages	Present	Rare
Perivascular lymphocytes	Present	Less common
Reactive astrocytes	Present	Less common
Sharp demarcation	Present	Rare
Response to steroids	Marked response	Response with varying degree

Modified from: Prayson R.A., Cohen M.L. *Practical Differential Diagnosis in Surgical Neuropathology*. 2000, Totowa, Humana Press.

Tumors: glioblastoma vs. metastatic carcinoma

- Metastatic tumors are often the major differential diagnostic consideration in the evaluation of a poorly differentiated high-grade neoplasm in the central nervous system.
- Metastases are the most common tumors in the CNS. However, spinal cord metastases are rare and are generally seen at the terminal stage of the disease process.
- The most common tumors to metastasize to the brain include lung, breast, melanoma, renal cell carcinomas, and choriocarcinoma.
- If one resorts to immunohistochemistry to distinguish a metastatic lesion from glioma, extra care needs to be taken not to confuse cross reactivity patterns of staining with certain markers.

Features	Glioblastoma	Metastatic carcinoma
Age	Peak at 3rd to 5th decade	Older
Multifocal	Less common	More common
Tumor border	Infiltrative	More discrete
Leptomeningeal involvement	Less common	More common, especially in hematologic malignancies
Fibrillary background	Present	Absent
Desmoplastic stroma	Absent	Present
Discrete cell borders	May be present	Absent
Vascular proliferation	More evident	Less evident
Perinecrotic pseudopalisading	May be present	Absent
GFAP	Positive	Negative
Cytokeratins	Can be positive	Positive, especially low-molecular weight keratin markers, e.g. CAM5.2

Tumors: gliosis vs. glioma

- One of the most challenging differential diagnostic problems in surgical neuropathology is to distinguish between gliosis or reactive astrocytosis and a low-grade glial tumor.
- In simple terms, gliosis is the brain's way of reacting to injury, insult, or to something that should not be there (e.g. tumor). Therefore, it is common to observe some degree of reactive gliosis adjacent to a tumor.
- In order to perform accurate interpretation, clinical and radiographic information should be available to pathologists. For example, a history of radiation may favor the presence of some gliosis.

Features	Gliosis	Glioma
Age	Any age	Peak 3rd to 5th decade
Location	Gray or white matter	White > gray matter
Gross	Firm	Firm, obliterate gray-white junction and may have cystic component
Hypervascularity	Evenly distributed	Unevenly distributed
Cellularity	Increased throughout	Increased cellularity is unevenly distributed
Distribution	Usually focal	Diffuse infiltration
Atypia	Binucleated cells, more eosinophilic cytoplasm with long tapered processes	High nuclear/cytoplasmic ratio, hyperchromatic, nuclear irregularity, and pleomorphism
Mitosis	Usually absent	Usually present
Calcification	None	May be present
Microcystic change	None	May be present
Satellitosis	None	May be present
Granulation	None	Can sometimes be seen in tumor

Tumors: pattern of immunohistochemical positivity in CNS tumors

- In addition to light microscopic examination, immunohistochemical staining has a useful role in differentiating different types of CNS tumors.
- The following information and examinations should be available to pathologists in order to perform accurate interpretation:
  - Light microscopic examination

- Neuroanatomic distribution
- Relevant immunohistochemistry examination
- Ultrastructure
- Aging changes
- Reaction to injury
- Neoplastic counterparts

Primary antibody	Tumors showing positivity
Glial fibrillary acidic protein (GFAP)	Astrocytoma, glioblastoma Ependymoma Subependymoma Anaplastic ependymoma Gliosarcoma Ganglioglioma Mixed glioma
Synaptophysin & neurofilament	Central neurocytoma Pineocytoma Medulloblastoma Neuroblastoma Ganglion cell tumor
Epithelial membrane antigen (EMA)	Meningioma Metastatic carcinoma
S-100 protein	Oligodendroglioma Anaplastic oligodendroglioma Neurofibroma Astrocytoma Melanoma Chordoma Neurilemoma
HMB-45	Melanoma
Vimentin	Meningioma Sarcoma
Cytokeratin	Metastatic carcinoma Choroid plexus papilloma Choroid plexus carcinoma Craniopharyngioma Chordoma Most germ cell tumors
Chromogranin	Pituitary adenoma Metastatic neuroendocrine tumors

Primary antibody	Tumors showing positivity
Alpha fetoprotein (AFP)	Embryonal carcinoma Endodermal sinus (Yolk sac) tumor
Placental alkaline phosphatase (PLAP)	Germinoma
Leukocyte common antigen (LCA) L-26 (B-cell marker) UCHL-1 (T-cell marker) Kappa and lambda light chains	Monoclonal staining pattern in lymphomas Polyclonal staining pattern in reactive inflammation and infections

Modified from: Vinters H.V., Farrell M.A., Mischel P.S., Anders K.H. *Diagnostic Neuropathology.* New York, Marcel Dekker, Inc.

Tumors: oligodendroglioma and its mimics

- Despite recent advances in immunohistochemical and molecular techniques, the oligodendroglioma still remains a tumor whose diagnosis is based on 'good old H&E'.
- The following are typical histological features of oligodendroglioma:
  - The cells appear to be easily spread into the cerebral cortex, resulting in prominent perineuronal satellitosis.
  - Calcifications, especially in a band-like pattern.
  - Germinal-like nodules of hypercellularity.
  - Admixed minigemistocytes.
  - Perinuclear halos.
- In addition to the above features, oligodendroglial-like components can be seen in the following tumors in which helpful differentiating features are provided below.

Features	Oligodendroglioma	DNET	Central neurocytoma	Clear cell ependymoma
Infiltration	Yes	Focal	No	No
Perineuronal satellosis	Yes	No	No	No
Minigemistocytes	Yes	No	No	No
Floating neurons	Yes	No	No	No
Cellular heterogeneity	May be present	Yes	No	May be present
Neuropil	No	No	Yes	No
Perivascular pseudorosettes	No	No	No	May be present

Continued

Features	Oligodendroglioma	DNET	Central neurocytoma	Clear cell ependymoma
GFAP	Minigemistocytes	Astrocytic areas	Weak/focal coexpression	Punctate cytoplasmic
Synaptophysin	No	May be present	Yes	No

DNET – dysembryoplastic neuroepithelial tumor.
Ref: Prayson R.A., Cohen M.L. *Practical Differential Diagnosis in Surgical Neuropathology*. 2000, Totowa, Humana Press.

Tumors: radiation change vs. high-grade glioma

- The major pathophysiological mechanisms underlying the use of radiotherapy include:
  1 inhibition of mitotic activity,
  2 chromosomal damage, and
  3 cell death.
- The effects of radiation therapy to the CNS can be acute, subacute, or chronic. Acute effects include headaches, vomiting, nausea, and focal neurological signs. Reactive astrocytosis and gliosis can develop during the subacute phase. Delayed effects, however, can develop months to years following treatment and include vascular changes and coagulative necrosis.
- It is not uncommon that radiation changes may be difficult to distinguish from recurrent glioma radiologically. Areas of radionecrosis can cause significant edema and enhance with contrast. In this situation, functional imaging, especially positron emission tomography (PET), may be indicated.

Features	Radiation changes	High-grade glioma
Edema	Present	Present
Contrast enhancement on imaging	Can be present	Present
Cell distribution	Even	Uneven
Vessels	Hyalinization	Vascular endothelial proliferation
Atypia	Reactive astrocytosis and bizarre cells	Present
High nuclear/cytoplasmic ratio	No	Yes
Perinecrotic pseudopalisading	None	Present
Necrotic without palisading	Can be present	Can be present
Calcification in necrosis	Can be seen	Very rare
Macrophages	Present	Less common
Long-term risk	Development of a secondary neoplasm	Most patients do not survive long term

Tumors: schwannoma vs. meningioma

- Schwannomas comprise at least 75% of cerebellopontine (CP) angle tumors, where they arise from the vestibular portion of the eighth cranial nerve. Such a tumor is termed an acoustic neuroma or vestibular schwannoma.
- Meningioma is the second most common tumor in the CP angle, accounting for 10–15% of tumors in this region.
- When confronted by a mass in the CP angle, the differential diagnosis usually lies between the above two, with a lower likelihood of exophytic brainstem glioma.
- The difficulty in differentiating between these two tumors pathologically usually arises when pathological specimens have overlapping features between Antoni A predominant schwannoma and fibroblastic meningioma.

Features	Schwannoma	Meningioma
Intracranial location	CP angle	Cerebral convexity, sphenoidal ridge, CP angle
Spinal location	Lumbar > cervical	Cervical > lumbar
Attachment	Nerve roots	Meninges
Spindle cells	Present	Present
Microcystic changes	Present	May be present
Antoni A	Present	Absent
True palisading	Present	May be present
Scattered atypical nuclei	Present	May be present
Hyalinized vessels	Present	Present
Perivascular hemosiderin	Present	Very rare
Psammoma bodies	Rare	May be present
S-100 protein	Strongly positive	May be positive
EMA	Focal	Diffuse

EMA – Epithelial membrane antigen.
Modified from: Prayson R.A., Cohen M.L. *Practical Differential Diagnosis in Surgical Neuropathology.* 2000, Totowa, Humana Press.

Viral CNS infections: cellular specificity and regional selectivity

- The essential histologic features of encephalitis include parenchymal damage (as evidenced by neuronophagia, demyelination), reactive astrocytosis, and inflammatory cellular infiltrates. In addition, inclusion bodies or cytomegalic cell changes can give important diagnostic clues on routine stains, especially when the involved cell type is considered.
- Every viral infection of the CNS usually features a fingerprint signature of selective vulnerability in the nervous system. Therefore, knowing cellular specificity as well as regional selectivity may help determine the etiologic viral agent.

Viral infections	Cellular specificity	Regional selectivity
HSV encephalitis	All cell types affected	Limbic system
VZV encephalitis	All cell types affected	Basal ganglia Central projection nuclei
CMV encephalitis	All cell types affected	Preference for periventricular area and superficial cortex, cauda equina and nerve roots
Poliomyelitis	Neurons	Motor neurons
SSPE	Large neurons, oligodendroglia	Low selectivity but usually spare cerebellum and spinal cord
PML	Oligodendroglia Astrocyte	Low selectivity
HIV encephalitis/ Leukoencephalopathy	Microglia/macrophages	Preference for white matter, basal ganglia
Rabies	Neurons	Preference for hippocampus, cerebellum
Tick-borne encephalitis	Neurons Ependyma	Preference for cerebellum, brainstem, spinal cord

HSV – herpes simplex virus, VZV – varicella zoster virus, CMV – cytomegalovirus, SSPE – subacute sclerosing panencephalitis, PML – progressive multifocal leukoencephalopathy.
Ref: Garcia J.H. Ed. *Neuropathology: The Diagnostic Approach.* 1997, St. Louis, Mosby.

Viral CNS infections: HIV-positive CNS biopsies

- Stereotactic brain biopsy is often required in HIV-infected patients who present with mass lesions, not responding to empiric anti-toxoplasma therapy.
- This procedure is often highly accurate and provides a safe diagnostic tool to ascertain the nature of mass lesions in HIV-infected patients.
- The three most common neuropathological diagnoses obtained from biopsies are progressive multifocal leukoencephalopathy, toxoplasmosis, and malignant lymphoma.
- HIV encephalitis and HIV leukoencephalopathy are increasingly recognized.

Diagnosis	Percentage
Progressive multifocal leukoencephalopathy (PML)	32
Toxoplasmosis	28
Malignant lymphoma	19
Necrosis of unclear significance	15
HIV encephalitis or leukoencephalopathy	2
Tuberculoma	2
Aspergilloma	2

Ref: Alesch F., Armbruster C., Budka H. Diagnostic value of stereotactic biopsy of cerebral lesions in patients with AIDS. *Acta Neurochir (Wien)* 1995; 134: 214–219.

Peripheral nervous system

Muscle biopsy: fiber types

- The adult muscle fiber is polygonal on transverse section. In infancy, fibers tend to be round. Extraocular muscles and some facial and pharyngeal muscle fibers remain round in adults.
- The functional unit of a muscle is a motor unit, which consists of multiple muscle fibers innervated by a single motor neuron. Therefore, all fibers within a single motor unit are of the same type. Because these fibers are distributed randomly across the muscle, normal muscle shows a checkerboard pattern of alternating light and dark fibers, as demonstrated on ATPase.
- Two major fiber types are recognized in muscle biopsies, and these correspond to some extent to the general physiologic subclassification of skeletal muscle cells. There is significant variability in the relative abundance of type 1 and type 2 fiber types among different muscles.

Features	Type 1 fibers	Type 2 fibers
Action	Sustained force	Sudden movement
	Tonic contraction	Purposeful motions
	Weight-bearing	
Physiology	Slow twitch	Fast twitch
Color	Red	White
Myoglobin content	High	Low
Lipid content	Abundant	Scant
Mitochondrial content	Abundant	Scant
Glycolytic enzymes and glycogen	Scant	Abundant
ATPase staining:		
• pH 4.2	Dark staining	Light staining
• pH 9.4	Light staining	Dark staining
NADH staining	Dark staining	Light staining

Muscle biopsy: neurogenic vs. myopathic features

- The technique for muscle biopsy can be either an open or closed (needle or punch) biopsy. Open biopsy yields a larger sample of tissue, allowing examination under light and electron microscopy as well as metabolic and molecular studies. Needle or punch biopsy has the advantage of obtaining specimens from different affected muscles.

- Muscle biopsy has greater diagnostic utility when the patient manifests with objective abnormalities on clinical examination, laboratory testing, or EMG. It is less useful or less sensitive in evaluating patients with subjective weakness, fatigue, or myalgias in the absence of objective abnormalities. In addition, biopsy of severely affected muscles should be avoided, as it is often impossible to determine the cause when there is widespread interstitial collagen deposit and fatty infiltration.
- Changes on muscle biopsy can occur in both neurogenic and myopathic processes.

Neurogenic features

1 Angular fibers
   - Atrophic fibers with a triangular shape on cross-section.
2 Target fibers
   - Cytoskeletal reorganization, which results in a central zone of disorganized filaments, best seen on NADH dehydrogenase staining.
3 Fiber type grouping
   - A group of adjoining fibers of the same histochemical type forms, and the normal checkerboard pattern of alternating light and dark fibers is lost.
4 Group atrophy
   - In chronic denervation, there is atrophy of the fibers of the type group.

Myopathic features

1 Basophilia
   - Regenerating muscle fiber has large internalized nuclei with prominent nucleoli, and the cytoplasm, laden with RNA, becomes basophilic.
2 Vacuolation
3 Fiber size variability
4 Muscle fiber splitting
   - Large fibers may divide along a segment, so in cross-section, a single large fiber contains a cell membrane traversing its diameter with adjacent nuclei.
5 Central nuclei
6 Myophagocytosis of necrotic muscle fibers
   - Characteristic but not pathognomonic for inflammatory myopathies.

NEUROPATHIC MUSCLE BIOPSY

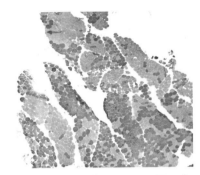

Myofiber grouping (ATPase at pH 9.4)

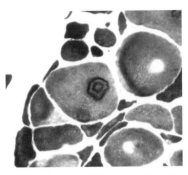

Target change (ATPase at pH 9.4)

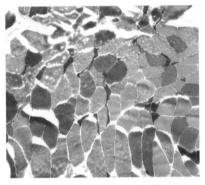

Angulated myofiber atrophy (non-specific esterase)

MYOPATHIC MUSCLE BIOPSY

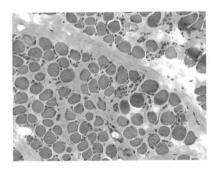

Endomysial fibrosis and fiber size variation (H&E frozen section)

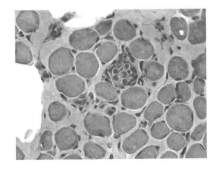

Endomysial fibrosis and fiber size variation (H&E frozen section)

Nerve biopsy: axonal vs. demyelinating neuropathy

- Indications for nerve biopsy are more limited than muscle biopsies. Often, the nerve biopsy does not give any further information, in addition to that obtained from clinical examination, laboratory testing, and electrophysiological studies.
- The sural nerve is most often biopsied. Biopsy of this nerve causes only a limited area of sensory loss on the lateral aspect of the ankle and foot. The superficial peroneal nerve is another nerve often biopsied because the underlying peroneus brevis muscle can also be biopsied under the same incision.
- The following are common indications for nerve biopsy:
  - Evaluation of amyloid neuropathy.
  - Evaluation of vasculitic neuropathy (muscle may be biopsied at the same time).
  - Suspected other autoimmune disorders, such as sarcoidosis.
  - Suspected infectious etiology.
  - To diagnose carcinomatous neuropathy, for example leukemia, lymphoma.
  - Evaluation of some hereditary neuropathy, for example Charcot-Marie-Tooth disease type 4, hereditary sensory and autonomic neuropathy, or giant axonal neuropathy.
  - As part of the investigation of chronic inflammatory demyelinating polyneuropathy (CIDP)

Features	Demyelinating neuropathy	Axonal neuropathy
Primary pathology	Dysfunction of Schwann cells or damage to the myelin sheath	Destruction of the axon with possible secondary disintegration of the myelin
Process	Usually segmental	Whole axon involved
Microscopic findings	Sequential episodes of demyelination and remyelination resulting in onion bulb appearance, new myelinated internodes shorter and thinner (seen best on teased nerve preparation)	Wallerian degeneration: breakdown and phagocytosis of axon and its myelin sheath (myelin ovoids), a regenerating cluster at the proximal stumps
Examples	Guillain-Barré syndrome Lead neuropathy Diphtheria neuropathy Leukodystrophies	Toxic, metabolic neuropathies Many hereditary neuropathies

NERVE BIOPSY: AXONAL VS. DEMYELINATING FEATURES

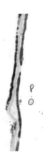

Wallerian degeneration

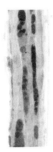

Wallerian degeneration (teased fiber preparation)

Segmental demyelination

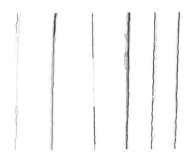

Segmental demyelination (teased fiber preparation)

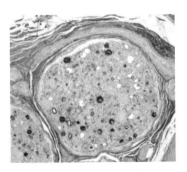

Loss of myelinated nerve fibers (toluidine blue, plastic section)

Onion bulb formation

- Onion bulb formation is caused by repeated bouts of demyelination and remyelination of peripheral nerves resulting in concentric arrays of Schwann cells and collagen surrounding individual axons.

Seen in:
1 Recurrent acquired demyelinating disorders
2 Hereditary hypertrophic neuropathies
   • Dejerine-Sottas sensory neuropathy (HMSN III)
   • Hypertrophic form of Charcot-Marie-Tooth disease
   • Refsum disease

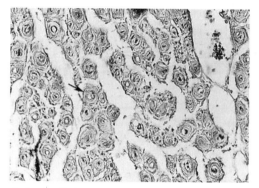

Onion bulb formation

Skin biopsy in neurological disorders

• Skin biopsy is not a common investigation used to evaluate patients
  with neurological disorders. However, it may be useful in diagnosing the
  following conditions.
• The most common indication for skin biopsy in patients with neurological
  disorders is to confirm the possibility of vasculitis, especially when they
  present with cutaneous lesions.

1 **Vasculitis**
   • Vasculitides can be classified into systemic necrotizing vasculitis, hypersensi-
     tivity vasculitis, giant cell vasculitis, and localized vasculitis.
   • The definite diagnosis of vasculitis can only be made on biopsy if transmural
     vessel wall inflammation is present.
   • Skin biopsy is usually considered in patients with suspected small vessel vascul-
     itis, especially when they present with cutaneous lesions.
2 Cerebral autosomal dominant arteriopathy with subcortical infarcts and leuko-
   encephalopathy (CADASIL)
   • The classic phenotype is for migraine to develop in the third and fourth decades
     in 40% to 60% of patients, strokes in the fourth and fifth decades, dementia in
     the sixth and seventh decades, and death usually in the seventh decade.

- The hallmark of the disease is the presence of granular osmiophilic material (GOM), seen adjacent to the basement membrane of the arteriolar smooth muscle cells on electron microscopy. The observation that GOM is detectable on skin biopsy suggests that this may be a useful diagnostic technique.

3 Small-fiber neuropathies

- Nerve conduction studies (NCS) assess only conduction of large myelinated nerve fibers. They are usually normal in patients with pure small-fiber neuropathies.
- Skin biopsy may show lower density of the intraepidermal nerve fibers (representing the terminals of C and A nociceptors) in patients with small-fiber neuropathies, while NCS or even nerve biopsies can be normal.
- Skin biopsy may allow an objective measurement of abnormality in patients with small-fiber neuropathies who mainly have subjective symptoms.

4 Dermatomyositis

- Dermatomyositis (DM) is a rare multisystem autoimmune disorder of adults and children that primarily affects skin and skeletal muscle. However, cutaneous disease does not always parallel muscle disease in its onset, activity, or response to therapy.
- Gottron papules are considered to be a pathognomonic skin lesion for dermatomyositis, while heliotrope rash with and without edema is very characteristic. Many other cutaneous lesions have been described to be associated with DM.
- In the absence of characteristic skin lesions, skin biopsy may be required in order to confirm the diagnosis. Salient features include vacuolar alteration of the basal cell layer of the epidermis, necrotic keratinocytes (apoptosis), vascular dilatation, and a sparse, superficial, perivascular lymphocytic infiltrate.

5 Storage disorders

- Skin or conjunctival biopsies are used to diagnose metabolic storage disorders more commonly in the pediatric population.
- Skin or conjunctival biopsy are helpful in diagnosing several types of metabolic storage disorders, including the following:
  - Neuronal ceroid lipofuscinoses: curvilinear and 'fingerprint' storage bodies.
  - Lafora disease: polyglucosan storage material
  - Neuroaxonal dystrophy: neuroaxonal spheroids (occasionally absent in peripheral nerves, in which cases skin biopsy can be negative)
  - Mucolipidoses: enzyme deficiencies in cultured fibroblasts
  - Mucopolysaccharidoses: enzyme deficiencies in cultured fibroblasts
  - Fabry disease: α-galactosidase deficiency in cultured fibroblasts
- Diagnostic findings from skin or conjunctival biopsy may be present in some of the multiple histological tissues contained within the biopsy. Diagnostic findings can be detected in peripheral nerve endings, fibroblasts (or fibroblast cultures), capillary endothelium, smooth muscle cells, and even sweat glands (skin biopsy only).

Chapter 2
Clinical Syndromes

Named syndromes   **97**

Motor and sensory signs and their localizations

- The following are useful neurological signs, commonly seen in clinical settings. Their common localizations are also provided as a quick guide.
- In the chart below, sensorimotor syndromes are divided into three broad categories:
  - Unilateral syndromes (sensory or motor symptoms on one side only) – suggests cerebral localization.
  - Bilateral and/or crossed syndromes with cranial/cerebral involvement (sensory or motor symptoms on either side with impairment of cranial nerves or mentation) – suggests brainstem localization.
  - Bilateral and/or crossed syndromes with NO cranial/cerebral involvement (sensory or motor symptoms on either side without impairment of cranial nerves or mentation) – suggests spinal cord localization.
- It is important for readers to be aware that the localizations listed below are common lesion locations for their correlate symptoms or signs. It is by no means the only localization for the symptoms/signs listed.

Motor and sensory symptoms or signs	Lesion localization
Unilateral syndromes	
Hemiparesis, including face, arm, and leg with hemisensory loss and aphasia or hemianopia	Contralateral (dominant) cerebral hemisphere involving a large area of motor, premotor, sensory cortices as well as corresponding language areas
Pure motor hemi-weakness	Subcortical lesion in the contralateral corona radiata, internal capsule, or the pons
Pure hemisensory loss	Contralateral ventroposterolateral nucleus of the thalamus
Ataxic hemiparesis	Contralateral posterior limb of the internal capsule or contralateral basis pontis
Dysarthria – clumsy hand syndrome	Basis pontis lesion in between its upper third and lower two-thirds
Weakness of isolated muscles of one extremity	Mononeuropathy, less likely to be mononeuritis multiplex or root lesions
Monoparesis	Brachial or lumbar plexus lesions, less commonly is the small cortical lesion

Motor and sensory symptoms or signs	Lesion localization
Bilateral or crossed syndromes with cranial/cerebral involvement	
Hemiparesis with contralateral LMN facial weakness and conjugate gaze deviation toward the weak extremities	Contralateral pontine lesion
Hemiparesis with ipsilateral loss of pain and temperature and a Horner syndrome and contralateral weakness of palate and tongue	Contralateral medullary lesion
Cruciate hemiplegia with weakness of the palate and tongue on the same side as the arm weakness	Paramedian medullary lesion ('arm' fibers decussate above 'leg' fibers decussation)
Quadriparesis with loss of facial movements but intact vertical eye movement (locked-in syndrome)	Bilateral ventral pontine lesions
Quadriparesis but preserved facial movements, but no tongue or palatal movement or speech	Bilateral medullary lesions
Bilateral arm weakness with relatively spared lower extremity function (man-in-the-barrel syndrome)	Lesions in the cerebral border zones
Quadriparesis with ventilatory support, diaphragmatic respiration	Bilateral C1-C4 lesions
Bilateral LMN arm weakness and UMN leg weakness	Bilateral C5-T1 lesions
Hemiparesis with contralateral loss of pain and temperature and preservation of vibration and joint position sense	Hemicord syndrome (Brown-Séquard syndrome)
Bilateral leg and/or arm weakness, associated with loss of pain and temperature but sparing of vibration and joint position sense	Anterior cord syndrome
Bilateral loss of vibration and joint position sense	Posterior columns
Spastic paraparesis	Commonly spinal cord lesions between lower cervical and thoracic levels NOTE: rarely can be central with a parasagittal lesion
Bilateral asymmetrical motor and sensory deficits in the lower lumbar and sacral segments, loss of pain and temperature in a saddle distribution, associated with bowel, bladder, and sexual dysfunction	Cauda equina lesions

Continued

Motor and sensory symptoms or signs	Lesion localization
Bilateral or crossed syndromes with NO cranial/cerebral involvement	
Mild motor weakness in lower extremities but marked loss of pain and temperature in the saddle distribution, associated with sphincter and sexual dysfunction	Conus medullaris lesion
Proximal muscle weakness without sensory changes	Myopathy, neuromuscular disorders, like myasthenia gravis

Clinical signs and symptoms

Alexia

- Alexia refers to an acquired inability to read.

Three types of alexia are recognized:
1 Alexia with agraphia
   - The patients cannot read and write and are not helped by spelling words aloud.
   - They perform as if truly illiterate.
   - It occurs with lesions in the left angular gyrus or left posterior inferior temporal lobe.
2 Alexia without agraphia
   - **A disconnection syndrome**
   - The patients often understand written words by spelling the words aloud and recognize the words from the letters they hear.
   - It occurs with lesions in the left medial occipital cortex and the splenium of the corpus callosum or lesions in the left lateral geniculate body and the splenium of the corpus callosum.
3 Frontal alexia
   - The deficits in frontal alexia involve the inability to name individual letters and disturbed comprehension of written language.
   - It occurs with lesions in the left frontal lobe.
   - Most patients with frontal alexia have Broca aphasia.

Amnesia associated with head injury

- Head injury is a frequent cause of amnesia, especially in young males.
- There are three distinct types of amnesia related to head injury.

1 **Post-traumatic amnesia (PTA)**
   - PTA refers to the period of amnesia following head trauma during which patients fail to acquire new information in normal and continuous fashion, despite being conscious and awake. Patients often deny memory problems, although it is apparent that they cannot learn new information.
   - Information is not encoded, and is not improved with cues.
   - The duration of PTA is a reliable marker of the severity of head injury, and also constitutes one of the best predictors of outcome.
2 Retrograde amnesia
   - Patients with head injuries often experience defective recall that occurred immediately before the injury. Information from the time closest to the injury is most likely to be lost, and the further back in time one goes, the less the impairment.
   - The extent of retrograde amnesia usually improves as the patients recover.
3 Anterograde amnesia
   - Moderate to severe head injuries often cause permanent damage to mesial temporal lobe structures (hippocampus), resulting in defective learning.
   - The impairment is usually centered on declarative knowledge and patients are usually sensitive to distraction, fatigue, and other influences that can produce suboptimal learning performance.

Aphasia

- Aphasia describes a difficulty in language.
- Aphasia should be differentiated from dysarthria, which implies slurred or poorly articulated speech with intact grammar and word selection.
- Nearly all aphasic states localize to the left hemispheric cortex. Exceptions include:
  - Left-handed persons (<50%) with language-dominant right hemispheres
  - Severe elevation in ICP or profound metabolic derangements with predominant anomia
  - Thalamic and/or basal ganglia lesions
- Aphasia is often associated with right hemiparesis.
- Acute onset aphasias are nearly always vascular in origin. Some types of epilepsy may also generate acute onset aphasias, though typically with return of function. Subacute and chronic etiologies include infectious/inflammatory pathologies, space occupying lesions, and several subtypes of dementia.
- Strictly speaking, most aphasic states exist on both a categorical and severity continuum. However, categorization is valuable both in attempting to localize a lesion and understanding language function.
- Essential elements in the evaluation of a patient with language difficulties include assessing:
  1 Speech output

2 Reading and writing
3 Repetition
4 Confrontational naming
5 Comprehension

Aphasia: type and localization

Aphasia subtype	Fluency	Compre-hension	Repetition	Anatomical localization	Vascular territory
Global	Impaired	Impaired	Impaired	Dominant perisylvian region	MCA
Mixed transcortical	Impaired	Impaired	Preserved, often with echolalia	Isolation of perisylvian language areas	Watershed zones between ACA, MCA, and PCA
Broca	Impaired	Preserved	Impaired	Broca area posterior, inferior, frontal gyrus	Superior division of MCA
Transcortical motor	Impaired	Preserved	Preserved	Isolation of Broca area from limbic language centers including prefrontal cortices and cingulated gyrus	ACA including watershed with MCA
Wernicke	Preserved, often with paraphasias and neologisms	Impaired	Impaired	Wernicke area posterior, superior temporal gyrus	Inferior division of MCA
Transcortical sensory	Preserved	Impaired	Preserved	Isolation of Wernicke area from posterior association cortices	Watershed area between MCA and PCA
Conduction	Preserved	Preserved	Impaired	Supramarginal gyrus, primary auditory cortex and insula, or the arcuate fasiculus	Branches of inferior or superior divisions of the MCA
Anomic	Fluent speech with good comprehension, but disturbance in retrieving object names either in spontaneous speech or confrontational naming			Variety of lesions, most frequently the dominant angular gyrus or dominant anterior temporal cortices	Branches of the inferior division of the MCA

MCA – middle cerebral artery, PCA – posterior cerebral artery, ACA – anterior cerebral artery.

Apraxia

- Apraxia refers to the inability to perform the movement on command when the disturbance could not be attributed to strength, coordination, sensory loss, or impaired comprehension.
- Apraxia is less predictable in left-handed individuals than in right-handed ones. Left-handers have right dominance for praxis regardless of which hemisphere is dominant for language. Apraxia in right-handed individuals is almost always associated with a left hemispheric lesion, although only about 50% of aphasic patients exhibit apraxia, suggesting that the right hemisphere compensates more readily for apraxia than for aphasia.

Three types of apraxia are recognized:
1 Limb-kinetic apraxia
  - Limb-kinetic apraxia refers to the loss of dexterity and coordination of distal limb movements that cannot be accounted for by weakness or sensory loss.
  - It is evident in pantomime, imitation, and use of objects.
  - It occurs contralateral to a hemispheric lesion.
2 Ideomotor apraxia
  - Ideomotor apraxia refers to the inability to perform a learned movement on command when the disturbance cannot be attributed to weakness, incoordination, sensory loss, or impaired comprehension.
  - It is obvious when asking patients to pantomime the use of objects.
  - This type of apraxia can occur with lesions in the inferior parietal lobe involving arcuate fasciculus, anterior callosal fibers, and frontal lobe.
3 Ideational apraxia
  - Ideational apraxia refers to the loss of the ability to pantomime the execution of an act that requires multiple steps to complete.
  - This type of apraxia is rare and occurs in diffuse brain lesions, such as head injury or dementia.

Ataxic gaits

- There are two major types of ataxic gait. One results from sensory ataxia and the other is associated with diseases of the coordinating mechanisms.
- It is possible that both types of ataxia may coexist in the same patient.

Gait of sensory ataxia	Gait of cerebellar disorders
Lesions usually involve the proprioceptive pathways in the spinal cord or peripheral nerve.	Lesions involve the coordinating mechanism in the cerebellum and its connections.
Romberg sign is present.	Romberg sign is absent. Unable to perform tandem gait.
Locomotion may not be abnormal when the eyes are open. The gait is usually irregular, jerky, with a broad base. Double tap feature may be present. The patient watches his/her feet and keeps his/her eyes on the floor while walking. When eyes are closed, staggering and unsteadiness increases and he/she may not be able to walk.	Ataxia that is present with eyes open and closed and may even increase when the eyes are closed. With a vermian lesion, there is staggering, unsteady, irregular, lurching with a wide-based gait. He/she may sway to any direction. If the lesion is in the cerebellar hemisphere, there is persistent swaying toward the involved side. Compass deviation may present.

Babinski sign and absent ankle jerks

- Can occur when one disease process affects both upper and lower motor neurons.
- Two common conditions can co-exist, resulting in this finding.

1 Subacute combined degeneration of the spinal cord
   - Low vitamin B$_{12}$ results in posterior column degeneration as well as peripheral neuropathy.
   - Manifestations include myelopathy, mental abnormalities, optic neuropathy, and peripheral neuropathy with loss of deep tendon reflexes.
2 Syphilitic taboparesis
   - Argyll-Robertson pupil is a useful diagnostic clue.
   - Tertiary syphilis characterized by obliterative endarteritis causing neuronal loss. Upper and lower motor neurons may be affected.
3 Friedreich ataxia (FRDA)
   - Centrally, there is degeneration of the posterior columns and pyramidal tracts.
   - Peripheral sensory neuropathy occurs due to loss of large myelinated fibers.
4 Amyotrophic lateral sclerosis
   - Upper and lower motor neuron involvement.
   - However, distinct from others because no peripheral sensory neuropathy.
5 Two common conditions at the same time (e.g. a diabetic patient with cervical cord lesion).
6 Metachromatic leukodystrophy
7 Adrenomyeloneuropathy

Bulbar vs. pseudobulbar palsy

- Weakness of bulbar muscles can be caused by lower or upper motor neuron lesions.
- The lesions are usually bilateral in order to result in clinically evident bulbar weakness.

Features	Bulbar palsy	Pseudobulbar palsy
Site of lesions	Lower motor neuron	Upper motor neuron

Causes	Nuclear lesions:
	  • Medullary infarction
	  • Medullary tumor
	  • Syringobulbia
	  • Demyelination
	  • Motor neuron disease
	Peripheral nerve lesions:
	  • Miller-Fisher syndrome
	  • Sarcoidosis
	  • Leptomeningeal infiltration by tumors
	  • Skull base tumor or metastasis
	  • Motor neuron disease
	Neuromuscular disorders:
	  • Myasthenia gravis
	  • Botulism
	Primary muscle disorders:
	  • Polymyositis
	  • Muscular dystrophy
		Supranuclear lesions:
		  • Stroke
		  • Demyelination
		  • Motor neuron disease
		  • Neurodegenerative disorders

Clinical features	Dysarthria (nasal) Dysphagia Wasted atrophic tongue Tongue fasciculations Absent gag reflex	Dysarthria (spastic, Donald-duck) Choking attacks Stiff, spastic tongue Exaggerated jaw jerk Exaggerated gag reflex Emotional lability

Coma

- The definition of coma rests on the definition of consciousness. For medical purposes, a descriptive approach defines coma as unarousable unresponsiveness (alteration of vigilance).
- Neuronal structures necessary for the maintenance of normal consciousness are the cerebral cortex, the ascending reticular activating system, and the connecting fibers of both structures. The functional or lesional disturbance of the ascending reticular activating system plays a definite role in the alteration of global consciousness.

- The part of the activating system sensitive for the maintenance of alertness lies in the pontomesencephalic tegmentum. Disturbances leading to coma must occupy both sides of the midline, be located at the pontomesencephalic junction, and be either acutely acquired or fairly large in extent.

Coma can result from the following lesions:

1 Coma with supratentorial lesions
   - In general, supratentorial lesions are unlikely to produce coma directly, provided the definition of coma excludes states of profoundly depressed cortical function.
   - Elevated intracranial pressure per se is not apt to cause coma.
   - More likely, supratentorial lesions cause coma by causing secondary alterations upon the brainstem, e.g. in cerebral herniation.
2 Coma with infratentorial lesions
   - Infratentorial lesions can cause coma in different ways.
   - Firstly, direct lesions in the paramedian pontomesencephalic recticular formation (e.g. pontine hemorrhage) can produce coma.
   - Secondly, infratentorial processes located outside the brainstem can lead to coma by pressure upon the reticular formation, either directly or by upward herniation through the tentorial notch.
3 Coma with diffuse brain disturbances
   - In general, prolonged diffuse encephalopathies are associated with depressions of cortical activities, but have preserved cycles of sleep and wakefulness.
   - Two possibilities can occur in patients with encephalopathy that may result in coma. One is diffuse cerebral edema with consecutive cerebral herniation. The other is anoxic, metabolic damage to a selective vulnerable area resulting in disintegrating cerebral functions down to the mesencephalic level.

Differentiation of coma from other conditions of altered responsiveness

- Several conditions of altered responsiveness must be distinguished from coma. The hallmark feature of coma is unarousable unresponsiveness with no established sleep-wake cycle and reduced cerebral metabolism.

1 Sleep
   - Sleep denotes physiological loss of consciousness. Its differentiation from coma is based on arousability.
   - Although it seems obvious, differentiation of initial stages of coma from physiological but exaggerated sleep due to prolonged sleep deprivation or states after intoxication with alcohol or CNS depressants can be difficult.

2 Locked-in syndrome (Pseudocoma or de-efferented state)
   - In patients with locked-in syndrome, there is no alteration of consciousness. The patient is completely paralyzed except for vertical eye movements and is able to communicate complex ideas by blinking Morse code.
   - Lesions are located in the ventral pons.
3 Akinetic mutism (sometimes called extrapyramidal locked-in syndrome)
   - In akinetic mutism, the patient is mute or speaks in fragments, and does not move spontaneously but moves secondary to exogenous stimuli. Communication is significantly reduced but not abolished.
   - The lesions responsible are located in the thalamus, basal ganglia, bilateral cingulate gyri, or posterior part of the third ventricle sparing the cortex.
4 Vegetative state (sometimes called apallic syndrome)
   - Patients with vegetative state have no signs of cortical function but have alternating periods of sleep and wakefulness. The eyes are opened periodically, but there are no signs of appreciation of the environment. Accompanying pyramidal signs help differentiate it from akinetic mutism.
   - No common patterns of lesions can be defined.
5 Nonconvulsive status epilepticus
   - This can be either complex partial status epilepticus or absence status epilepticus.
   - This condition is more common than suspected and the diagnosis is often missed.
6 Frontal lobe disease
   - Lesions are usually prefrontal and bilateral.
   - Patients exhibit long delays between a stimulus and reaction.
7 Others
   - Transient unresponsiveness in the elderly (idiopathic recurrent stupor)
   - Pseudocoma or hysterical coma
   - Vegetative depression
   - Catatonia

Neurological conditions associated with lack of awareness

- A coma is the state in which a patient can not be aroused by any stimulus, however vigorous or painful (unarousable unresponsiveness). The patient in coma elicits no response to external stimulus or inner need, and lacks both wakefulness and awareness.
- Persistent vegetative state (PVS) is defined as that condition where a vegetative state is present 1 month after an acute traumatic or nontraumatic brain injury, or lasting for at least 1 month in patients with degenerative or metabolic disorders or developmental malformations.

- Brain death is declared when brainstem reflexes, motor responses, and respiratory drive are absent in a normothermic, nondrugged comatose patient with a known irreversible massive brain lesion and no contributing metabolic derangements.

Condition	Persistent vegetative state (PVS)	Coma	Brain death
Self-awareness	Absent	Absent	Absent
Suffering	No	No	No
Motor function	No purposeful movement	No purposeful movement	None, except spinal reflexes
Sleep-wake cycles	Intact	Absent	Absent
Respiratory function	Normal	Variable	Absent
EEG activity	Polymorphic delta/theta activity with occasional slow alpha	Polymorphic delta and theta activity	Electrocerebral silence
Cerebral metabolism	Reduced by 50% or more	Reduced by 50% or more	Absent
Life expectancy	Usually 2–5 years	Variable	Death within 2–4 weeks (Harvard criteria)
Neurologic recovery	Nontraumatic: rare after 3 months Traumatic: rare after 12 months	Usually recovery, or PVS, or death within 2–4 weeks	No recovery

Ref: Ashwal S., Cranford R. Medical aspects of the persistent vegetative state. The multi-society task force on PVS. *N Engl Med J* 1994; 330: 1499–1508.

Confabulation

- Confabulation refers to the production of erroneous answers by patients with memory defects and represents a failure of error recognition rather than a desire to deliberately mislead. It should be distinguished from prevarication in which the patient attempts to deliberately mislead the examiner.

- Studies of patients with confabulation demonstrated that it most likely reflects impairment of executive function. Confabulation frequently co-exists with other evidence of executive dysfunction, such as preservation and apathy.
- Functional imaging in patients with confabulation showed abnormalities of orbital and medial frontal regions that resolve in concert with resolution of confabulation.

Two types of confabulation are described:

1 Confabulation of embarrassment
   - The amnesic patient provides incorrect answers based on personal past experience. Patients respond to questions with answers derived from the past. The answers are usually coherent and possible, but incorrect.
   - It typically occurs in the acute stage of Wernicke-Korsakoff syndrome.
2 Fantastic confabulation
   - A more rare and colorful syndrome, may be viewed as a delusional disorder.
   - Patients have impaired judgement and current amnesia or recent amnesia, and spontaneously describe impossible, adventurous, and often gruesome experiences.
   - Most patients have obvious frontal lobe syndromes, for example in post-traumatic encephalopathy and degenerative dementias.

Disconnection language syndromes

- Disconnection language syndromes result from interruption of connections between functional language cortices and other areas of the cortex.
- These syndromes are infrequently encountered, though typically result from vascular insult.

Syndrome	Associated deficit	Localization
Ideomotor apraxia	Able to utilize left hand without compromise, except for functions suggested by verbal command	Left frontal cortex and adjacent corpus callosum
Pure word deafness	Unable to interpret or repeat verbal words, though reads and hears sounds without compromise	Deep, dominant temporal lobe or bilateral primary auditory cortex
Alexia without agraphia	Able to write but not read	Splenium of corpus callosum disconnecting right occipital cortex from left language centers

Dysarthria

- Dysarthria refers to impairment in motor aspects of speech.
- Abnormalities include disturbances in rate (too slow, too fast, or bursts), volume (hypophonia, megaphonia), tone, pitch, and timing of articulation.
- Mixed dysarthria can occur in a disorder that affects more than one type of motor dysfunction, for example mixed spastic-ataxic dysarthria in multiple sclerosis or mixed spastic-flaccid speech in amyotrophic lateral sclerosis.
- Speech therapy should be considered in all patients with dysarthria, regardless of etiology and type.

Types of dysarthria	Features	Disorders
Flaccid	Hypernasality Imprecise consonant Monopitch	LMN lesions, such as myasthenia gravis
Spastic	Strained-strangled voice, slow rate, imprecise, harsh voice	UMN lesions, such as stroke with pseudobulbar palsy
Ataxic	Excess stress, irregular rate and rhythm, distorted vowels	Multiple sclerosis
Hypokinetic	Monopitch, short rushes of speech, inappropriate silence, variable rate	Parkinson disease
Hyperkinetic	Imprecise consonants, prolonged intervals, excess loudness varations, harsh voice	Huntington disease
Dystonic	Strained-strangled voice, monopitch, irregular articulation, distorted vowels	Spasmodic dysphonia
Mixed	Mixed features of the above	Multiple sclerosis Amyotrophic lateral sclerosis

Dysphagia

- The descending motor pathway for swallowing closely follows that for articulation. Corticobulbar fibers travel to the nuclei of the 9th and 10th cranial nerves with bilateral innervation. Motor fibers from the 10th nucleus supply the soft palate and pharynx, which are required for swallowing. The adjacent 9th nucleus sends motor fibers to the middle constrictor of the pharynx and stylopharyngeus.

- Any lesions affecting the above pathway usually cause difficulty with swallowing. However, neurogenic dysphagia often have difficulty with solids and more so liquids, as opposed to mechanical dysphagia, due to obstruction of the esophagus when difficulty swallowing solids starts first and predominates.
- Dysphagia is frequently accompanied by dysarthria. Indeed, the causes often overlap, but not invariably so.

1 **Brainstem lesions**
   1.1 Vascular lesions
       ▪ Most common.
       ▪ Examples include lateral medullary lesion (Wallenberg syndrome), pontine lesion affecting corticobulbar fibers, or cerebellar hemorrhages compressing medulla.
   1.2 Nonvascular lesions causing multiple cranial neuropathies
       ▪ Infections related, for example Lyme disease, diphtheria, poliomyelitis, tetanus, etc.
2 Bilateral cerebral hemispheric lesions
   ◆ Other physical signs, including altered consciousness, often present.
   ◆ Less commonly, opercular syndrome and putaminal lesions can also cause dysphagia.
3 Motor neuron disease
   ◆ Amyotrophic lateral sclerosis
   ◆ Progressive bulbar palsy
   ◆ Postpolio syndrome
4 Neuromuscular junction disease
   ◆ Most common in this category is myasthenia gravis.
   ◆ Botulism is an important differential diagnosis.
5 Myopathy
   ◆ Not a common cause (e.g. polymyositis, inclusion body myositis).
6 Local pathology
   ◆ Mechanical lesions in the pharynx and esophagus
7 Others
   ◆ Anticonvulsants
   ◆ Paraneoplastic syndromes

Dysphonia/aphonia

- Phonation is a function of the larynx and the vocal cords. Sound is produced by air passing over the vocal cords, while the pitch is altered by changes in tension of the membranous part of the vocal cords, brought about by the intrinsic laryngeal muscles.
- All muscles are supplied by the laryngeal branches of the tenth cranial nerve. The recurrent laryngeal nerve supplies all muscles except the cricothyroid muscle, which is innervated by the external laryngeal nerve, arising from nucleus ambiguus.
- Paralysis of vocal cord can be visualized by indirect laryngoscopy showing the inability to abduct on attempted phonation.

Common causes of dysphonia:

1 **Recurrent laryngeal nerve palsy**
   - Recurrent laryngeal nerve carries motor, sensory, and parasympathetic fibers. The nerve divides into an internal branch, which supplies sensation to the vocal cords and subglottic region, and an external branch, which provides motor function to four intrinsic laryngeal muscles, including the thyroarytenoid, the lateral and posterior cricoarytenoid, and the transverse and oblique arytenoid.
      - Following thyroid surgery: the most frequent post-thyroidectomy complication is recurrent laryngeal nerve (RLN) damage with subsequent vocal cord palsy.
      - Aortic or carotid aneurysm
      - Bronchogenic carcinoma: Pancoast tumor
2 Medullary lesion
   - Lesions in the medulla involving nucleus ambiguus can cause dysphonia, commonly occurs as part of lateral medullary syndrome.
   - Other causes include syringobulbia, tumors.
3 Local lesions in the vocal cord
   - Polyps
   - Tumors
4 Functional dysphonia

Excessive daytime sleepiness (EDS)

- Excessive sleepiness can result from both physiological and pathological causes.

1 **Voluntary sleep deprivation**
   - The most common cause of EDS and is increasingly common.

- Sleep deprivation and sleepiness because of lifestyle and habits of going to sleep and waking up at irregular hours can be considered to result from disruption of the normal circadian and homeostatic physiology.

2 Primary sleep disorders

  2.1 **Obstructive sleep apnea (OSA)**

    ▪ **The second most common cause of EDS, but the most common cause of pathological sleepiness**

    ▪ Most patients are usually overweight middle-aged men.

    ▪ Complications include hypertension and cardiac arrthythmias.

    ▪ Hypoventilation results in frequent arousals.

  2.2 Narcolepsy

    ▪ The two most common features of narcolepsy are sleep attacks and cataplexy.

    ▪ The important feature is that most patients feel fresh on awakening from sleep attacks, contrary to OSA.

3 Medication related hypersomnia

- Common cause of EDS and probably under-recognized.
- Examples include benzodiazepines, antipsychotics, anticonvulsants, narcotic analgesias, and antihistamines, etc.

4 Restless legs syndrome (RLS)

5 General medical conditions

- Several systemic diseases, such as hepatic, renal, and respiratory failure or electrolyte abnormalities can cause metabolic encephalopathies resulting in EDS.
- Other examples include hypothyroidism, congestive cardiac failure, anemia, upper airway resistance syndrome.

6 Neurological causes

- Neurological conditions are not the common causes of EDS. EDS associated with neurological diagnosis usually results from metabolic encephalopathies.
- Focal brain lesions causing EDS include tumors or vascular lesions affecting reticular activating system, hypothalamus, or bilateral paramedian thalamus.
- Certain neurodegenerative conditions can cause EDS, such as Alzheimer disease, Parkinson disease and multisystem atrophy, etc.
- Neuromuscular causes of EDS include myotonic dystrophy (EDS from nocturnal hypoventilation and reticular activating system dysfunction).

7 Idiopathic hypersomnolence

8 Klein-Levin syndrome: rare cause, but an interesting condition

- A rare cause of EDS, characterized by episodes of hypersomnolence for 16–18 hours, followed by enhanced appetite.
- Exact cause is not known, but is thought to be a limbic-hypothalamic dysfunction.

Frontal release signs

- The terms frontal release signs and primitive reflexes are used for responses that are present in some patients with advanced dementias, diffuse encephalopathies, normal-pressure hydrocephalus, and cerebral neurodegenerative disorders. They are usually diffuse, but often affect primarily the frontal lobes or the frontal association areas.
- The significance of these release signs is debatable. In general, any single one of these reflexes may be present in persons without severe central nervous system disorders, but the presence of a combination of several such signs is correlated with poorer neurological prognosis.
- The primitive reflexes do not have great localizing value, suggesting instead the presence of diffuse and widespread dysfunction of the hemispheres.

1 Exaggeration of the muscle stretch reflexes
   - For example, grasp reflex of the hands and feet, Hoffmann, Trömner, and Babinski signs.
   - Some of these reflexes are normally found in infants, disappear in childhood, but return in cerebral disease.
2 Glabellar or orbicularis oculi reflex
   - When repeated stimuli are directed to the glabella, the blink response normally stops after the first few taps. In corticospinal tract disease, extrapyramidal disease or diffuse CNS disorders, the reflex is exaggerated and the blinks continue with repeated stimuli (Myerson sign).
3 Orbicularis oris reflex
   - This reflex can be elicited by a minimal tap to either upper or lower lip or even sweeping the tongue blade across the lips. If such stimulation produces puckering and protrusion of the lips, the response is called a snout reflex.
4 Sucking reflex
   - This reflex is normally present in infants, in whom the stimulation of the lips is followed by sucking movements of the lips, tongue, and jaw.
   - An exaggerated response of sucking reflex is called the mastication reflex.
5 Head retraction reflex
   - This reflex is a quick, involuntary backward jerk of the head that follows a brisk tap of the upper lip while the head is bent slightly forward.
   - It is normally absent in adults but can be seen in patients with bilateral supracervical lesions and those with diffuse CNS disorders.
6 Palmomental reflex
   - There is ipsilateral contraction of the mentalis and orbicularis oris muscles following stimulation of the thenar eminence of the hand or palm.

Hemifacial sensory loss

- Acute onset of facial paresthesias presenting as numbness, tingling, or an ill-defined discomfort is frequently encountered in clinical practice.
- Cutaneous sensation from the face is carried to the brainstem by trigeminal nerve. After entering the pons, the fibers form the spinal tract of the trigeminal nerve, which ascends ipsilaterally in the trigeminothalamic tract terminating in the thalamus. Spinothalamic tract also joins the medial lemniscus and terminates at the posterior thalamic nuclei. The cortical projection then ends in the postcentral cortex in a somatotopic arrangement.
- The etiologies vary from anxiety related to serious intracranial lesions. Accompanied physical findings usually give a clue to lesion localization.

1 **Nonspecific or anxiety**
  - When the paresthesias last for seconds or minutes, related to stress, or nervousness in young persons, no specific pathology is often identified.
  - Perioral paresthesias may be related to hyperventilation.
2 **Multiple sclerosis**
  - This diagnosis should be considered in all young patients who present with a persistent sensory impairment in the infraorbital area corresponding to the maxillary division of the trigeminal nerve.
3 Herpes zoster infection
  - Herpes zoster infection of the trigeminal nerve (e.g. herpes zoster ophthalmicus) can cause dysesthesia, which often follows after several days of hypesthesia to pain or light touch sensation.
4 Cavernous sinus lesions
  - Patients usually present with numbness over the first divisions of the trigeminal nerve, associated with diplopia or peri-orbital pain.
  - If patients also demonstrate proptosis, chemosis, headache, and fever, cavernous sinus syndrome should be strongly considered. Septic cavernous sinus thrombosis is a life-threatening condition and requires immediate assessment and evaluation.
  - If diplopia is a main feature, associated with retro-orbital pain, Tolosa-Hunt syndrome is a possibility. It is a low-grade inflammatory process of unknown etiology involving a cavernous sinus.
5 Bell palsy
  - Patients may complain of abnormal sensations over the paretic facial muscles.
6 *Lateral medullary lesion (Wallenberg syndrome)*

- Patients usually present with hypalgesia and thermoanesthesia over the entire half of the face, accompanied by hypalgesia and thermoanesthesia over the contralateral half of the trunk and extremities.
- Other associated findings in lateral medullary syndrome include dysphagia, dysarthria, vertigo, ipsilateral cerebellar findings, and Horner syndrome.

7 Others
- Chronic frontal or maxillary sinusitis
- Progressive dental pathology
- Numb chin syndrome: a paraneoplastic syndrome, associated with lymphoma, breast, and prostate carcinoma.

Gait abnormalities

- Normal gait requires a complex neural integration of vision, proprioception, vestibular, and motor function.
- Due to the complex integration and multimodal requirements, analysis of gait abnormalities is extremely high yield and in some cases diagnostic.
- Gait is composed of antigravity support, stepping, maintenance of equilibrium, and propulsion.
- Gait evaluation should include natural, tandem, heel, and toe gait as well as observation of arising from a seated position, turns, and resistance to external forward and backward pushing.

1 **Parkinsonian and festinating gait**
- Characterized by short, shuffling steps, absent or reduced arm swing, stooped posture, hesitation, freezing, and en bloc turning.
- Arms are typically flexed and held in advance of the body, legs are stiff and bent at the hips and knees. Feet may barely clear the floor.
- Festination ('hasten') refers to the tendency in these patients to accelerate during ambulation in an apparent attempt to keep up with their center of gravity.
- Festination occurs both forwards and backwards and may result in falls and injury in unassisted patients.

2 **Sensory ataxia gait**
- Due to pathology involving proprioceptive sensory modalities or occasionally bilateral parietal lobe lesions.
- Awkward foot placement with inability to rapidly correct.
- Coarse movements of legs with stamping of feet, which are placed far apart to correct for instability. Frequent visual checks of foot placement.
- Gait is achieved as patient flings legs forward and outward abruptly in steps of variable length and height. Ataxia markedly enhanced with the deprivation of visual cues.

- ◆ Romberg sign present.
- ◆ Frequently seen in tabes dorsalis, Friedreich ataxia, subacute combined posterior column degeneration, syphilitic meningitis, and chronic sensory polyneuropathy.

3 **Steppage (equine) gait**
- ◆ Regular and even steps with the advancing foot held with the toes down. Walking accomplished with excessive flexion at the hip lifting the foot abnormally high in an effort to clear the foot off of the ground.
- ◆ Frequently accompanied by a foot slap.
- ◆ May be unilateral or bilateral and occurs as a result of chronic axonal neuropathies such as Charcot-Marie-Tooth disease, muscular atrophy, poliomyelitis, and paralysis of the pretibial and peroneal musculature.

4 **Cerebellar gait**
- ◆ Wide based with separation of the legs.
- ◆ Unsteadiness with irregularity of steps and lateral veering.
- ◆ Steps are uncertain with variable length, some very short and others longer than intended. Observed in patients with cerebellar stroke, multiple sclerosis, cerebellar tumors, and cerebellar degeneration.

5 Normal pressure hydrocephalus gait
- ◆ Few distinguishing features, frequently but inaccurately, referred to as 'apraxic.'
- ◆ Cardinal features include shuffling, widened base, and diminished cadence.
- ◆ An important diagnosis requiring further evaluation especially in the setting of unexplained, progressive dementia and urinary incontinence.

6 Spastic gait (hemiplegic/paraplegic)
- ◆ Characterized as slow, stiff, and scraping.
- ◆ Patients hold the affected limb stiffly without flexion at the hip, knee, and ankle. Leg is propelled outwards and forwards in a semi-circular pattern known as circumduction.
- ◆ The foot frequently wears down the shoe on the outer soles and toes.
- ◆ Often the result of stroke or as a major manifestation of cerebral palsy.

7 Waddling (gluteal, Trendelenburg) gait
- ◆ Seen with weakness in the gluteal muscles and the resultant failure to stabilize the weight-bearing hip during ambulation.
- ◆ Exaggerated outward bulging of the weight-bearing hip with a concomitant hip drop and truncal tilt to the opposite side.
- ◆ Observed in progressive muscular dystrophies, spinal muscular atrophy, and inflammatory myopathies.

8 Dystonic/choreoathetotic gait
- ◆ A gait with superimposition of involuntary muscle movements.
- ◆ Gait occurs with continuous, irregular movements of the face, neck, arms, and hands and, when severe, the trunk and proximal joints.

- Movements include head-jerking, facial grimacing, tongue protrusion. Twisting and squirming movements of the trunk and limbs are seen as the arms and hands are alternatively flexed, extended, pronated, and supinated.
- Seen in focal axial dystonias, congenital athetosis, Huntington chorea, and Oppenheim dystonia.

9 Reeling (drunken) gait
- Tottering gait with lateral leering and frontward/backward tipping, giving the appearance of being on the verge of losing balance and falling.
- Able to momentarily correct, unlike cerebellar gait.
- Marked variability.

10 Toppling gait
- A general term used in describing gaits characterized by frequent tottering and falling.
- Often the result of lateral medullary syndrome with falls to the side of the lesion, vestibular neuronitis with falls to the affected side, or midbrain strokes with frequent backwards falls.
- Apparently a disorder of balance, in particular a decrement in 'righting' reflexes.

11 Hysterical gait
- Broad category of abnormal gait patterns including hysterical monoplegia, hemiplegia, paraplegia, as well as astasia-abasia.
- Astasia-abasia refers to patients unable to stand or walk but retaining normal leg movements while supine. When placed on their feet, they are able to make only a few, if any, steps before crumpling down. Almost always hysterical.

Hearing loss: Rinne and Weber tests

- The bedside examination of hearing loss may include tuning fork tests of air and bone conduction.
- Tuning forks at a frequency of 256 Hz or 128 Hz **should not be used** because the vibrations they produce by bone conduction may be mistaken for sounds. Therefore, the 512-Hz tuning fork is the lowest useful frequency.
- Although tuning fork tests allow the examiner to screen for a conductive versus a sensorineural loss, the tests do not evaluate the degree of impairment or the effects of that impairment on speech understanding.
- Two standard tuning fork tests are the Rinne and Weber tests.

Weber test	Rinne test
Signal transmitted by bone conduction is localized to the better-hearing ear or the ear with the greatest conductive deficit.	Comparing the patient's hearing sensitivity by bone versus air conduction.

Weber test	Rinne test
The stem of vibrating fork is placed on the skull in the midline and the patient is asked to indicate in which ear the sound is heard.	The stem of the fork should be placed firmly on the mastoid, as near to the posterosuperior edge of the ear canal as possible. The stem cannot touch the auricle. Then, the fork is held 2.5 cm lateral to the tragus.
Lateralization to the poorer-hearing ear indicates an element of conductive impairment in that ear.	Positive Rinne test: air conduction is better than bone conduction.
Lateralization to the better-hearing ear indicates a sensorineural hearing loss in the opposite ear.	Negative Rinne test: bone conduction is heard better than air conduction

Hemiplegia

- Hemiplegia refers to weakness or paralysis involving the arm and the leg, and sometimes the face on one side of the body.
- Hemiplegia is the commonest form of paralysis and is attributable to a lesion in the corticospinal pathway on the side opposite to the paralysis.
- The corticospinal tract starts from fibers of the motor, premotor, supplementary motor, and parietal cortices converging in the corona radiata and descending through the posterior limb of the internal capsule, cerebral peduncle, basis pontis, and medulla. 75% of corticospinal tract fibers decussate at the lower end of the medulla, and the rest descend ipsilaterally as uncrossed ventral corticospinal tracts.
- The somatotopic organization of the corticospinal system is important clinically. In the cortex, leg representation is located parasagittally, while face representation is situated more laterally. Once the fibers converge in the internal capsule, the axons subserving the face are situated more anteriorly in the posterior limb, while those for hand and arm are situated in the central part, and those for foot and leg, more posteriorly.
- Hemorrhagic or ischemic vascular lesions are the most common cause of hemiplegia, followed by trauma. Other causes include tumors, demyelination, abscess, meningoencephalitis, etc.

Location of lesions producing hemiplegia:

Lesion localization	Pattern of hemiplegia
Cerebral cortex Corona radiata Internal capsule	Weakness or paralysis of the contralateral leg, arm and lower face

Continued

Lesion localization	Pattern of hemiplegia
Upper brainstem	Weakness or paralysis of the contralateral leg, arm, and face
+ Ipsilateral oculomotor nerve palsy	Midbrain: Weber syndrome
+ Ipsilateral abducens and facial palsy	Lower pons: Millard-Gubler syndrome
Medulla	Weakness of the contralateral leg and arm with ipsilateral pharyngeal or laryngeal weakness
Lower medulla	Weakness of the contralateral or ipsilateral arm and leg, with sparing of the face and tongue
Lateral column of the cervical spinal cord	Ipsilateral hemiplegia

Intracranial hypotension

- The normal lumbar CSF pressure is between 60 and 200 mm H_2O. Intracranial hypotension is considered when the initial lumbar CSF pressure is below 60 mm H_2O.
- Symptoms of intracranial hypotension include:
  - Positional headache: the most characteristic symptom. Patients experience headache in the erect position, relieved by supine position.
  - Headache can also be precipitated by cough, straining, the Valsalva maneuver, or jugular venous compression.
  - Nausea, vomiting, dizziness.
  - Watery rhinorrhea, salty taste, or fullness in the ear: symptoms suggesting the location of CSF leaks.

1 **Technical error** (artifactually low intracranial pressure)
   - Due to incomplete penetration of the subarachnoid space by the needle
2 **CSF fistulae**
   2.1 **Previous lumbar puncture**
      - The most common cause of CSF fistula.
      - Persistent hole is created from previous LP resulting in leakage of CSF into the subdural and extradural spaces.
   2.2 Neurosurgical procedures
   2.3 Trauma
   2.4 CSF rhinorrhea
   2.5 CSF otorrhea
3 Spontaneous intracranial hypotension (Schaltenbrand syndrome)
   - This condition refers to the occurrence of the typical postural headache, insidious, subacute in onset, without prior head or spinal injury or lumbar puncture due to a cryptic CSF leak.
   - The condition is self-limited within a few weeks to months.

- It is the diagnosis of exclusion requiring the exclusion of the site of CSF leak.
- In some case reports, the sites of CSF leak were later identified with more advanced diagnostic technology.

4 Spinal subarachnoid block
  - Causes include tumor, disc, or arachnoiditis
5 Severe dehydration
  - Seen in infants, manifest by sunken fontanelle.

Kyphoscoliosis in neurological disorders

- The most common deformities of the chest and spine are scoliosis, kyphosis, or a combination of the two.
- Kyphosis results in anterior concavity of the thoracic spine and thereby leads to shortening of the chest.
- Scoliosis is the lateral curvature of the spine with convexity to one side. Scoliosis can be functional or structural. Functional scoliosis is a compensatory posture to a number of conditions; for example, shortening of one leg, sciatica, or painful arthritis. Functional scoliosis usually disappears on bending, but structural scoliosis caused by deficiency, absence, or disease of the vertebrae remains unaltered when bending.

The following neurological disorders can have prominent kyphoscoliosis:
1 Neurofibromatosis
  - The typical clinical picture includes multiple circumscribed areas of increased skin pigmentation, accompanied by dermal and neural tumors of various types.
  - Scoliosis is usually seen, which can be associated with other bony abnormalities, including bone cysts, pathological fractures, and bone hypertrophy.
2 Friedreich ataxia
  - Although gait ataxia is usually the presenting symptom, pes cavus and kyphoscoliosis can precede other neurological symptoms.
3 Poliomyelitis
  - Asymmetrical atrophic, areflexic paralysis of muscles of the trunk and limbs represents a likely etiology of kyphoscoliosis associated with polio.
4 Extrapyramidal syndromes
  - Kyphosis can be seen in Parkinson disease, sometimes called camptocormia.
  - Scoliosis can be seen in truncal dystonia.
5 Syringomyelia – kyphoscoliosis is usually mild
6 Others
  - Cerebral palsy
  - Marfan syndrome
  - Spina bifida
  - Tethered cord

Lhermitte sign

- Forward flexion of the neck results in a burst of electric-shock-like paresthesias shooting into all four limbs, or down the center of the back. Sometimes, this may occur only in lower limbs or even on one side only.

Seen in:
1 **Multiple sclerosis**
2 Subacute combined degeneration of the spinal cord
3 High cervical cord compression from cervical spondylosis
4 Cerebellar ectopia
5 Early stage of radiation myelopathy

Monoplegia

- Monoplegia refers to weakness or paralysis of all the muscles of one leg or arm. However, examination of patients who complain of weakness of one limb often discloses an asymptomatic weakness of another, and the condition is actually hemiparesis, in which the etiology can be different from monoplegia.
- Monoplegia can be caused by upper and lower motor neuron lesions. Evidence of muscular atrophy is helpful in further localizing the lesion.

1 Monoplegia without muscular atrophy
   - Localizes to a lesion of the cerebral cortex.
     - **Thrombotic or embolic vascular lesions** are the most frequent cause.
   - Subcortical lesions are unlikely to cause monoplegia.
   - Often associated with other upper motor neuron findings including spasticity, increased reflexes, Babinski sign.
2 Monoplegia with muscular atrophy
   - More frequent than monoplegia without muscular atrophy.
   - Can be caused by:
     - **Disuse atrophy**, in which reflexes are retained and nerve conduction study is normal or denervation of muscles in which there are visible fasciculations and reduced reflexes.
   - Complete atrophic brachial monoplegia is uncommon and only parts of a limb are usually affected. Other common causes include:
     - Brachial plexus trauma in infants
     - Poliomyelitis in a child
     - Syringomyelia
     - Amyotrophic lateral sclerosis in adults

Muscular wasting of the small hand muscles

- Intrinsic hand muscles (small muscles of the hand) include the thenar and hypothenar eminences and dorsal interrossei.
- The ulnar nerve innervates the flexor pollicis brevis (thenar eminence), hypothenar eminence, and dorsal interossei.
- The median nerve innervates the remainder of the thenar muscles.
- Etiology is different between bilateral and unilateral wasting of the small muscles of the hand.

Causes of BILATERAL wasting of the small muscles of the hands:
1 **Age-related**
2 **Associated with rheumatoid arthritis**
3 Cervical causes:
   - **Cervical spondylosis**
   - Syringomyelia
   - Bilateral cervical ribs
4 Motor neuron disease
5 Peripheral nerve causes:
   - Combined bilateral medial and ulnar nerve lesions or bilateral ulnar nerve lesions
   - Chronic inflammatory demyelinating polyneuropathy (CIDP)
   - Charcot-Marie-Tooth disease

Causes of UNILATERAL wasting of the small muscles of the hand:
1 **Ulnar neuropathy**
   - Focal compression
   - Overuse
   - Associated with rheumatoid arthritis
2 C8-T1 nerve root compression
3 Brachial plexus trauma, infiltration
4 Pancoast tumor
5 Combined medial and ulnar nerve lesions

Neck stiffness

- Neck stiffness is not an uncommon finding on examination, especially in the emergency room setting.
- Although neck stiffness may raise the possibility of meningeal irritation, many elderly patients, children, and chronically ill patients may have a stiff neck that does not represent central nervous system involvement.

- In the presence of neck stiffness along with other findings of meningeal irritation (such as Kernig or Brudzinski signs), and in the absence of signs of increased intracranial pressure, lumbar puncture should be performed to define the etiology. If acute bacterial meningitis is suspected, antibiotics must be initiated before cultures become positive.
- In the presence of neck stiffness in patients with depressed consciousness, the possibility of a mass lesion with rupture or herniation needs to be excluded before lumbar puncture is performed.

1 **Neurological causes**
  1.1 **Meningeal irritation** – usually indicates a neurological emergency. Therefore, the following conditions should be excluded:
  - *Infection*, e.g. bacterial meningitis
  - *Neoplasia*, e.g. leptomeningeal carcinomatosis
  - *Subarachnoid hemorrhage* (triad includes sudden onset of headache, depressed consciousness, and stiff neck/meningismus)
  1.2 Axial rigidity/stiffness
  - Extrapyramidal syndromes, including Parkinson disease, Parkinson-plus syndrome (e.g. progressive supranuclear palsy)
  - Dystonia, e.g. cervical dystonia, generalized dystonia
  - Stiff-man or stiff-person syndrome
  1.3 Secondary paravertebral muscle spasm due to cervical spine disease or radiculopathy.
2 Non-neurological causes
  2.1 *Cervical spine traumatic injury* – locked facet, fracture/dislocation, severe muscle spasm. Of course, the possibility for this to result in significant neurological injury must not be overlooked.
  2.2 Degenerative cervical spine disease
  2.3 Muscle sprain
  2.4 Part of the spectrum seen in catatonia

Palatal myoclonus

- 'Palatal tremor' is perhaps a better term.
- A rhythmic contraction (60–180/min) affecting the palatal and pharyngeal structures.
- Often associated with synchronous movements of the ocular muscles, diaphragm, head, and neck.
- Persists in sleep.

Differential localizations:

1 **Gullain-Mollaret triangle lesion**
   - Pathway between the red nucleus, inferior olivary nucleus, and dentate nucleus.
   - Case reports with vascular, traumatic, neoplastic, and demyelinating lesions
2 Rare localizations
   - Cortical palatal myoclonus
   - Epileptic palatal myoclonus (secondary to epilepsia partialis continua)
3 Psychogenic palatal tremor (recently reported)

Paraplegia

- Paraplegia refers to paralysis of both lower extremities.
- If the onset is acute, it may be difficult to differentiate a spinal cause from a neuropathic process. This is because acute spinal shock results in early abolition of reflexes and flaccidity, and increased tone and hyperreflexia develop only with time.
- All spinal causes of paraplegia also apply to quadriplegia, with the lesion being in the cervical rather than the thoracic or lumbar segments of the spinal cord.

1 **Spinal cord lesion**
   - Paralysis and weakness affect all muscles below a given level.
   - If the lesions are bilateral, bowel and bladder function are often affected.
   - The most common cause of ACUTE paraplegia is:
     - *Spinal cord trauma*, associated with fracture dislocation of the spine.
   - Less common causes include:
     - *Hematomyelia from AVM*
     - *Infarctions* of the cord
     - *Myelitis.*
   - In adults, the most common causes of CHRONIC OR SUBACUTE paraplegia are:
     - **Multiple sclerosis**
     - **Tumors.**
   - In children, congenital cerebral disease from periventricular leukomalacia accounts for a majority of cases of infantile diplegia.
2 Peripheral nerve lesions
   - Motor involvement tends to be in distal groups rather than proximal ones.
   - Sensory loss, if present, follows a peripheral nerve pattern rather than a dermatomal pattern.
   - Sphincter functions are usually preserved and sensory loss is usually in the distal segments.

3 Cauda equina lesions
4 Bilateral medial frontal lobe lesions or parasagittal lesions (e.g. falcine meningioma)
5 Pseudotumor cerebri (benign intracranial hypertension)

Pes cavus

- The intrinsic muscles of the sole of the foot run along the longitudinal arch of the foot. The short muscles of the foot are particularly responsible for the management of the arch and any dysfunction of these muscles may result in pes cavus.
- In addition, increased height of the longitudinal arch can be associated with dorsal contracture of the metatarsophalangeal joints resulting in pes cavus.
- In most cases, pes cavus is not associated with any neurological conditions.

1 **Isolated finding with no association with neurological disorders**
   ◆ Most common.
2 Friedreich ataxia
   ◆ Most common inherited autosomal recessive ataxia.
   ◆ Predominant features include ataxia, clumsiness, dysarthria, peripheral neuropathy and dorsal column dysfunction.
3 Charcot-Marie-Tooth disease (CMT) or hereditary motor sensory neuropathy (HMSN)
   ◆ Most common form of inherited peripheral neuropathy.
   ◆ The hallmarks of this syndrome are genetic transmission, symmetry of affection, slow progression, degeneration of functionally related systems of fibers, and axonal myelin fiber loss.
4 Syringomyelia
5 Spina bifida

Pyramidal versus extrapyramidal syndromes: spasticity vs. rigidity

- The terms pyramidal, corticospinal, and upper motor neuron are often used interchangeably. The pyramidal tract, strictly speaking, designates only those fibers that course longitudinally in the pyramid of the medulla.
- The term 'extrapyramidal' refers to all the motor pathways except pyramidal ones. The term is imprecise and includes the basal ganglia and the cerebellum, which function very differently in the control of movement and posture.
- Different clinical features and signs distinguish between pyramidal and extrapyramidal syndromes. They are often helpful in disease localization and when considering pathological process.

- These clinical signs may be seen in isolation or combination.
- Rigidity is an extrapyramidal sign.
- Spasticity is a pyramidal sign.
- Etiologies for both phenomena are vast and include vascular, hereditary, demyelinating, and neurodegenerative conditions.

Features	Pyramidal	Extrapyramidal
Characteristic of the muscle tone alteration	Spasticity (clasp-knife effect)	Plastic (equal throughout passive movement-rigidity), or intermittent (cogwheel rigidity)
Distribution of hypertonus	Flexors of arms Extensors of legs	Generalized, but predominates in flexors of limbs and of trunk
Shortening and lengthening reaction	Present	Absent
Involuntary movements	Absent	Can be present, including tremor, chorea, myoclonus, etc.
Tendon reflexes	Significantly increased	Normal or slightly increased
Clonus	Present	Absent
Babinski sign	Present	Absent
Paralysis of voluntary movements	Present	Absent or slight

Ref: Modified from Adams and Victor, *Principles of Neurology*, 7th edition.

Recurrent falls: neurological causes

- Although falling is not a common cause for neurological referral, there are special circumstances that affect postural control mechanisms for which neurological evaluation is warranted.
- Orthostatic hypotension is identified as a factor in 5–10% of falls and should always be considered as a treatable non-neurological cause.
- Intoxication with medications, alcohol, or drugs should also be considered as a common non-neurological cause of recurrent falls.
- Drop attacks are defined as sudden lapses of postural tone and collapse without loss of consciousness. Drop attacks are rare causes of recurrent falls.
- Subdural hematoma is always a concern as a complication in patients with recurrent falls. A low threshold for imaging is appropriate in this group of patients.

1 Neurological disorders that affect the postural control
　1.1 Parkinson disease
　1.2 Other akinetic-rigid syndromes
　　▪ Parkinson-plus syndromes
　　▪ Progressive supranuclear palsy
　　▪ Multiple system atrophy
2 Cerebellar degeneration
　　▪ Patients with ataxia have poorly coordinated postural synergies.
　　▪ Ataxic patients commonly present with falls.
3 Sensory deficits
　3.1 Sensory deficits affecting proprioception
　　▪ These patients usually have a positive Romberg test and complain of increasing unsteadiness in the dark.
　　▪ Severe peripheral neuropathy can result in unsteadiness.
　3.2 Vestibular dysfunction
　　▪ Patients with bilateral vestibular deficits are particularly unsteady in stance.
　3.3 Visual impairment
4 Recurrent falls associated with dementia
　◆ The pathophysiology of falls in this context is not well understood.
　◆ There may be a failure of attention or integrative control of posture at a high level.

Romberg sign

- The Romberg is a test of proprioceptive function. The patient is asked to stand with the feet closely approximated, first with his/her eyes open, and then closed. The position of the body as a whole and that of the feet, shoulders, and head should be noted, as should any tremors, swaying or lurching.
- Slight swaying with the eyes shut may occur in some normal individuals. The test is 'positive' when the patient is able to stand with his/her feet together while his/her eyes are open, but sways or falls when they are closed.
- Any lesions along the proprioceptive pathway can result in a positive Romberg test. The peripheral sense organs are located in the muscle, tendons, and joints. The first cell body is situated in the dorsal root ganglion, going without a synapse to the ipsilateral fasiculi cuneatus and gracilis to the lower medulla where the synapse occurs. Following a decussation of the internal arcuate fibers, the impulses ascend in the medial lemniscus to the thalamus, terminating in the parietal lobe, posterior to those that convey touch.
- In a false Romberg test, seen in conversion reaction, the patient sways from the hips instead of from the ankles. He/she may sway through a wide arc and it may seem inevitable that he/she will fall, but he/she is usually able to regain his/her balance and resume the upright position.

Conditions commonly causing a positive Romberg test:

1 **Posterior column dysfunction**
   - Posterior cord compression
   - Multiple sclerosis
   - Subacute combined degeneration of the spinal cord
   - Tabes dorsalis
2 **Sensory polyneuropathy**
   - Idiopathic
   - Diabetes mellitus
3 Intracranial lesions
   - Less common.
   - Associated features involving surrounding structures are usually present, for example, other brainstem findings.

Scapular winging

- Scapular winging is seen in weakness of the serratus anterior, trapezius and rarely, rhomboid muscles.
- In serratus anterior weakness, the winging at rest is negligible and worsens with shoulder flexion. These patients may have difficulty abducting the shoulder >90 degrees. The vertebral scapular border lies close to the midline (medial translocation) and its lower border rotates medially.
- In trapezius weakness, the winging is present at rest and worsens with shoulder abduction. Findings become less prominent with abduction >90 degrees. The scapula is farther from midline (lateral translocation). The levator scapulae is prominent due to atrophy of the trapezius.

Causes:

1 Isolated or combined neuropathies:
   - **Long thoracic nerve neuropathy** (most common) causes serratus anterior weakness. It is usually due to acute or chronic neck trauma, and is described in workers carrying heavy, angular loads on the shoulder (hod carrier palsy).
   - Spinal accessory nerve neuropathy causes trapezius weakness.
2 C5, 6 radiculopathy
3 Proximal brachial plexopathy
4 Myopathies: rare, usually occur as part of diffuse conditions.
5 Spinal muscular atrophy

Temperature-sensitive neurological conditions

- Patients with certain neurological diagnoses will report subjective or objective changes in their neurological symptoms based on temperature.

1 Worsened by a rise in body temperature:
  • Multiple sclerosis
  • Myasthenia gravis
  • Eaton-Lambert syndrome
  • Febrile seizures
2 Worsened by a low body temperature:
  • Paramyotonia

Upper vs. lower motor neuron distinctions

• Upper motor neuron lesions describe pathologies of the descending motor pathway from the cortex through spinal cord, proximal to the anterior horn cells. Lower motor neuron lesions are the direct result of loss of function of anterior horn cells or their axons in anterior roots and peripheral nerves.
• Differentiation between upper and lower motor neuron lesions is an important aspect of neurological localization.
• Nerve conduction study and electromyography are useful tools in confirming lower motor neuron lesions, further localizing the lesion, and providing clues on underlying pathophysiology. In lower motor neuron lesion, EMG is abnormal with fibrillations, fasciculations, and positive sharp waves, while the tests are usually normal in upper motor neuron lesions.

Sign or symptom	Upper motor neuron	Lower motor neuron
Paralysis or paresis	Yes, although muscles affected in groups, not individual muscles	Yes, with individual muscles affected
Effect on residual movement	Increased degree of co-contraction of antagonistic muscles	No evidence of co-contraction of antagonistic muscles
Muscle tone	Increased	Decreased
Reflexes	Increased	Decreased or absent
Clonus	May be present	Absent
Babinski sign	Present	Absent
Fibrillations	Absent	May be present
Fasiculations	Absent	May be present
Muscle atrophy	Absent (early)	Present

Named syndromes

Alien limb syndrome

- Failure to recognize ownership of one's limb when visual cues are removed; a feeling that one body part is foreign.
- The hand is most frequently affected, but any limb or combinations may occur.
- Patients have apraxia, problems with bimanual coordination and display non-goal directed activities.

Causes:
1 Corticobasal ganglionic degeneration (CBGD)
   - Cortical reflex myoclonus is frequent.
2 Infarcts: the following lesions have been reported.
   - Corpus callosum
   - Mesial frontal lesions
   - Combination of posterior corpus callosum and thalamic lesions
3 Others
   - Alzheimer disease
   - Anterior communicating artery rupture
   - Corpus callosotomy
   - Corpus callosal tumors
   - Bifrontal penetrating injury

Balint syndrome

- Balint syndrome refers to a syndrome consisting of:
   1 Psychic paralysis of gaze
   2 Optic ataxia
   3 Disturbance of visual attention, particularly in the peripheral visual field.
   4 Simultagnosia
- Almost invariably associated with large bilateral parietal lobe lesions.

1 Etiology:
   - **Bilateral watershed infarct** between the middle and posterior circulation is the most common cause.
2 Signs and symptoms:
   - Psychic paralysis of gaze: inability to voluntarily look into the peripheral field.

- Optic ataxia: clumsiness or inability to manually respond to visual stimuli, with mislocation in space when pointing to visual targets.
- A disturbance of visual attention: resulting in dynamic concentric narrowing of the effective field.
- Simultagnosia: an inability to recognize the whole picture despite the ability to perceive its parts.
- Inferior altitudinal field defect: not part of Balint syndrome, but upper banks of occipital cortex are usually involved.

3 Treatment:
- According to the etiology of stroke.

Cavernous sinus syndrome

- The cavernous sinus is a small but complex structure consisting of a venous plexus, carotid artery, cranial nerves, and sympathetic fibers, surrounded by a dural fold.
- The third, fourth cranial nerves, as well as the first and second divisions of the trigeminal nerve (V1 and V2), lie along the lateral wall of the cavernous sinus, whereas the sixth cranial nerve, internal carotid artery, and the third-order oculosympathetic fibers from the superior cervical ganglion lie more medially.
- According to the anatomy described above, cavernous sinus involvement would be suggested by any combination of unilateral third-, fourth-, or sixth-nerve dysfunction, accompanied by hypesthesia of the forehead, cornea, or cheek, or by Horner syndrome. Various degrees of pain may be involved. Complete interruption of all three ocular motor nerves would result in total ophthalmoplegia, ptosis, and/or mydriasis.
- Although the classical syndrome of cavernous sinus results from aneurysm or carotico-cavernous fistula, the most common causes of cavernous sinus lesions include tumors, trauma, and infections.
- Except for sparing of V2, lesions of the superior orbital fissure are clinically difficult to distinguish from those of cavernous sinus, and the differentials are similar. In orbital apex syndrome, patients present with third-, fourth-, and sixth-nerve palsies, V1 distribution sensory loss, oculosympathetic paresis, and visual loss due to optic nerve involvement.

1 **Tumors**
- Most common cause.
- The most common neoplastic lesion in the cavernous sinus is caused by direct invasion from nasopharyngeal carcinoma. Metastatic lesions are the second most common.

2 **Trauma**
  - Trauma is reported to be the most common cause of cavernous sinus syndrome when surgical cases are included.
3 **Infections or cavernous sinus thrombophlebitis**
  - Thrombophlebitis of the cavernous sinus is potentially a lethal condition, caused by bacterial or fungal invasion, complicating sinusitis in patients with poorly controlled diabetes or immunosuppression.
  - Rhinocerebral mucormycosis is a common cause in poorly controlled diabetics.
  - Aspergillosis arises most commonly as a result of hematogenous spread, and occasionally by direct extension of infection from the paranasal sinuses, middle ear, or orbit in immunocompromised patients.
  - Actinomycosis gains access to the cavernous sinus by direct extension from the ear, sinus, and less commonly, hematogenous spread. Most patients are immunocompetent.
4 Tolosa-Hunt syndrome
  - Tolosa-Hunt syndrome is a recurrent painful ophthalmoplegia due to nonspecific granulomatous inflammation in the anterior cavernous sinus, superior orbital fissure, or orbital apex.
  - Rare cause of cavernous sinus syndrome.
  - The diagnosis is based on findings of painful ophthalmoplegia, accompanied by variable deficits of cranial nerves in the cavernous sinus, excellent response to corticosteroid therapy, and exclusion of other causes.
5 Carotico-cavernous fistula (CCF)
  - CCF usually result from traumatic laceration of the carotid artery or from rupture of an aneurysm into the surrounding venous sac, establishing a direct communication between internal carotid artery and the venous spaces of the cavernous sinus.
  - Pulsating exophthalmos, orbital pain, and, eventually, restriction of eye movements due to orbital congestion.
6 Other rare causes
  - Aneurysm of the internal carotid artery
  - Inflammatory pseudotumors

Central pontine myelinolysis (CPM): causes

- Central pontine myelinolysis (CPM) is a demyelinating disease of the pons, frequently associated with demyelination of other areas of the central nervous system. The term 'osmotic demyelination syndrome' is used for pontine and extrapontine myelinolysis (CPM/EPM).
- The etiologies of CPM/EPM vary. However, almost all cases are related to severe illnesses, with chronic alcoholism being the most common underlying condition. A significant high percentage of CPM/EPM cases were also observed among liver transplant patients.

- The role of hyponatremia and its correction in the pathogenesis of CPM is unclear, although multiple factors are most likely involved. It is important to recognize that CPM/EPM may be seen when plasma sodium levels are high, low, or normal.
- CPM/EPM should be considered in patients suffering from chronic alcoholism, electrolyte disturbances, liver transplantation, or other chronic diseases when presenting with massive mental status changes as well as brainstem symptoms despite negative CT or MRI. MRI findings may lag behind clinical presentation, up to weeks in some cases.

Disease	Percentage of CPM/EPM cases
Chronic alcoholism, including liver transplant patients	41%
Electrolyte disturbances, particularly hyponatremia, but also hypernatremia	32%
Pulmonary infections, including pneumonia, abscess, and tuberculosis	10%
Malignant tumors, especially of the lungs and GI tract	6%
Diseases of the CNS, including hemorrhage, infection, inflammation, and tumors	7%
Non-alcoholic liver disease	5%

Ref: Lampl C., Yazdi K. Central pontine myelinolysis. *Eur Neurol*, 2002; 47: 3–10.

Cerebellopontine angle syndrome

- The two most common adult tumors in the cerebellopontine angle region are vestibular schwannoma and meningioma.

Schwannoma	Meningioma
Involvement of cranial VIII early: originating from vestibular division, later causing pressure on the acoustic component. Later, involves cranial nerves V, IX, X	May initially present with facial palsy. Late involvement of cranial VIII
Positive for S-100 staining Negative EMA staining	Positive for epithelial membrane antigen staining (EMA)
No desmosomes Presence of Luse bodies **Presence of Antoni type A, B tissue** (characteristic feature)	Elongated intertwined cell processes, joined by desmosomes

Other causes:
- Craniopharyngioma
- Glomus jugulare tumor
- Aneurysm of the basilar artery
- Large intra-axial brainstem or cerebellar tumors

Geschwind syndrome

- A consistent personality alteration seen in some patients with complex partial seizures.
- Clinical features include:
  - circumstantiality,
  - hypergraphia,
  - altered sexual status, and
  - intensified cognitive and emotional states.

Horner syndrome

- Horner syndrome results from damage to ocular sympathetic fibers at any level along the symapathetic pathway; central, preganglionic, or postganglionic neurons.
- Features of Horner syndrome includes:
  - Mild ptosis: paresis of Müller muscle
  - Miosis: paralysis of pupillary dilator muscle
  - Ipsilateral anhidrosis
  - Apparent enophthalmos
  - Heterochromia iridis: usually in congenital cases
  - Lower eyelid reverse ptosis
- Pharmacologic testing:
  - Confirm the diagnosis of Horner syndrome by instillation of 4–10% cocaine solution in each eye, which will dilate normal eyes only.
  - Once the diagnosis is confirmed, 1% hydroxyamphetamine can be used to differentiate central and preganglionic from postganglionic lesions. Because hydroxyamphetamine stimulates the release of norepinephrine from sympathetic postganglionic nerve terminals, it will fail to dilate the pupil in patients with postganglionic lesions.
- Differentiation of lesions is clinically useful because central and preganglionic lesions are likely to have more serious causes than postganglionic lesions.

The oculosympathetic pathway consists of a three-neuron arc. The first-order neurons of the sympathetic pathway originate in the posterior hypothalamus, descend to the intermediolateral gray column of the spinal cord, and synapse at the ciliospinal center of Budge at spinal levels C8 to T2. Preganglionic second-order neurons arise from the intermediolateral column, leave the spinal cord by the ventral spinal roots, and enter the rami communicans. They join the paravertebral cervical sympathetic chain and ascend through this chain to synapse at the superior cervical ganglion. **Postganglionic third-order neurons** originate in the superior cervical ganglion, entering the cranium with the internal carotid artery. The fibers join the ophthalmic division of the trigeminal nerve within the cavernous sinus, reaching the ciliary muscle and pupillary dilator muscle by means of the nasociliary nerve and the long posterior ciliary nerves.

1 Central lesions:
  • Vascular events, e.g. Wallenberg syndrome
  • Tumor, e.g. brainstem tumor
2 Preganglionic lesions:
  • Apical lung tumor (Pancoast tumor)
3 Postganglionic lesions:
  • Neck trauma
  • Spontaneous dissection of the carotid artery
  • Cluster headaches

Kluver-Bucy syndrome

• Due to bilateral lesions of the amygdala.
• Characterized by:
  • chronic amnesia,
  • distractibility,
  • hyperorality,
  • hypersexuality,
  • affective dyscontrol, and
  • socially inappropriate behavior.

Etiologies include:
1 Herpes simplex encephalitis
2 Pick disease
3 Anoxic-ischemic lesions in the anterior medial temporal lobe
4 After bilateral temporal lobectomy
5 Rarely seen in:
  • Alzheimer disease
  • Huntington disease
  • Creutzfeldt-Jakob disease

Orbitofrontal syndrome

- Behaviorally, the outstanding feature of orbitofrontal syndrome is disinhibition and impulsiveness. Patients lack social judgement, make tactless and socially inappropriate comments. Sexual preoccupation and inappropriate sexual comments are frequent, but overt sexual aggression is rare.
- The patients' insight into their own behavior is limited.
- A variety of mood changes have been described in these patients, including emotional lability, mania, and depression.
- Most patients with orbitofrontal syndrome have a normal neurological examination as well as minimal neuropsychological deficits. Therefore, careful observation of the above symptoms is of utmost importance. Anosmia can be the only physical finding.

Common etiologies of orbitofrontal syndrome:
1 **Traumatic brain injury: most common**
   - The most common injury to the orbitofrontal cortex results from closed head trauma with contusion of the inferior frontal cortex and adjacent white matter connections by the irregular bony surface of the anterior fossa.
2 Subfrontal neoplasm
   - The second most common etiology.
   - Neoplasm may arise from adjacent structures including pituitary fossa, olfactory groove, or sphenoidal ridge.
   - In these locations, the following are particularly frequent:
     - Meningioma
     - Chromophobe pituitary adenoma
3 Others
   - Aneurysm of the anterior communicating artery
   - Frontotemporal dementia

Thoracic outlet syndrome

- It is difficult to make the diagnosis of true thoracic outlet syndrome (TOS), as the condition is poorly defined and there are no specific neurological or electrophysiological studies that can be used to definitively confirm the diagnosis.
- True compression and dysfunction of the brachial plexus is rare, and even recognized experts in the field have seen few cases.
- The term 'thoracic outlet syndrome' is often used loosely in describing patients with chronic shoulder/limb pain.

> • Loss or reduction of the radial pulse during various maneuvers [such as tilting the head back and toward the affected side (Adson test) or abducting and externally rotating the shoulder (Wright maneuver)] is not entirely reliable.

1 Etiology:
- The condition is usually caused by a **fibrous band** traversing the brachial plexus.
- Cervical ribs are commonly associated with TOS, but also are present in many asymptomatic persons.
- Abnormal insertion of the scalene muscles is often proposed as a rationale for surgery. However, the low response rate to this procedure casts doubt as to there being a causal relationship.
2 Signs and symptoms (may be neurological and/or vascular):
- Patients usually present with weakness, pain, and numbness in the hand, in a pattern consistent with median and ulnar nerve (posterior trunk) involvement.
- In another type of thoracic outlet syndrome, patients can present with numbness, tingling, and pain without demonstrable neurological deficit. The symptoms may depend on arm and shoulder position.
- Aching pain is usually reported in the shoulder, upper back, and/or upper arm.
- Compression of the subclavian vein results in vascular congestion of the arm.
- Compression of the subclavian artery can result in distal limb ischemia.
3 Diagnosis:
- Electrophysiological investigations demonstrate reduced sensory action potentials in the little finger and medial forearm, and denervation changes in many intrinsic hand muscles (in both ulnar and median nerves) and sometimes in the muscles of the forearm that contain a C8 component.
- Some patients can have normal studies.
4 Treatment:
- Physiotherapy over a period of several months.
- In some centers, a removal of the first rib has been performed through a transaxillary approach, although the response is not consistent.
- Surgical section of the scalene muscles rarely improves symptoms.

Tolosa-Hunt syndrome

> • Tolosa-Hunt syndrome refers to a granulomatous inflammation at the superior orbital fissure or in the cavernous sinus, causing multiple cranial nerve palsies and severe pain.

1 Etiology:
   - A low-grade, granulomatous, noninfectious, inflammatory process adjacent to the cavernous sinus or within the superior orbital fissure lasting weeks or months.
   - Differential diagnosis includes tumor, infection, aneurysm, or carotico-cavernous fistula.
2 Signs and symptoms: according to the structures located at the superior orbital fissure.
   - CN V1 distribution: steady, unremitting retro- and supraorbital pain
   - CN III, IV, VI: painful ophthalmoplegia
   - CN V: diminished corneal reflex
   - CN V2: diminished sensation and pain in the V2 distribution
   - Less commonly: optic nerve and oculosympathetic pathway involved
3 Treatment:
   - The pain and diplopia dramatically improve with systemic corticosteroids.
   - Spontaneous remission has been reported.

Wernicke encephalopathy and Korsakoff syndrome

- Wernicke encephalopathy is the neurological manifestation of thiamine deficiency.
- Not all patients with Wernicke encephalopathy and Korsakoff syndrome exhibit the complete triad (or tetrad) of
   - (dietary deficiency),
   - oculomotor abnormalities,
   - cerebellar dysfunction, and
   - altered mental status.
- Therefore, it is important to administer large doses of parenteral thiamine to all patients with undiagnosed altered mental status, oculomotor disturbances, and ataxia.
- This condition is treatable if promptly recognized and evaluated. However, patients usually progress to stupor and coma if untreated.

1 Etiology:
   - The condition is caused by thiamine or vitamin B_1 deficiency. These are usually associated with nutritional deficiency, most commonly and classically in alcoholism, but they can also be seen in hyperemesis gravidarum or cancer.
2 Pathology:
   - Wernicke encephalopathy is characterized by neuronal loss, demyelination, and gliosis in periventricular gray matter regions.

- Structures commonly involved include medial thalamus, mamillary bodies, periaqueductal gray matter, cerebellar vermis as well as oculomotor, abducens, and vestibular nuclei.

3 Symptoms and signs:
- Onset is usually abrupt but insidious onset can occur.
- In the classical syndrome, patients present with encephalopathy, ophthalmoplegia, and ataxia in the setting of nutritional deficiency. The complete triad or tetrad of symptoms are present in only one-third of reported cases.
- The most common ocular abnormality is nystagmus. Others include abducens nerve palsy, oculomotor nerve palsy, horizontal and vertical gaze palsy.
- Ataxia is usually cerebellar.
- Cognitive impairment mainly involves global confusion with defective immediate and recent memory.
- The major long-term complication of Wernicke encephalopathy is Korsakoff amnesic syndrome. This syndrome is primarily a disorder of anterograde greater than retrograde amnesia. Language is not usually affected, although patients may exhibit disorientation due to recent memory impairment. Confabulation and lack of insight are also common.

4 Diagnosis:
- Based on suggestive clinical history and physical findings as described above.
- CT may demonstrate symmetrical low density abnormalities in the diencephalon and periventricular regions, which enhance after contrast injection. Gross hemorrhages are uncommon.
- MRI findings of increased T2W signal intensity in the diencephalon, midbrain, and periventricular regions can be seen and are very suggestive of the diagnosis when present in alcoholics.

5 Treatment:
- Prompt treatment with large doses of parenteral thiamine administration.
- Ocular abnormalities usually improve within hours to days, and ataxia and confusion within days or weeks.
- Gastrointestinal absorption of thiamine is unreliable in alcoholics and malnourished patients. Therefore, oral administration is usually not recommended.

Chapter 3
Vascular Neurology

Evaluation for stroke

Is it a stroke? Differential diagnosis

- Stroke is a clinical diagnosis. By definition, it is a clinical syndrome, characterized by rapidly developing clinical symptoms and/or signs of focal, and at times global, loss of cerebral function, lasting more than 24 hours, and with no apparent cause other than that of vascular origin.
- The clinical differentiation of 'stroke' from 'not a stroke' is accurate more than 95% of the time if there is a clear history of focal brain dysfunction of sudden onset, and if there is a residual focal neurological deficit present at the time of examination.
- The absence of persistent neurological deficit by no means excludes a stroke in patients who have suffered a sudden decline in neurological function. It may represent a delay in presentation, signs that have resolved, or subtle signs that have been missed. In patients without obvious focal neurological signs, look specifically for visuospatial-perceptual dysfunction.
- The presence of papilledema and unexplained fever in uncomplicated stroke should call into question the accuracy of the diagnosis.

1 **Epileptic seizures**
   - Epileptic seizures are one of the most common causes of misdiagnosed stroke. The usual scenario is a patient with postictal confusion, stupor, coma, or hemiparesis in whom the preceding seizure was unwitnessed or unrecognized.
   - Careful history is the most important tool to differentiate recurring seizures from stroke.

2 **Intracranial lesions**
   2.1 Tumors
   - Intracranial tumors can cause symptoms and signs mimicking stroke, although the progression of symptoms are usually slower, days to weeks or months, associated with headache, seizures, or papilledema.
   - Occasionally, tumors can give rise to sudden focal neurological deficits when they cause Todd paralysis from seizures or intratumoral hemorrhage.
   2.2 Subdural hematoma
   - Rarely, can present with abrupt onset of focal neurological signs.

3 Metabolic encephalopathy
   - Various metabolic abnormalities may present with focal neurological symptoms and signs, although they generally cause subacute evolution of altered consciousness with or without systemic disturbances.
   - Examples include hyponatremia, hepatic failure, Wernicke-Korsakoff syndrome, hypoglycemia, hyperglycemia, and hyperosmolarity.

4 Head injury
   - Head injury and stroke may co-exist or predispose to each other.
   - For example, head injury may cause intracranial hemorrhage, dissection, or herniation resulting in ischemic stroke, while stroke may predispose patients to head injury from falls.

5 Encephalitis, cerebral abscess, or empyema
   - Clues are patients with focal neurological deficits, associated with altered consciousness, and fever.

6 Functional symptoms and signs
   - Clues are that the history tends to be vague and inconsistent and may disclose evidence of social disruption or personality disturbance or a past history of functional disorders or unexplained somatic symptoms.
   - The causes can be hysterical conversion (unconscious) or malingering (conscious).
   - Examinations are usually very helpful in confirming the suspicious. For those with apparent weakness, there are no hard signs of upper motor neuron deficits. Voluntary efforts are inappropriate and intermittent. Sensory loss tends to be inconsistent in location and incompatible with normal sensory anatomy as well as intermittence.
   - It is important to note that it is not uncommon for patients with an organic problem to have a functional overlay as well, as if to try and draw attention to their underlying problem.

7 Others
   - Multiple sclerosis
   - Peripheral lesions

Focal vs. nonfocal: Neurological symptoms of transient ischemic attack or stroke

- The anatomical location as well as the nature of neurological symptoms of a TIA or stroke reflect the area of the brain that has been deprived of blood supply or compromised by hemorrhage or edema.
- Focal neurological symptoms are those which arise from a disturbance in an identifiable focal area of the brain. On the other hand, non-focal symptoms are not anatomically localizing and therefore should not be interpreted as a TIA or stroke because there are seldom due to focal cerebral ischemia.
- TIA/stroke symptoms are usually 'negative', representing a loss of function.

Focal neurological symptoms suggestive of TIA or stroke	Non-focal neurological symptoms
Motor symptoms • Weakness or clumsiness • Heaviness on one side of the body • Bilateral arm or leg weakness • Dysphagia	• Generalized weakness or sensory disturbances • Light-headedness • Fainting episodes • Blackouts • Incontinence of urine or feces • Confusion • Lack of concentration • Inability to focus
Speech and language disturbances • Difficulty understanding or expressing spoken language • Difficulty reading or writing • Difficulty calculating	
Sensory symptoms • Altered feeling on one side of the body or part of it	Any of the following symptoms, if isolated, is unlikely to represent focal brain dysfunction. • Dysarthria • Vertigo (some case reports of isolated vertigo resulting from stroke, although very rare indeed) • Dysphagia • Diplopia
Visual symptoms • Loss of vision in one eye • Loss of vision in part of both eyes • Total blindness • Double vision • Tilted images	
Vestibular/cerebellar symptoms • Spinning sensation (vertigo) • Sensation of imbalance or unsteadiness • Veering to one side	
Behavioral or cognitive symptoms • Difficulty dressing, combing hair, etc. • Geographical disorientation • Difficulty in recognition (e.g. familiar faces) • Amnesia (not always)	

Clues to the etiology of TIA or stroke from physical examination

- Neurological examination is primarily aimed to localize the brain lesion, although some patients with TIA or minor stroke may not have any positive findings after a few days.
- Often, neurological as well as general physical examination findings; in addition to pertinent history, may give some clues as to the cause of the patient's TIA or stroke.

Physical signs	Possible causes
Impaired consciousness, but the stroke seems mild – consider other causes, which may have focal features masquerading as stroke	Chronic subdural hematoma Cerebral vasculitis Intracranial venous thrombosis Hypoglycemia Sedative drugs Comorbid medical conditions Mitochondrial disorders
Horner syndrome (not part of lower brainstem stroke where it might be expected)	Internal carotid artery dissection
Clubbing of fingers	Infective endocarditis Right-to-left shunt Pulmonary AVM Carcinoma
Splinter hemorrhages	Infective endocarditis Cerebral vasculitis
Scleroderma	Systemic sclerosis
Livedo reticularis	Systemic lupus erythematosus (SLE) Polyarteritis nodosa Cholesterol emboli Sneddon syndrome
Petechiae/purpura/bruises	Thrombotic thrombocytopenic purpura Fat embolism Cholesterol emboli Antiphospholipid syndrome
Red flush skin	Polycythemia vera
Thrombosed veins/needle tracks	Intravenous drug use with or without right-sided endocarditis
Lax skin	Ehler-Danlos syndrome Pseudoxanthoma elasticum
Orogenital ulcers	Behçet disease
Café-au-lait spots	Neurofibromatosis

Craniocervical bruits

- Many structures in the neck area can cause local bruits. Of those, the most important is the local bruit over the carotid bifurcation, which is predictive of some degree of carotid stenosis. However, a very severe or tight stenosis may not cause a bruit at all.
- Carotid bruits are neither specific nor sensitive in the diagnosis of carotid stenosis of sufficient severity to make surgery worthwhile. However, listening for carotid bruits is a useful physical sign in patients with or having risk factors for stroke or transient ischemic attack.

Causes of head and neck bruits
1 Bruits over carotid bifurcation
   - Common carotid or internal carotid artery stenosis.
   - External carotid artery stenosis can also cause a bruit.
2 Ophthalmic bruits (heard best with bell of stethoscope over closed eyelids)
   - Due to retrograde flow along ophthalmic artery in presence of significant internal artery stenosis.
3 Cranial bruits
   - May be heard in locations overlying dural or superficial cerebral arteriovenous malformations.
4 Occipital bruits
   - May occasionally be heard in cases of vertebral-basilar stenosis.
5 Diffuse neck bruits
   - Always think of thyrotoxicosis; other physical signs may be evident, including exophthalmos, sweating, tachycardia, etc.
   - Hyperdynamic circulation during pregnancy, hemodialysis, anemia.
6 Bruits over supraclavicular area
   - Subclavian artery stenosis.
   - Vertebral artery stenosis.
   - May occur in young normal individuals.
7 Bruits transmitted from other adjacent structures: usually from the heart and major vessels
   - Aortic stenosis.
   - Aortic regurgitation.
   - Coarctation of the aorta.
   - Venous hums: continuous and roaring sounds, which are obliterated by light pressure over the ipsilateral jugular vein.

Stroke types

Cerebral hemorrhage

Etiology of primary intracranial hemorrhages based on the patient's age and location

- Age is an important factor in determining the particular cause of hemorrhage in an individual patient.
- AVMs are the leading cause in the young, and degenerative small vessel disease is the most common cause in the elderly and middle-aged. Amyloid angiopathy is also a common cause of lobar hemorrhage in the elderly.
- The relative importance of some causes also depends on the location of hemorrhages.

Age (years)	Basal ganglia, thalamus	Lobar	Cerebellum/brainstem
Below 50	• AVMs • Lipohyalinosis or microaneurysms • Moyamoya syndrome • Amphetamines and cocaine	• AVMs • Saccular aneurysm • Tumors • Intracranial venous thrombosis • Infective endocarditis	• AVMs • Lipohyalinosis or microaneurysms • Tumors
50–69	• Lipohyalinosis or microaneurysms • AVMs • Atherosclerotic moyamoya syndrome	• Lipohyalinosis or microaneurysms • AVMs • Saccular aneurysm Tumors • Amyloid angiopathy • Intracranial venous thrombosis	• Lipohyalinosis or microaneurysms • AVMs • Tumors • Amyloid angiopathy
70 or over	• Lipohyalinosis or microaneurysms • Tumors • AVMs	• Lipohyalinosis or microaneurysms • Amyloid angiopathy • Saccular aneurysm • Tumors • AVMs • Intracranial venous thrombosis	• Lipohyalinosis or microaneurysms • Amyloid angiopathy • Tumors • AVMs

Ref: Warlow C.P., Dennis M.S., van Gijn G., *et al. Stroke: A Practical Guide to Management.* 1996. Blackwell Science. Oxford.

Subarachnoid hemorrhage (SAH): causes

- Subarachnoid hemorrhage is the result of bleeding from arteries and veins that are located close to the brain surface, with the accumulation of blood in the basal cisterns and surrounding subarachnoid space.
- SAH is a serious condition. In nonselected hospital series, the mortality is 50% after three months, although specialized neurosurgical centers usually publish more optimistic figures.

1 **Traumatic subarachnoid hemorrhage**
   - Most common cause of subarachnoid hemorrhage.
2 Nontraumatic subarachnoid hemorrhage or spontaneous SAH
   2.1 **Saccular aneurysm**
      - About 85% of all spontaneous subarachnoid hemorrhages are due to the rupture of an intracranial aneurysm.
      - 85% of aneurysms are distributed in the carotid circulation, with 35% in the anterior communicating and anterior cerebral arteries, 30% in the internal carotid artery at the origin of the posterior communicating artery, and 20% in the middle cerebral artery. The posterior circulation accounts for 15% of aneurysms, and the distribution is 10% at the top of the basilar artery and basilar-superior cerebellar artery junction and 5% in the vertebral artery at the origin of the posterior inferior cerebellar artery.
   2.2 Non-aneurysmal pretruncal subarachnoid hemorrhage (perimesencephalic SAH)
      - Accounts for 10% of all SAHs.
      - This is a benign but mysterious condition, with the center of hemorrhage around the midbrain or pons.
      - The presenting symptom is usually explosive headache with the normal angiogram.
      - The prognosis is good and patients recover and, without exception, go on to live a normal life. There is no risk of rebleeding and no incidence of vasospasm.
3 Others
   - Arterial dissection
   - Cerebral arteriovenous malformations
   - Metastasis of cardiac myxoma
   - Cocaine abuse
   - Sickle cell disease
   - Coagulation disorders
   - Undetermined: can be up to 20% in some series.

Intracerebral hemorrhage (ICH)

- Intracranial hemorrhage accounts for approximately 15% of all strokes and its cause is hypertension in 50–70% of cases.
- ICH is the cause of 11% of all stroke deaths, and it carries a mortality rate of 50% in which half of the deaths occur within the first 2 days.
- The majority of hemorrhages are located deep in the cerebral hemispheres.
- Rupture of AVMs is the leading cause of ICH in young adults (less than 50 years) followed by hemorrhage of undetermined cause, hypertension, and drug abuse.

1 *Hypertensive intracerebral hemorrhage*
   - The most common cause of ICH, accounting for 50–70% of all cases.
   - The pathogenesis involves the rupture of small parenchymal perforating arteries, commonly lenticulostriate, thalamostriate, and paramedian basilar arteries, as a result of lipohyalinosis (hypertension-induced degenerative changes in the vessel walls). This is usually followed by fibrinoid necrosis and formation of local outpouching of arterial walls, called microaneurysms.
   - The history of hypertension does not have to be present, as 50% of patients do not have a history of chronic hypertension.
   - The preferential locations for hypertensive hemorrhage include putamen (most common), followed by thalamus, cerebellum, and pons, respectively.
2 *Non-hypertensive intracerebral hemorrhage*
   2.1 Cerebral amyloid angiopathy
      - Referred to a form of cerebral angiopathy with deposits of amyloid in the media and adventitia of small and medium-sized arteries of the cerebral hemispheres. These arteries are located in the superficial layers of the cerebral cortex and leptomeninges. Therefore, hemorrhages usually occur in the superficial layer, subcortical, or lobar locations with a lesser tendency to affect the basal ganglia and brainstem.
      - It affects 50% of people older than 70 years of age in whom histological features of Alzheimer disease are also found. It accounts for 10% of all ICHs.
      - It also has a tendency to produce recurrent ICHs over periods of months to years.
   2.2 Vascular malformations
      - Vascular malformations are responsible for 4–8% of all ICH cases.
      - The risk of bleeding is highest in arteriovenous malformations, lowest in venous angiomas, and intermediate in cavernous angiomas.
      - The preferential locations are usually in the subcortical white matter, less frequently deep in the basal nuclei.

2.3 Oral anticoagulants
- Oral anticoagulants increase the risk of ICH between 8 and 11 times.
- Patients may present with gradual and slow progression of neurological deficits, suggesting a slow bleeding into parenchyma.
- The mortality rate from anticoagulant-related hemorrhages can be as high as 65%, especially if patients are unconscious on admission.

2.4 Brain tumors
- Brain tumors are found in 2–10% of cases of all ICHs, especially if the tumor is highly malignant (glioblastoma) or metastatic.
- Commonly metastatic tumors that are prone to hemorrhage include:
  - bronchogenic carcinoma,
  - melanoma,
  - choriocarcinoma, and
  - renal cell carcinoma.

2.5 Medications and toxins
- Examples include amphetamines, phenylpropanolamine, and cocaine.
- The majority of hemorrhages are lobar.
- Associated transient elevation of blood pressure may predispose to hemorrhage, and the possibility of drug-induced angiopathy has been proposed.

2.6 Vasculitis
- Rare cause of ICHs.
- Primary isolated CNS angiitis usually causes ischemic infarction, with hemorrhages only on rare occasions.

Multiple intracerebral hemorrhages

- Multiple hemorrhages are rare. Patients with intracerebral hemorrhage and a history of hypertension rarely have multiple bleeds, as the etiology is thought to be lipohyalinosis and microaneurysms.
- Multiple hemorrhages, either at the same time or separated by days, are suggestive of amyloid angiopathy.

1 Local conditions
1.1 **Amyloid angiopathy**
- Most common.
- The etiology is assumed that the arteries affected by amyloidosis are so fragile that minor injury may cause a hemorrhage.

1.2 Cerebral vasculitis
- Can be very difficult to diagnose as most tests are often negative.
- Biopsy may be needed to confirm the diagnosis.
- Patients do not have to manifest systemic vasculitis.

1.3 Hemorrhages from tumors
- The hemorrhages may be multiple sites from a primary intracerebral tumor or from multiple locations of metastatic tumors.

1.4 Head injury

2 Systemic conditions: usually as a result of a defect in homeostasis
2.1 Disseminated intravascular coagulation (DIC)
2.2 Thrombocytopenia
2.3 Clotting disorders, e.g. hemophilia

Primary intraventricular hemorrhage

- Intraventricular hemorrhage is usually associated with either subarachnoid hemorrhage from a ruptured aneurysm (most often in the anterior communicating artery) or intracerebral hemorrhage.
- In both conditions, the outcome is worse with intraventricular rupture than without, and an intraventricular blood volume of more than 20 ml is almost invariably fatal.
- The outcome of primary intraventricular hemorrhage without a detectable cause is much better than if it is associated with SAH or intraparenchymal hemorrhage.

1 **Occult arteriovenous malformations**
- Idiopathic intraventricular hemorrhage is often speculatively attributed to occult AVMs in the ependymal wall or choroid plexus.
- Rupture of the dural fistula of the superior sagittal sinus can also result in intraventricular hemorrhage.

2 Uncommon aneurysms
- Aneurysms of the posterior inferior cerebellar artery and anterior inferior cerebellar artery.

3 Tumors
- Pituitary tumors
- Ependymoma
- Meningioma

4 Others
- Brain abscess
- Moyamoya syndrome
- Lacunar infarction
- Cocaine, amphetamine

Intracranial aneurysms: description and types

- An aneurysm is a focal dilatation of an artery. There are many different types of aneurysm, as listed below. The most frequent aneurysm in the CNS is the berry aneurysm.
- At present, the definite diagnosis of aneurysm is made on conventional angiography.
- An organized hematoma from a vessel that has bled is called a **pseudoaneurysm**. There are no vessel walls, and the hematoma is confined by the adventitia.
- The diagnosis of aneurysm should not be missed. Subarachnoid hemorrhage (SAH), a complication of ruptured aneurysm, carries a significant mortality and morbidity. 15% of patients with SAH die before reaching the hospital. Rebleeding occurs in 20% of patients within 2 weeks, in 30% by 1 month, and in 40% by 6 months. Rebleeding is associated with an increased mortality of more than 40%.

1 **Saccular or Berry aneurysm**
   - The most common type of aneurysm
   - Forms as a result of congenital weakness in the media and elastica of the arterial wall. Common locations are at branching points where the parent vessel is curving including:
     - Anterior cerebral/anterior communicating artery
     - Internal carotid/posterior communicating artery
     - Middle cerebral artery
     - Posterior inferior cerebellar artery
   - Arterial stress (age and hypertension) are important risk factors in the growth of aneurysms.
2 Fusiform aneurysm
   - Atherosclerotic dilatations, usually of the vertebral and basilar artery.
3 Mycotic aneurysm
   - Results from endocarditis with septic emboli to the vasa vasorum with secondary destruction of the vessel wall so that all is left is the intima.
   - Tends to be peripheral in the middle cerebral artery distribution, and multiple peripheral aneurysms should suggest the diagnosis.
4 Neoplastic aneurysm
   - Results from tumor emboli and subsequent growth of tumor through the vessel wall.
   - Occurs in atrial myxoma and choriocarcinoma.
5 Dissecting or traumatic aneurysm
   - May occur after the trauma or spontaneously.

Intracranial aneurysms: locations and associations

- Overall prevalence of saccular aneurysm in the general population is 9.6 per 100,000.
- Peak incidence is in the 6th decade of life. Rare in children and adolescents.
- Multiple in 15–20% of cases, especially in mirror locations.
- Aneurysms that rupture are usually more than 7–8 mm.
- Aneurysms that are larger than 25 mm (giant aneurysms) more often behave like space-occupying lesions.
- 85–95% of aneurysms involve the circle of Willis and 5–15% are located in the vertebrobasilar circulation.

The most common locations are:
1 The anterior communicating artery (30%)
2 The junction of posterior communicating with internal carotid artery (25–30%)
3 The bifurcation of internal carotid and middle cerebral artery (20–25%)
4 The tip of the basilar artery (5–10%)
5 Infratentorial – posterior inferior cerebellar artery, body of the basilar, anterior inferior cerebellar artery (1–3%)

Associations:
1 Polycystic kidney disease (PKD)
   - Autosomal dominant.
   - 10–30% of patients with PKD have intracerebral aneurysms.
2 Fibromuscular dysplasia
   - 25% of patients have aneurysms.
3 Family history
   - Aneurysms found in 9.5% of patients with a family history of intracranial aneurysms.
4 Coarctation of aorta; anomalies of the circle of Willis
5 Moyamoya disease
6 Ehler-Danlos syndrome
7 Neurofibromatosis type 1
8 Other possible associations: sickle cell disease, Marfan syndrome, vasculitis, tumors, infections.

Risk of hemorrhage:
- 0.5% annual risk of aneurysmal rupture – no prior history and aneurysm <10 mm
- up to 6% annual risk of aneurysmal rupture – aneurysm >25mm

- *Factors predisposing to rupture*:
  - Increasing age
  - Female gender
  - Hypertension
  - Alcohol
  - Smoking
  - History of spontaneous dissections

Intracranial aneurysms: patterns of hemorrhage from a ruptured aneurysm

- The distribution of extravasated blood on brain CT is an invaluable guide in determining the presence and the site of an offending aneurysm, and therefore in planning the order and the extent of angiography, especially in elderly patients in whom surgical repair is not always indicated.
- Identifying the source of hemorrhage from the scan is very helpful if more than one aneurysm is found, because there is a significant difference in management between a ruptured and an unruptured aneurysm.

The following patterns of hemorrhage can occur in combinations.

1 Brain parenchyma
  - Intracerebral hematomas usually give a good indication of the site of the ruptured aneurysm.
  - Aneurysms from the posterior circulation rarely give rise to intraparenchymal hematomas.

Location of hematoma	Location of aneurysm
Midline or paramedian frontal areas	Anterior cerebral or anterior communicating artery
Frontal lobe, not close to the midline	Ophthalmic artery
Between the frontal horns	Anterior communicating artery
Medial part of the temporal lobe	Posterior communicating artery
Lateral fissure	Middle cerebral artery

2 Subarachnoid cisterns
  - The pattern of hemorrhage is less specific for the site of the aneurysm, especially if the hemorrhage is diffuse. However, the source can sometimes be inferred if the hemorrhage remains confined to one or is most dense in a single cistern.

3 Intraventricular hemorrhage
  - Intraventricular hemorrhage occurs mostly with aneurysms of the anterior communicating artery, which can bleed through the lamina terminalis to fill the third and lateral ventricles.

- Rupture of an aneurysm at the posterior inferior cerebellar artery may preferentially fill the fourth and the third ventricle from the back.
4 Subdural hematomas
  - Subdural hematomas develop with aneurysmal rupture in 2–3%, most often associated with subarachnoid blood, but sometimes as the only manifestation.

Abrupt severe headache: 'worst headache of my life'

- The abrupt onset of a severe headache may not be caused by subarachnoid hemorrhage (SAH), but also by other conditions including meningitis, encephalitis, or intracerebral hemorrhage, etc.
- In one study, about 25% of patients with sudden headache in general practice prove to have SAH. This is because a headache with a more common cause, such as migraine or tension headache, can also arise suddenly and become severe.
- Although most patients with a sudden severe headache do not have SAH, SAH should always be considered in differential diagnosis, and suspected cases must all be investigated to exclude this diagnosis. **Missed SAH can be fatal!**

1 Sudden onset of severe headache WITH neck rigidity
  1.1 **Subarachnoid hemorrhage**
    - Headache is the cardinal feature in SAH, classically occurring in a split second, 'like a blow on the head' or 'an explosion inside the head', reaching a maximum within seconds. The headache is generally diffuse and poorly localized but tends to spread within minutes or hours to the back of the head, neck, and back as blood tracks down the spinal subarachnoid space.
    - Consider subarachnoid hemorrhage whenever a patient complains of the sudden onset of '*the worst headache of my life*'.
  1.2 **Meningitis/encephalitis**
    - The headache in meningitis/encephalitis can be less abrupt, with subacute onset over 1–2 days, although sudden abrupt severe headache can occur.
    - Other clues to suggest this possibility include high fever, tachycardia, and skin rash.
    - Frequently, when clinical differentiation between meningitis and SAH alone is not possible, neuroimaging and CSF examination should be considered.

1.3 Stroke
- Cerebellar stroke may give rise to sudden severe headache, nausea, and vomiting, but is usually associated with other symptoms or signs including vertigo, ataxia.
- Intraventricular hemorrhage, either primary or secondary, may also mimic SAH.

2 Sudden onset of severe headache WITHOUT neck rigidity
2.1 **Migraine**
- Migraine headache can sometimes occur suddenly, be severe, and is associated with photophobia, vomiting, confusion, and mild fever.
- However, the headache in migraine is more likely to be unilateral, throbbing, not so rapid in onset and follows the resolution of focal positive neurological symptoms of migraine aura.
- Vomiting, in general, tends to occur well into migraine attack, in contrast to SAH, which usually occurs soon after the onset.

2.2 Post-traumatic headache
- Immediately after a head injury, there is often headache due to soft-tissue damage.
- Post-trauma, intracranial vessels dilate, giving rise to a pulsating headache, which is worse with head movement, sneezing or exertion.
- Either type of post-concussive headache tends to resolve over hours to days.

2.3 Thunderclap headache
2.4 Benign orgasmic or exertional headache
2.5 Others
- Idiopathic stabbing headache
- Carotid or vertebral artery dissection
- Pheochromocytoma
- Reactions while on monoamine oxidase inhibitors

Cerebral ischemia/infarction

Causes of transient focal neurological symptoms (in addition to TIA)

- As the symptoms of TIA usually resolve within 15–60 minutes (within 24 hours by definition), the diagnosis of TIA is almost always based entirely on the clinical history. However, the history may not be entirely clear in some patients, resulting in uncertainty for the clinician.
- The following clues suggest that the symptoms may be attributed to TIA:
  - Focal neurological or monocular symptoms.
  - 'Negative' symptoms, representing a loss of function.

- ◆ Abrupt onset, but resolves gradually and completely.
- ◆ No warning, antecedent symptoms may occur but are rare.
- ◆ Following recovery, a few physical signs may be elicited, e.g. asymmetric reflexes.
- ◆ TIAs often recur, although very frequent stereotyped attacks raise the possibility of an alternative diagnosis.
- ◆ Loss of consciousness is unlikely to be due to TIA; it is more likely to be syncope or epilepsy.
- It is important to be aware that there are many conditions that can clinically mimic TIA and some are both serious and treatable.

1 **Migraine with aura** (classical migraine)
   - ◆ **Most common cause of TIA-mimics** (52%).
   - ◆ Migraine with aura differs from TIA in that it usually starts in younger patients who may have a family history of migraine.
   - ◆ Aura commonly consists of positive symptoms of focal cerebral and retinal dysfunction that develop gradually over 5–20 minutes. Symptoms may also evolve, spread over a period of time in a 'marching' fashion.
2 **Epilepsy** (29%)
   - ◆ Partial seizures can be distinguished from TIAs because they usually cause sudden positive sensory or motor phenomena, which spread quickly to adjacent body parts over 1 minute.
   - ◆ Positive sensory symptoms can sometimes occur in TIA (e.g. tingling). However, they tend to arise in an affected body part at the same time while the symptoms of seizures spread from one to the other.
   - ◆ Negative symptoms can also occur in seizures, such as Todd paralysis, and a history of a seizure is crucial to confirm this diagnosis.
3 Transient global amnesia (TGA, 17%)
   - ◆ TGA is a very characteristic syndrome, which typically occurs in the middle-aged or the elderly.
   - ◆ The manifestations include a sudden memory deficit of current information (anterograde), and the patient often cannot recall more distant events (retrograde amnesia). However, there is no loss of personal identity.
4 Intracranial lesions, not ischemia
   - ◆ Intracranial lesions, such as tumor or demyelination, can cause focal brain dysfunction mimicking TIAs.
   - ◆ However, onset is usually gradual over several days or weeks and not abrupt like TIAs.

5 Metabolic disorders
   - Hypoglycemia, hypercalcemia, and hyponatremia are well-recognized causes of TIA-like symptoms.
   - Differentiation is usually not difficult as associated symptoms are usually evident, for example hunger and profuse sweating in hypoglycemia.
   - Encephalopathy or mental status change may be present.
6 Peripheral lesions
   - TIA symptoms in the extremities can sometimes mimic entrapment neuropathy.
   - Symptoms of entrapment neuropathy are usually precipitated by any posture, movement, associated with positive sensory symptoms, such as pain or tingling.
7 Others
   - 'Funny turns' is the term used to describe transient episodes of only non-focal symptoms not due to any identifiable conditions.
   - Myasthenia gravis, e.g. diplopia
   - Psychological causes. Clues are that attacks are usually emotionally based.

Cerebral embolism: causes

- About 95% of ischemic strokes and TIAs are due to embolic or thrombotic consequences of atherothrombosis and intracranial small vessel disease. Of these, 20% of causes are due to embolism from the heart.
- The source of embolism is usually located in the heart and the large vessels (including aorta, carotid, or vertebral arteries).

1 **Cardiac sources**: most common source of cerebral embolism
   - Embolic material of cardiac origin is often composed of fragments of thrombus that originate from either the left atrium or atrial appendages in the case of atrial fibrillation, or the left ventricle as a result of mural thrombus formation after recent or remote myocardial infarction.
   - These materials are mechanically unstable at the site of final occlusion and are prone to spontaneous fragmentation.
     1.1 Atrial fibrillation (AF)
        - The most important cardiac risk factor for cerebral embolism.
        - In the setting of rheumatic AF, the risk of cerebral embolism is 17-fold higher than in control populations, while the risk is 5-fold in nonrheumatic AF.
        - AF is present in 16% of all ischemic strokes, but it has a causal role in the 10% that are associated with atrial thrombi.

1.2 Myocardial infarction (MI)
- Recent MI, especially transmural and of the anterior wall, carries up to 5% risk of cerebral embolism within the first 30 days, largely as a result of fresh mural thrombus formation.

1.3 Bacterial endocarditis
- Infected mitral and aortic valvular vegetations are a major source of cerebral embolism.
- Emboli usually present subacutely, mimicking an encephalopathy, rather than with the most typical acute and focal deficits.

1.4 Prosthetic heart valves
- Mechanical heart valves carry a risk of cerebral embolism of approximately 3% per year, even in the presence of chronic oral anticoagulation. The risk is higher in mitral than with aortic valves.
- INR should be kept in the range of 2.5–3.5.

1.5 Mitral valve prolapse
- The presence of mitral valve prolapse is not more common among young patients with unexplained ischemic stroke than in control subjects.

1.6 Patent foramen ovale (PFO) and interatrial septal aneurysm
- In patients with an otherwise unexplained ischemic stroke, the prevalence of PFO, as detected by air contrast echocardiography with Valsalva maneuver, increases significantly to 40–50%. Interatrial septal aneurysm presents in 28% of patients with undetermined cause of stroke.
- Possible mechanisms in this setting include thrombus formation in the right atrium, deep vein thrombosis with paradoxical embolus, and atrial vulnerability.

1.7 Other cardiac sources
- Atrial myxoma
- Calcified mitral and aortic valves

2 **Arterial sources:** artery-to-artery mechanism of embolism

2.1 Ulcerated aortic atheroma
- Embolization risk increases in plaques between 4 and 5 mm in thickness and in those with mobile components on transesophageal echocardiogram (TEE), ulceration of more than 2 mm or more, and with non-calcified hypoechoic features suggesting superimposed thrombus.

2.2 Carotid artery atheroma
- Cerebral embolism is assumed to be a stroke mechanism in cases of tight stenosis and acute occlusion of the extracranial internal carotid artery.

2.3 Vertebral artery
- The vertebral artery is prone to trauma at the level of the C1–C2 junction, where extreme head rotation and hyperextension may occur leading to dissection.

▪ The emboli usually travel to the ipsilateral PICA, but also into the basilar artery and distal branches.

3 Unidentified source of emboli

♦ In some patients, the embolic source is not identified, although the clinical history and stroke pattern supports the embolic etiology.

♦ Emboli, as small as 2 mm, may occlude the artery without being detected by current diagnostic technology.

Stroke in a young person (under age 40 years)

- Embolism is the most common cause (31%), usually arising from a previously known cardiac source.
- Interestingly, uncertain etiology is the second most common category (27%), which could be related to migraine, oral contraceptive use, or undiagnosed hypercoagulable states. Many types of hypercoagulable states are increasingly recognized.

1 **Cerebral embolism** (31%)

1.1 Cardiac source: most commonly from previously known cardiac lesions. Emboli can originate from the heart due to structural lesions or dysrhythmias.

▪ Structural lesions: emboli usually arise from valvular lesions, most commonly mitral valve; mitral stenosis being the most common. Others include prosthetic valves and infective endocarditis.

▪ Dysrhythmias: most common atrial fibrillation.

1.2 Paradoxical emboli: For paradoxical emboli to occur, there has to be a right-to-left shunt. So the DDx comes from that:

▪ ASD, VSD with right-to-left shunt

▪ Patent foramen ovale with shunt

▪ Pulmonary AVM

1.3 Other structural sources, for example, aortic atherosclerotic plaques.

2 **Unknown etiology (27%)**. Surprisingly, this is the second most common cause of stroke in the young. Probably the majority of causes are related to hypercoagulable states that are undiagnosed at the time.

♦ Idiopathic.

♦ Migraine? – called migrainous infarction.

♦ Oral contraceptive pills – not proven.

♦ Oral contraceptive pills + smoking?

There is an increased risk of stroke in patients who have migraine and are taking oral contraceptive pills.

3 Arteriopathy: divided into narrowing of the lumen due to deposition (athero-sclerosis) and vessel wall problems.

    3.1 Cerebrovascular atherosclerosis (18%)

    3.2 Non-atherosclerotic arteriopathy (19%) – suggests vessel wall problems – so the DDx may be generated from the following conditions:

        ▪ Dissection

        ▪ Fibromuscular dysplasia (most common in middle-aged female, ICA)

        ▪ Inflammation, e.g. Takayasu arteritis, any forms of CNS vasculitis

        ▪ Radiation-induced arteriopathy

4 Hypercoagulable state: an uncommon etiology of ischemic stroke but increas-ingly recognized, particularly in the young.

Recommended tests, although diagnostic yield is low.
- Protein C & protein S
- Antithrombin III
- Plasminogen
- Activated protein C resistance
- Factor V Leiden mutation
- Anti-cardiolipin antibody or lupus anticoagulant

---

5 Don't forget venous thrombosis as another possible etiology of infarction in a young person.

- About 95% of ischemic strokes and TIAs are due to the embolic or thrombotic consequences of atherothrombosis affecting large or medium-size arteries, intracranial small vessel disease, or embolism from the heart.
- Another 5% of cases are due to rare or unusual causes.

Unusual causes of TIA or stroke

1 Arterial trauma or dissection

- Ischemic strokes or TIAs, particularly in young and middle-aged patients, are increasingly being found to be due to arterial trauma and dissection.
- Penetrating neck injuries are more likely to damage the carotid than the better protected vertebral arteries.
- Blunt trauma usually causes intimal tearing or dissection with complicating thrombosis or embolism, while traumatic rupture of an atheromatous plaque, vasospasm, or delayed aneurysm is rare.
- Internal carotid artery is more vulnerable to a direct blow to the neck, whereas vertebral arteries are more prone to rotational and hyperextension injuries at the level of the atlas and axis.

- Cervical dissection is usually traumatic or coincides with trivial neck movement, although it can be spontaneous. Helpful clues to suggest dissection include:
  - pain in the face around the eye and neck,
  - Horner syndrome,
  - carotid bruits for ICA dissection and
  - pain in the occiput and neck for vertebral dissection.
2 **Inflammatory vascular disorders**
  - CNS vasculitis may cause not just thrombosis within arteries but also rupture of any affected arteries, causing subarachnoid or intracerebral hemorrhage and intracranial venous thrombosis.
  - Clues to diagnosis may be lacking, and some cases may require conventional angiography or even biopsy for diagnosis.
3 Migraine
  - To make a diagnosis of migrainous stroke, there should be no reason to suspect that stroke has been caused by anything else, particularly ones which can be confused with migraine, such as dissection.
  - Most often, a migrainous stroke causes a homonymous hemianopsia and seldom results in severe disability.
4 Hematological
  - Occasionally, ischemic stroke can be due to underlying hematological disorders.
  - The disorders are usually the conditions which predispose individuals to prothrombotic or hypercoagulable states, including polycythemia, hemoglobinopathies, or coagulation abnormalities, etc.
5 Connective tissue disorders
  - 5.1 Fibromuscular dysplasia is an uncommon segmental disorder of small and medium-sized arteries. It is more common in females and tends to affect more than one artery. Renal arteries are often involved, as well as the mid-high cervical portion of the ICA and vertebral artery at the level of C1–2.
  - 5.2 Ehler-Danlos syndrome
  - 5.3 Pseudoxanthoma elasticum
  - 5.4 Marfan syndrome
6 Others
  - 6.1 Stroke in association with acute myocardial infarction
    - Possibilities include embolism from left ventricular thrombus, low-flow state, arrhythmias, or instrumentation-related complications, etc.
  - 6.2 Infections
    - These organisms usually cause stroke by inducing inflammation and secondary thrombosis of arteries and veins.
    - Examples include tuberculosis, syphilis, fungal, herpes zoster, and HIV.
    - Bacterial agents are less likely to cause stroke.

6.3 Female sex hormones – oral contraceptives (in conjunction with smoking)

6.4 Pregnancy and puerperium

6.5 Moyamoya syndrome: is a radiologically defined syndrome of severe stenosis or occlusion of distal ICAs, with frequent additional involvement of the circle of Willis or proximal arteries.

Venous versus arterial infarcts

- Venous infarcts are uncommon, and are frequently misdiagnosed as arterial infarcts, intracerebral hemorrhages, or tumors.
- The possibility of venous infarction is often not even considered.
- Cerebral venous disease consists of a spectrum, varying from the effects of sinus thrombosis, without any parenchymal change, to purely parenchymal lesions due to cortical vein thrombosis without sinus thrombosis. The clinical presentation as well as radiological findings depend on the balance of these components.
- The key differentiating features between arterial and venous infarcts are that the venous infarcts do not usually fit the usual site of arterial infarcts or the symptoms cannot be explained by any specific arterial territory. The lesions are usually more swollen beyond the low density area on the CT and they often contain hemorrhage.

Features	Arterial infarcts	Venous infarcts
Shape	Wedge or rounded	Wedged if cortical Rounded if deep
Number occurring simultaneously	Usually single	May be multiple
Density on CT	Early: mildly hypodense Later: more hypodense	Early hypodensity and persists
Margins on CT	Early: indistinct Clear distinction after several days	Early distinction
Swelling	Develops after a few days, up to two weeks	Marked swelling, appears very early
Hemorrhage	Infrequent, more likely to be peripheral and with larger lesions	Frequent and central finger-like lesions
Additional signs	Hyperdense artery sign	Empty delta sign

Ref: Modified from Warlow C.P., Dennis M.S., van Gijn J., *et al. Stroke: A Practical Guide to Management.* Blackwell Science. Oxford. 1996: p.160.

Intracranial venous thrombosis: causes

- Intracranial venous thrombosis is an under-recognized condition. This diagnosis should be considered in any patients with primary intracerebral hemorrhage.
- The diagnosis of venous infarction should be strongly suspected if:
  - The patient is a young woman.
  - Hemorrhage is preceded by other manifestations.
  - Hemorrhage is in parasagittal area, especially bilateral.
- Extensive hemorrhage in intracerebral venous thrombosis is uncommon and is often secondary to infarction caused by obstruction of cortical veins. It is usually preceded by an ischemic phase, manifested by focal deficits or seizures.

1 Infectious causes
  - Intracranial infection
  - Local infection, for example, tonsillitis and otitis
  - Systemic infections, for example, septicemia, endocarditis, encephalitis
2 Trauma: may be associated with infection
  - Head injury, with or without fractures
  - Procedure-related, e.g. neurosurgical procedures
3 Neoplasia
  - Tumors obstructing the venous drainage predisposing to thrombosis
  - Tumors with associated hypercoagulable state
4 Medical conditions
  - Oral contraceptives, e.g. estrogens
  - Pregnancy, puerperium
  - Medical disorders associated with hypercoagulable state
    - Myeloproliferative disorders
    - Protein C, S deficiency
    - Antithrombin III deficiency
    - Factor V Leiden heterozygous or homozygous
    - Disseminated intravascular coagulation
  - Connective tissue diseases
  - Autoimmune disorders
  - Heart disease, e.g. congestive cardiac failure

Stroke syndromes

Large vessel syndromes

Ocular stroke

- Branches of the ophthalmic artery supply both the retina and the optic nerve. The central retinal artery supplies the retina, whereas the posterior ciliary artery supplies the optic nerve.

Features	Retinal ischemia	Optic nerve ischemia
Artery involved	• Central retinal artery or its branch	• Posterior ciliary artery
Etiology	• Carotid occlusive disease • Cardiac or aortic arch emboli • Hyperviscosity state • Hypoperfusion from high-grade stenosis	• Intrinsic atherosclerosis • Temporal arteritis • Carotid disease is a rare cause
Symptoms	• Amaurosis fugax 'shade being pulled down' over the eye	• Unilateral visual loss, maximally in the temporal field or inferior altitudinal pattern
Signs	• Hollenhorst plaques may be present • Roth spot in the case of infective endocarditis • Optic atrophy in chronic cases • Segmental retinal infarct in branch occlusion	• A pale, swollen disc, associated with flame hemorrhages around the disc • Afferent pupillary defect

Neurological symptoms and arterial territory

- Cerebral vascular anatomy can be divided into two main parts, the anterior (carotid) and posterior (vertebrobasilar) systems. In each system there are three components: the extracranial arteries, major intracranial arteries, and the small deep perforating arteries. Large intracranial arteries have important anastomotic connections over the pial surface or at the base of the brain. The deep perforating arteries are usually end-arteries with limited anastomotic potentials.
- Localization by arterial territory is difficult because there can be individual variations in arterial anatomy, different patterns of arterial disease affecting collateral circulations, and the fact that one function can be served by both circulations but at different levels. Therefore, the information in the table on page 132 is provided as a guide. Bear in mind that individual variations may occur.

Symptoms	Arterial territory		
	Carotid	Either	Vertebrobasilar
Aphasia	+++		
Monocular visual loss	+++		
Unilateral weakness		+++	
Unilateral sensory loss		+++	
Dysarthria		+++	
Apraxia		+++	
Ataxia (except in ataxic hemiparesis)			+++
Dysphagia (in majority)			+++
Diplopia			+++
Vertigo			+++
Bilateral simultaneous visual loss			+++
Bilateral simultaneous weakness			+++
Bilateral simultaneous sensory disturbances			+++
Cross motor/sensory symptoms			+++
Facial sensory disturbances			+++

Ref: Modified from Warlow C.P., Dennis M.S., van Gijn J., *et al. Stroke: A Practical Guide to Management.* 1996. Blackwell Science. Oxford.

The anterior (carotid) system

- The cerebral vascular anatomy can be divided into two main parts, the anterior (carotid) and posterior (vertebrobasilar) systems.
- For each system, there are three components: the extracranial arteries, the major intracranial arteries, and the small superficial and deep perforating arteries.
- These groups of arteries at different levels have functional characteristics and can cause different symptoms and signs.
- The carotid circulation starts with the common carotid artery and terminates into anterior and middle cerebral arteries.

1 **Common carotid artery (CCA)**
   - Anatomy: the left common carotid artery usually arises directly from the left side of the aortic arch, whereas the right CCA arises from the brachiocephalic artery. At the level of the thyroid cartilage, they divide into the internal carotid artery (ICA) and the external carotid artery (ECA).
   - Lesions: the CCA is closely associated with ascending sympathetic fibers.
     - Therefore, lesions of the CCA may cause ipsilateral Horner syndrome, with involvement of sudomotor fibers of the face.
     - Carotidynia – a syndrome characterized by tenderness over the artery and pain referred to the ipsilateral frontotemporal region – may occur.

2 **Carotid bifurcation**
   - Anatomy: The carotid bifurcation is usually at the level of thyroid cartilage. It contains the carotid body. The ICA is usually posterior to the ECA. The carotid body and carotid sinus receive their blood supply from the ECA. The bifurcation is also the most common site for the atheroma to develop. The carotid body responds to an increase in the PaO_2, blood flow, and arterial pH, a decrease in $PaCO_2$ or temperature. It has a modulatory role on pulse rate, blood pressure, and hypoxic ventilatory drive. Stretching the wall of carotid sinus will increase the depth and rate of respiration.
   - Lesions:
     - Atheroma at the bifurcation is the common site for cerebral emboli and is the common location for carotid endarterectomy.
     - Carotid sinus hypersensitivity is probably an under-recognized cause of collapse and syncope in the elderly.

3 External carotid artery (ECA)
   - Anatomy: ECA starts from the carotid bifurcation and has many branches including ascending pharyngeal, superior thyroid, lingual, occipital, facial, internal maxillary, superficial temporal, and posterior auricular arteries.
   - Lesions: in patients with stroke, the branches of ECA are the possible sites of anastomosis with intracranial ICA.
     - ECA can be affected by giant cell arteritis.
     - Chronic ECA occlusion may occasionally result in amaurosis fugax due to failure of perfusion through ECA-ICA collaterals.

4 **Internal carotid artery**
   - Anatomy: the ICA ascends through the foramen lacerum in the skull base.
   - Lesions:
     - 78% of cases of ICA occlusion were associated with ipsilateral infarction. The mechanisms may be artery-to-artery embolism, low flow, or local arterial thrombosis.
     - Around the origin of the ICA, there are hypoglossal and superior laryngeal nerves, which may be damaged during carotid endarterectomy.
     - ICA dissection may be due to trauma, inflammation, or occur spontaneously.

5 Carotid siphon
   - Anatomy: the S-shape carotid siphon lies within the venous plexus of the cavernous sinus, adjacent to cranial nerves III, IV, V1, V2, and VI, which run in the lateral wall of the sinus. Persistent trigeminal artery, a congenital variant, may arise from the ICA at this level and links with the basilar artery.
   - Lesions:
     - Atheromata can affect the carotid siphon.
     - Aneurysm at this level can cause oculomotor nerve palsy, and rupture may result in carotico-cavernous fistula.

6 Supraclinoid internal carotid artery
- Anatomy: the supraclinoid portion of the ICA lies in the subarachnoid space and is close to the oculomotor nerve. The ophthalmic artery, the only branch from the supraclinoid ICA, enters the orbit through the optic foramen.
- Lesions:
  - Amaurosis fugax may be due to emboli passing through ophthalmic artery.
  - The combination of ocular and cerebral hemisphere ischemic attacks on the same side is a strong indicator of a severe ipsilateral internal carotid artery stenosis or occlusion.

7 Posterior communicating artery (PCoA)
- Anatomy: it arises from the dorsal aspect of the ICA and tracks caudally to join the posterior cerebral artery (PCA).
- Lesions:
  - Aneurysms at this level may present with painful oculomotor nerve palsy.
  - PCoA may be absent in some patients.

8 Anterior choroidal artery
- Anatomy: although a small artery, branching before the ICA terminates into ACA and MCA, it supplies various important structures, including: globus pallidus, anterior hippocampus, uncus, posterior limb of internal capsule, rostral midbrain, cerebral peduncle, lateral geniculate nucleus, and part of optic radiation.
- Lesions:
  - Isolated occlusion of anterior choroidal artery is usually a result of intrinsic disease of the artery rather than thrombosis or infarction.
  - It produces contralateral hemiparesis, hemisensory loss sparing proprioception, disturbance of language and visuo-spatial function, and a hemianopia.

Posterior (vertebrobasilar) system

- The cerebral vascular anatomy can be divided into two main parts, the anterior (carotid) and posterior (vertebrobasilar) systems.
- The vertebrobasilar system develops quite separately from the carotid system and is subject to many more changes during fetal development.

1 **Precerebral vertebral artery**
- Anatomy: the right vertebral artery arises as the first branch of the right subclavian artery, which arises from the innominate artery, while the left vertebral artery arises as the first branch of the left subclavian artery, which comes out directly from the aortic arch. The major branch outside the skull is the single, midline anterior spinal artery, formed by a contribution from both vertebral arteries.
- Lesions:
  - The origin of the vertebral artery can be affected by atheroma, which can be the site of occlusion or the source of emboli.

- Vertebral dissection may occur following trauma or even other trivial injuries.
- Takayasu arteritis may also affect the vertebral artery.

2 Intracranial vertebral artery
- Anatomy: the fourth segment of the vertebral artery is intracranial, until the two arteries unite to form the basilar artery at the pontomedullary junction.
- Lesions:
  - Vertebral occlusion may result in lateral medullary as well as inferior cerebellar infarction.
  - Subclavian steal syndrome occurs when there is hemodynamically significant stenosis of the subclavian artery proximal to the origin of the vertebral artery. The pulse and blood pressure will be lower in the affected arm, and exercise increases the flow away from the hindbrain, which may cause the symptoms of hypoperfusion.

3 Posterior inferior cerebellar artery (PICA)
- Anatomy: the PICAs usually arise from the intracranial vertebral arteries although one may be absent in 25% of patients. The PICA may supply the lateral medulla, but more frequently there are direct branches from the vertebral artery between the ostium of the PICA and the origin of the basilar artery.
- Lesions:
  - Classic Wallenberg syndrome is relatively infrequent in clinical practice. Rather, patients with PICA infarction usually present with vertigo, ataxia, headache, nystagmus, and ipsilateral lateropulsion.
  - Isolated vertigo can occur from PICA infarction, although most cases of isolated vertigo are peripheral in origin.

4 Basilar artery
- Anatomy: branches from the basilar artery are the perforating branches, supplying the base of the pons and the paramedian pontine tegmentum.
- Lesions:
  - Locked-in syndrome is due to bilateral infarction or hemorrhage, at the base of the pons.
  - The 'top of the basilar syndrome' is a syndrome due to embolus impacted in the rostral basilar artery, resulting in bilateral infarction of the rostral brainstem and of the PCA territories. The syndrome consists of pupillary abnormalities, vertical gaze palsy, ptosis, hallucinations, hemiballismus, cortical blindness, and amnesia.
  - Dolichoectasia of the basilar artery can cause mass effect to the brainstem and the development of in situ thrombus.

5 Anterior inferior cerebellar artery (AICA)
- Anatomy: AICAs originate from the caudal part of the basilar artery, supplying the rostral medulla, cerebellar, and basis pontis. They also give branches to labyrinthine and internal auditory arteries.

♦ Lesions:
  ▪ Isolated occlusion of the AICA, often secondary to atherosclerosis of the basilar artery or dolichoectasia, is relatively rare, but causes infarction of both cerebellum and pons. Signs include ipsilateral Horner syndrome, limb ataxia, facial palsy, nystagmus, trigeminal sensory loss, and dysarthria.
  ▪ Occlusion of the internal auditory artery can cause unilateral deafness.
6 Superior cerebellar artery (SuCA)
  ♦ Anatomy: SuCAs arise from the basilar artery before its terminal bifurcation. It supplies the dorsolateral midbrain, superior cerebellum, and superior cerebellar peduncle.
  ♦ Lesions:
  ▪ SuCA infarction, often as a result of emboli, causes ipsilateral Horner syndrome, limb ataxia, tremor, contralateral spinothalamic deficits, upper motor neuron facial palsy. Isolated cerebellar infarction may occur. (Vertigo is not common in SuCA infarction.)
7 Posterior cerebral artery (PCA)
  ♦ Anatomy: PCAs are usually the terminal branch of the basilar artery. The P1 segment passes around the cerebral peduncle lying between the temporal lobe and upper brainstem before giving off branches to supply inferoposterior temporal lobes and parieto-occipital lobes.
  ♦ Lesions:
  ▪ PCA infarction, often embolic subsequent to the embolus at the basilar bifurcation, usually causes homonymous hemianopia with hemiparesis. Other signs include alexia with or without agraphia (with left PCA infarction), aphasia, disorders of language, and amnesia.

Anterior cerebral artery (ACA)

- The anterior cerebral artery arises as the medial branch of the bifurcation of the ICA, at the level of the anterior clinoid process.
- The proximal A1 segments of the ACAs pass medially and forward over the optic nerve or chiasm and corpus callosum to enter the interhemispheric fissure, where they are linked by the ACoA. The distal 'post-communicating' segments run together in the interhemispheric fissure and then continue backwards as the pericallosal and callosomarginal arteries.
- Clinical features of ACA infarcts include predominant leg weakness (more than the arm), and are often marked distally, in contrast to MCA infarcts. There is often no sensory deficit. Frontal lobe dysfunction may be present, including urinary incontinence. Bilateral leg weakness may occur with bilateral ACA infarcts, although it needs to be differentiated from spinal cord or brainstem lesions.

Different types of ACA infarctions:

1 **Embolic ACA infarction**
   - Most cases of ACA infarcts are related to either cardiogenic embolism or artery-to-artery embolism from an occluded or stenosed ICA.
2 Non-embolic ACA infarction
   - Isolated infarction of the ACA territory is comparatively rare, other than when due to vasospasm in complicating subarachnoid hemorrhage.
   - May also occur (unilateral or bilateral) when subfalcine herniation occurs in cases of severe unilateral cerebral edema.
   - This rarity may be due to the possible collateral supply from the ACoA if one ACA is occluded.
3 Bilateral ACA infarction
   - Not common, it can occur in the setting of both ACAs receiving their supply from the same carotid artery via the ACoA, or due to the crossover of distal branches in the interhemispheric fissure.
   - Bilateral ACA infarction should always prompt a search for an aneurysm, which may have bled recently.
4 Recurrent artery of Heubner infarction
   - The recurrent artery of Huebner is an inconstant branch of the ACA, that, if present, usually arises around the level of the ACoA.
   - It supplies the head of caudate nucleus, the inferior portion of the anterior limb of internal capsule, and the hypothalamus.
   - The deficits usually depend on the extent of capsular supply. Weakness of the face and arm with dysarthria is said to be characteristic.

Middle cerebral artery (MCA)

- The first segment of the MCA tracks laterally between the upper surface of the temporal lobe and the inferior surface of the frontal lobe until it reaches the Sylvian fissure. The lenticulostriate arteries arise from the proximal part of the MCA stem.
- In the Sylvian fissure, the MCA usually bifurcates into superior and inferior divisions. The superior division usually supplies the large part of the frontal and parietal lobes, including the orbitofrontal, frontal, pre-Rolandic, Rolandic, anterior parietal, and posterior parietal branches. The inferior division supplies parts of the temporal and occipital lobes, including angular, tempero-occipital, anterior/middle/posterior temporal, occipital, and temporopolar branches. The MCA terminates as multiple medullary perforating arteries in the subcortical white matter.

1 **MCA main stem infarction**

- Occlusion of the MCA stem is almost always symptomatic. In most cases, it occurs in the proximal stem involving lenticulostriate arteries, resulting in ischemia of both the deep and superficial territory of the MCA. Typically, patients have contralateral hemiparesis, sensory deficit, hemianopia, and deficits of higher cortical function. Exact symptoms may vary if there is a collateral supply. Distal stem occlusion usually spares the leg, as the cortical leg area is supplied by ACA.
- In Caucasians, the mechanism of occlusion tends to be an embolus or extension of a proximal thrombus, while atheroma in situ is common in Asians.

2 **Lenticulostriate arteries infarction** (deep perforating arteries infarction)

- Lenticulostriate arteries usually arise from the proximal part of the MCA stem.
- They supply the lentiform nucleus, lateral head of the caudate nucleus, anterior limb of the internal capsule, part of the globus pallidus.
- Mechanisms of infarctions are divided equally among cardiogenic embolism, stenosis or occlusion at the ICA, or occlusion or stenosis at the MCA stem.
- Typically, patients present with predominant contralateral weakness with the severity equally between the arm and leg. Sensory deficit is less and cortical deficits are usually transient.
- Occlusion of a single lenticulostriate artery results in lacunar infarct, thought to be secondary to local vasculopathies rather than embolism.

3 Middle cerebral artery cortical branch infarction

- The mechanisms are usually due to embolism or low flow secondary to proximal vascular lesions. Local disease is unlikely except in the context of vasculitis. There are no significant collaterals between individual cortical branches.
- Typically, with superior division involvement, patients present with contralateral hemiparesis and hemisensory loss greater in the face and arm than in the leg.
- Hemianopia, fluent aphasia, and higher cortical sensory deficits may occur if the inferior division is occluded.

4 Middle cerebral artery medullary perforating arteries infarction

- MCA medullary perforating arteries arise from the cortical arteries of the surface of the hemispheres. They then descend to supply the subcortical white matter, for example, centrum semi-ovale. They are functional end arteries and their distal fields are part of the internal border zone.
- The majority of infarcts of perforating arteries are from the occlusion, secondary to local vasculopathies. Large vessel disease and embolism are unlikely causes.
- Typically, patients present with the classical lacunar syndromes depending on the location of the perforating arteries involved.

Clinical deficits suggesting posterior circulation involvement

- The clinical deficits which point to the lesion being in the distribution of the vertebrobasilar system are provided below.
- Although there are some clinical syndromes, due to well-localized lesions within the vertebrobasilar system (e.g. Wallenberg syndrome, Millard-Gubler syndrome) in clinical practice, such syndromes are less likely seen in pure form.
- The presence of higher cortical functional deficits should not exclude the possibility of posterior circulation involvement, as there can be variations in vascular anatomy among individuals.

Any of the following syndromes are considered to be due to posterior circulation dysfunction.

1 Ipsilateral cranial nerve palsy (single or multiple) with contralateral motor and/ or sensory deficit
2 Bilateral and/or motor sensory deficit
3 Disorder of conjugate eye movement (either horizontal or vertical)
4 Cerebellar dysfunction without ipsilateral long-tract deficit
5 Isolated hemianopia or cortical blindness

The following syndromes and signs may present in posterior circulation diseases, although they have no specific localizing value.

1 Horner syndrome
2 Nystagmus
3 Dysarthria
4 Hearing impairment

Moyamoya syndrome

- Moyamoya syndrome is a radiologically defined syndrome of severe stenosis or occlusion of one or, more often, both distal internal carotid arteries with frequent additional involvement of parts of the circle of Willis and sometimes of the proximal cerebral and basilar arteries.
- As a result, numerous tiny collaterals develop from the lenticulostriate, thalamoperforating, and pial arteries, looking like a puff of smoke in the basal ganglia region on a cerebral angiogram.
- This disease is more common, although not restricted, in Japanese and other Asians.
  - Clinical presentation in young adults usually includes alternating hemiparesis, early morning headache, choreiform movements, seizures, and intellectual decline.

> • In adults, the most common symptom is hemorrhagic, caused by SAH, subependymal, or intraventricular hemorrhage.

Causes:
1 Familial cause: in approximately 10% of patients.
2 Acquired causes resulting in occlusion of the arteries at the case of the brain.
   • Basal meningeal or nasopharyngeal infections
   • Congenital heart disease
   • Down syndrome
   • Fibromuscular dysplasia
   • Irradiation: post-cranial
   • Neurofibromatosis
   • Sickle cell disease
   • Tuberous sclerosis
   • Vasculitis
   • Young females with smoking and oral contraceptive use

Lacunar syndromes (LACS)

> • The occlusion of a single, deep perforating artery results in a restricted area of infarction, known as a 'lacune'. In fact, 'lacune' is a pathological term and should be used only with clinico-pathological correlation. The term 'small deep infarct' is preferred when the imaged area of infarction is within the territory of a single perforating artery.
> • The clinical syndromes from lacunar infarction vary from clinically silent (e.g. lentiform nucleus) to severe hemiparesis.
> • By definition, a lacunar syndrome is a result of a single vascular event with no evidence of visual field deficit or brainstem disturbance and no new disturbance of higher cortical functions.

Different types of lacunar syndromes are recognized.
1 **Pure motor stroke**
   • The most common lacunar syndrome, defined as a complete or incomplete paralysis of the face, arm, and leg on one side, unaccompanied by sensory signs, visual field defects, dysphagia, and agnosia. In the case of brainstem lesions, there is no vertigo, diplopia, ataxia, or nystagmus.
   • The anatomical location for pure motor stroke is in the area where the motor tracts are packed together, such as internal capsule and pons.

- Partial pure motor stroke is recognized when face and arm or arm and leg are involved. The lesions are usually situated in the corona radiata or the junction between it and the capsule.

2 **Sensorimotor stroke**
  - Second most common lacunar syndrome. Most cases report different lesion locations, including posterior limb of internal capsule (31%), corona radiata (22%), thalamus (9%), and genu of the internal capsule (7%).

3 **Pure sensory stroke**
  - Less frequent than the pure motor or sensorimotor stroke.
  - It is controversial if objective sensory deficits need to be present in order to diagnose pure sensory stroke.
  - Most cases are due to small infarcts in the thalamus.

4 **Ataxic hemiparesis, clumsy-hand-dysarthria syndrome, homolateral ataxia, and crural paresis**
  - These syndromes are less accepted as 'lacunar' and there are significant variability in clinical findings in all case reports.
  - Most cases suggest lesions in the contralateral basis pontis, although variations of each syndrome are associated with other lesion locations.

Brainstem and cerebellar syndromes

Midbrain syndromes

- In midbrain infarcts, the most commonly affected region is the medial midbrain, and the most frequently involved artery is the paramedian artery, followed by the posterior cerebral artery, and the territory intermediate between the two. Involvement from the superior cerebellar artery is rare.
- Patients with medial midbrain infarcts have localizing clinical features that are linked to the involvement of the third nerve or its nucleus. Paramedian infarcts involve the nuclear portion of the oculomotor nerve, while more lateral infarcts are associated with fascicular involvement of the third nerve with or without ataxia or hemiparesis.
- Rostral or caudal midbrain lesions have less localizing neurologic signs. Vertical gaze impairment suggests the involvement of the rostral dorsal midbrain, such as Parinaud syndrome.
- Locked-in syndrome, classically due to bilateral ventral pontine lesions, can occur with midbrain lesions as well as bilateral lesions in the internal capsules.

Syndrome	Structures involved	Physical signs
Weber syndrome	• Rootlets of oculomotor nerve • Cerebral peduncle	• Ipsilateral oculomotor nerve palsy • Contralateral UMN paralysis, including lower face
Benedikt syndrome	• Rootlets of oculomotor nerve • Red nucleus	• Ipsilateral oculomotor nerve palsy • Contralateral Holmes tremor • Contralateral hemianesthesia may occur
Claude syndrome	• Rootlets of oculomotor nerve • Red nucleus • Brachium conjunctivum	• Ipsilateral oculomotor nerve palsy • Contralateral Holmes tremor • Contralateral ataxia
Nothnagel syndrome	• Oculomotor nerve fascicles • Brachium conjunctivum • Superior and inferior colliculi	• Ipsilateral or bilateral oculomotor nerve palsy • Contralateral ataxia • Vertical gaze palsy may present
Parinaud or dorsal midbrain syndrome	• Pretectal region	• Upgaze paralysis • Large pupil, light-near dissociation • Lid retraction (Collier sign) • Convergence retraction nystagmus on upward gaze
Wall-eyed or WEBINO syndrome	• Bilateral lesions involving rostral MLF	• Exotropic gaze • Absence of eye adduction
Vertical one-and-a-half syndrome	• Bilateral lesions in the mesencephalic-diencephalic junction • Bilateral riMLF • Premotor fibers to the contralateral SR and ipsilateral IO subnucleus	• Bilateral impairment of downgaze (one) • Monocular paralysis of elevation (half)
Locked-in syndrome	• Ventral mesencephalon	• Mute • Quadriplegia • Preservation of consciousness • Preserved vertical eye movements and blinking
Top of the basilar syndrome	• Mesencephalon • Thalamus • Part of temporal and occipital lobes	• Hemianopia or cortical blindness • Balint syndrome • Vertical gaze abnormalities • Impaired vergence • Light-near dissociation • Somnolence, memory disturbances, hallucinations

Syndrome	Structures involved	Physical signs
Peduncular hallucinosis	• Tegmental lesions • Cerebral peduncle lesions	• Nonstereotyped, colored, vivid hallucinations • Somnolence

UMN – upper motor neuron, MLF – medial longitudinal fasciculus, riMLF – rostral interstitial nucleus of medial longitudinal fasciculus, SR – superior rectus, IO – inferior oblique, WEBINO – wall-eyed bilateral internuclear ophthalmoplegia

Pontine syndromes

- The functional anatomy of the pons is best understood by dividing it into two portions, a dorsal pontine tegmentum and a ventral 'belly' of the pons, or basis pontis. The basis pontis is composed mainly of nerve fiber bundles, predominantly corticospinal and corticopontocerebellar fibers passing through the pons. The tegmentum contains medial lemniscus, spinothalamic, trapezoid body, central tegmental tract, medial longitudinal fasciculus, tectospinal, and descending sympathetic fibers.
- The blood supply of the pons is derived from the basilar artery, including paramedian vessels (supplying the medial basis pontis and the tegmentum) and both short and long circumferential arteries (supplying the ventrolateral region of the basis pontis and lateral tegmentum).
- Different pontine syndromes are described below. Most cases are due to ischemic infarction from small vessel disease.

Syndromes	Structures involved	Physical sign
Basal pontine syndromes		
Millard-Gubler syndrome	• Caudal basis pontis • Facial nucleus or fascicles • Corticospinal tract • Abducens nucleus	• Ipsilateral LMN facial paralysis • Contralateral UMN weakness • Ipsilateral sixth nerve palsy
Rostral basal pontine syndrome	• Trigeminal sensory and motor tract • Corticospinal tract	• Ipsilateral trigeminal sensory and motor signs • Contralateral UMN weakness
Pure motor hemiparesis	• Corticospinal tract	• Contralateral UMN weakness
Ataxic hemiparesis	• Corticospinal and corticopontocerebellar tracts	• Contralateral UMN weakness • Contralateral appendicular ataxia

Continued

Syndromes	Structures involved	Physical sign
Clumsy hand-dysarthria syndrome	• Junction of the upper third and lower two-thirds of the pons	• Ipsilateral UMN facial paralysis • Severe dysarthria • Dysphagia • Contralateral hand paresis and clumsiness
Locked-in syndrome	• Ventral half of the pons bilaterally involving all corticospinal tracts and corticobulbar tracts	• Paralysis of all motor activity • Aphonia • Preservation of vertical gaze and blinking
Crying and laughter	• Discrete lesion in basis pontis although precise location is unclear	• Sudden onset of involuntary crying and rarely laughter

Tegmental pontine syndromes

Syndromes	Structures involved	Physical sign
Medial tegmental syndrome	• Abducens nucleus and fascicles • Genu of the facial nerve • Medial lemniscus	• Ipsilateral sixth nerve palsy • Lateral gaze paralysis • Ipsilateral LMN facial paralysis • Contralateral loss of kinesthesia and discriminative touch
One-and-a-half syndrome	• MLF • Abducens nucleus (dorsal paramedian tegmentum)	• Ipsilateral lateral gaze paralysis • Internuclear ophthalmoplegia
Caudal tegmental pontine syndrome (Foville syndrome)	• Corticospinal tract • Paramedian pontine reticular formation (PPRF) • Abducens nucleus • Facial nucleus or fascicles	• Ipsilateral LMN facial paralysis • Ipsilateral conjugate gaze paralysis • Contralateral UMN weakness
Rostral tegmental pontine syndrome (Raymond-Cestan syndrome)	• Medial lemniscus • MLF • Spinothalamic tract • Corticospinal tract • Cerebellar fibers	• Internuclear ophthalmoplegia • Ipsilateral ataxia • Contralateral UMN weakness • Hemisensory loss
Extreme lateral tegmental pontine syndrome (Marie-Foix syndrome)	• Brachium pontis • Spinothalamic tract • Corticospinal tract	• Ipsilateral ataxia • Contralateral UMN weakness • May include: Horner syndrome, palatal myoclonus, and contralateral spinothalamic sensory loss

Lateral versus medial medullary syndrome

- Vascular lesions in the medulla are best suited to anatomico-clinical correlation.
- The medulla receives its blood supply from vertebral, anterior spinal, posterior spinal, and posterior inferior cerebellar arteries. The lateral medulla receives its blood supply from the vertebral artery, and a dorsally variable supply from the PICA, whereas the paramedian territory receives its blood supply from vertebral and anterior spinal arteries.
- There are other variants of medullary syndromes, in addition to lateral and medullary syndromes, although they rarely occur. These include dorsal medullary syndrome, and Babinski-Nageotte syndrome, which is a combined lateral and medial medullary syndrome.

Features	Lateral medullary syndrome (Wallenberg)	Medial medullary syndrome
1 Artery	• Vertebral artery • Medial branch of PICA (rare)	• Anterior spinal artery • Paramedian branches of vertebral artery
2 Frequency	The most common brainstem syndrome	Less common
3 Structures involved	• Spinal trigeminal nucleus • Spinothalamic tract • Nucleus ambiguus • Vestibular nuclei • Inferior cerebellar peduncle • Descending sympathetic tract	• Medial lemniscus • Pyramid • Hypoglossal nerve nucleus and rootlets
4 Clinical features	• Loss of pain and temperature in ipsilateral face and contralateral half of the body • Ipsilateral loss of gag reflex • Ipsilateral Horner syndrome • Hoarseness • Hiccups • Dysphagia • Dysarthria • Vertigo • Lateropulsion	• Contralateral UMN weakness • Contrateral loss of kinesthesia and discriminative touch • **Ipsilateral LMN tongue weakness**
5 Bilaterality	Not reported	May occur bilaterally, although rare

Specific differentials

- It is important to consider the use of illicit drugs as a cause of stroke, especially in the young.
- Various drugs can produce immediate and long-term effects on the vascular network that may predispose patients to stroke. In addition, patients who are drug users may have increased risk of blood-borne infections including infective endocarditis, syphilis, or HIV, which can also cause stroke.

Illicit drugs and stroke

1 **Cocaine**
   - Crack, the most popular form of cocaine, is inhaled or smoked and has a high power of addiction.
   - The mechanisms of cocaine-related stroke are multiple:
     - Cocaine-induced hemorrhagic stroke is associated with more than 50% of cases with AVM and aneurysms, secondary to severe hypertension.
     - Cocaine-induced vasoconstriction due to increased monoamine activity can result in ischemic stroke.
     - Vasospasm as a result of severe hypertension or SAH may cause ischemic stroke.
     - Cocaine-associated vasculitis: rare.
     - Cocaine-induced arrhythmias resulting in cardioembolic stroke.
2 **Amphetamine and psychostimulant drugs**
   - Amphetamine and psychostimulants can cause severe hypertension, AVM rupture, and vasculitis as possible mechanisms of stroke, and are more likely to cause intracranial hemorrhage rather than ischemic stroke. However, AVMs in amphetamine users are uncommon and amphetamine-induced vasculitis is often found only at autopsy.
3 Phenylpropanolamine (PPA)
   - PPA is a drug structurally related to amphetamine, although less potent. It can be found in over-the-counter medications including nasal decongestants, cough and cold remedies.
   - Potential stroke mechanisms include hypertension and vasculitis.
4 Phecyclidine (PCP) and lysergic acid diethylamide (LSD)
   - PCP can cause hypertension leading to hypertensive intracranial hemorrhage.
   - Lysergic acid diethylamide has been related to ischemic stroke with possible vasculitis.
5 Opiates and barbiturates
   - Heroin can cause intracranial hemorrhage and SAH as a result of mycotic aneurysm in the setting of infective endocarditis.

- Infectious endocarditis is usually the main cause of ischemic stroke in heroin addicts, with the most common pathogens being Staphylococcus aureus and Candida albicans.
- Heroin-induced vasculitis is another possible mechanism.

6 Alcohol
- The relationship between alcohol and stroke is not clear. Light to moderate alcohol intake decreases low-density lipoprotein, cholesterol, and high-density lipoprotein, whereas heavy alcohol consumption increases triglyceride and blood pressure.
- It seems that heavy alcohol intake may have significant impact on stroke risks. Moderate alcohol consumption may decrease the risk of cerebral infarction, but the stroke risk is higher in heavy drinkers than in abstainers. Acute intoxication is related to an increased risk of both ischemic and hemorrhagic strokes.

Perioperative stroke

- The risk of stroke during the perioperative period may increase, especially in certain types of surgery, for example cardiac surgery.
- The possible mechanism for perioperative stroke may be related to the type of surgery, hemodynamic instability during surgery causing low-flow state, additional trauma to blood vessels, complications from anesthesia, or patients' underlying comorbid conditions, etc.

1 **Cardiac surgery**
- Cardiac surgery is complicated by stroke in about 2% of cases, the risk being greater for valvular rather than coronary artery bypass surgery.
- A more diffuse neurological syndrome, postoperative confusion, soft neurological signs, and neuropsychological impairments, is much more common than a focal stroke, but it usually resolves in days or weeks.
- Possible mechanisms for these complications include embolization during surgery, embolus after surgery from thrombus on suture lines, prosthetic materials, complicating MI, arrhythmias, cholesterol embolization syndrome, etc.

2 Instrumentation of the coronary arteries and aorta
- These procedures may result in dislodging valvular or atheromatous debris or thrombus causing cerebral ischemia. Thrombus may also form on an intra-arterial catheter tip.

3 Neurosurgery
- Depending upon the area of neurosurgical intervention, both hemorrhagic and ischemic complications can occur.

- Carotid endarterectomy may result in distal infarction due to hypoperfusion or by embolism of dislodged atheromatous debris.
4 General surgery
  - General surgery is less frequently complicated by stroke than cardiac surgery.
  - There are numerous mechanisms, for example, postoperative hypotension, hemostatic defect, positional trauma, dissection, complications related to anesthesia, etc.
  - Stroke may have happened anyway, particularly in elderly patients with multiple vascular risk factors undergoing surgery.

Chapter 4
Paroxysmal Disorders

Seizures and epilepsy

International classification of epileptic seizures

I Partial seizures

  A Simple partial seizures

    1 With motor signs

    2 With somatosensory or special sensory symptoms

    3 With autonomic symptoms or signs

    4 With psychic symptoms

  B Complex partial seizures

    1 Simple partial onset followed by impairment of consciousness

    2 With impairment of consciousness at onset

  C Partial seizures evolving to secondarily generalized seizures

    1 Simple partial seizures evolving to generalized seizures

    2 Complex partial seizures evolving to generalized seizures

    3 Simple partial seizures evolving to complex partial seizures evolving to generalized seizures

II Generalized seizures (convulsive or non-convulsive)

  A Absence seizures

    1 Typical absences

    2 Atypical absences

  B Myoclonic seizures

  C Clonic seizures

  D Tonic seizures

  E Tonic-clonic seizures

  F Atonic seizures (astatic seizures)

III Unclassified epileptic seizures

International classification of epilepsy syndromes

I Localization-related epilepsies and syndromes

  A Idiopathic, with age-related onset

    1 Benign childhood epilepsy with centrotemporal spikes

    2 Childhood epilepsy with occipital paroxysms

  B Symptomatic: related to area of onset and clinical and EEG features

II Generalized epilepsies and syndromes

  A Idiopathic, with age-related onset

    1 Benign neonatal familial convulsions

    2 Benign neonatal convulsions

    3 Benign myoclonic epilepsy in infancy

    4 Childhood absence epilepsy

    5 Juvenile absence epilepsy

    6 Juvenile myoclonic epilepsy

    7 Epilepsy with generalized tonic-clonic seizures on awakening

  B Cryptogenic and/or symptomatic epilepsy syndromes

    1 West syndrome (infantile spasms)

    2 Lennox-Gastaut syndrome

    3 Epilepsy with myoclonic-astatic seizures

    4 Epilepsy with myoclonic absences

  C Symptomatic-epileptic seizures as the presenting or dominant feature

III Epilepsies and syndromes undetermined as to whether they are focal or generalized

  A Both generalized and focal seizures

    1 Neonatal seizures

    2 Severe myoclonic epilepsy in infancy

    3 Epilepsy with continuous-spike waves during slow-wave sleep

    4 Acquired epileptic aphasia (Landau-Kleffner syndrome)

  B Without unequivocal generalized or focal features

IV Special syndromes

  A Situation-created seizures

    1 Febrile convulsions

    2 Seizures related to identifiable situations

  B Isolated, apparently unprovoked epileptic events

  C Epilepsies with specific modes of seizure precipitation

  D Chronic, progressive epilepsia partialis continua of childhood

Signs and symptoms suggestive of a seizure

- Although there are no 'hard and fast' rules, many signs and symptoms should lead the examiner to strongly consider seizure versus syncope, migraine, TIA, etc.
- A careful history is the most critical aspect of evaluating a seizure and should include an accurate description of the event (preferably including witnesses), characteristics at onset, temporal progression, and post-event state.
- Below are features that are consistent with a seizure.

1 **Drowsiness and confusion following the event**
2 **Stereotypical motor activity**
3 **Loss of memory for the event**
4 **Physical trauma, especially oral lacerations**
5 **Bladder or bowel incontinence**
6 Muscle aches and pains
7 Distortions in sensations including olfactory, gustatory, auditory, visual, and tactile

8 Positive family history
9 History of head trauma or other CNS pathology including meningitis, encephalitis, and stroke

Common causes of status epilepticus

- Defined as a state of continuous epileptic activity greater than 5 minutes or with a frequency that prevents neurological return to baseline interictally.
- In most cases, patients should be monitored on continuous EEG telemetry in an ICU setting until stabilized.
- May be convulsive or non-convulsive.
- Convulsive status epilepticus is a medical emergency.
- Non-convulsive status epilepticus may be absence or complex partial.

1 **Anti-epileptic drug non-compliance or withdrawal (most common in emergency department: 20% of children and 20% of adults with status epilepticus)**
   - Check serum levels of prescribed anticonvulsants.
   - Review compliance history, medication quantity, or refill history with reliable friends and family or pharmacy (especially useful for newer AEDs where serum levels may not be commonly available).
2 **Fever, systemic infection** (**35% of children**, rare in adults)
   - If no source, or in infants, consider work-up for CNS infection (see below).
3 *Stroke* (rare in children, **25% of adults**)
   - Associated with risk factors such as hypertension, smoking, vascular disease.
   - History of acute focal neurologic deficit(s).
   - Neuroimaging work-up – MRI with DWI if available.
4 *Metabolic abnormalities* (10% of children and adults)
   - Assess chemistry panel with particular attention to sodium, calcium, and glucose.
   - Common in ICU and critically ill patients.
   - Common in patients with large volume shifts.
5 *Meningitis, encephalitis* (5% of children, 10% of adults)
   - History of antecedent coryza or febrile illness. Check for stiff neck.
   - Higher suspicion in immunocompromised patients.
   - Evaluate with lumbar puncture and neuroimaging, do not delay antibiotic treatment when suspicion is high.
6 *Hypoxia* (5% of children, 10% of adults)
7 *Alcohol withdrawal* (rare in children, **15% of adults**)
   - Review social history.
   - Check blood alcohol level.
8 Congenital (10% of children, rare in adults)

- Due to cerebral dysgenesis, cortical dysplasia, heterotopias, or known congenital syndromes.
- Neuroimaging work-up – MRI more sensitive.
9 *Traumatic brain injury* (3.5% of children, 5% of adults)
   - Children suffering nonaccidental trauma may present with seizures and altered mental status but parents offer no history of head injury.
   - Neuroimaging work-up – CT scan is sufficient acutely.
10 *Brain tumors* (rare in children, 5% of adults)
   - Review history, especially gradual onset of focal neurologic deficit.
   - Neuroimaging work-up – use contrast enhancement.
11 *Intracranial hemorrhage*
   - As in stroke.
   - Neuroimaging work-up – CT is sufficient acutely.
12 Undetermined etiology – fairly rare.

Work-up of new onset seizure

- Classification of seizures include epilepsy (recurrent seizures), isolated (single), febrile convulsions, and acute symptomatic.
- Epilepsy is typically divided between primary (idiopathic) and secondary (with a presumed cause).
- There are many different causes of seizures, many of which do not imply epilepsy.
- Lifetime incidence of seizures in the general population is approximately 1%.
- Important clues to etiology can be gleaned by considering the patient's age (see seizures as a function of age).

Common causes of symptomatic and single seizures	
1 Alcohol/drug withdrawal	~21%
2 Cerebrovascular disease	~15%
3 Trauma	~15%
4 *Neoplastic disease*	~14%
5 *Infection*	~10%
6 Metabolic	~8%
7 *Eclampsia*	~6%
8 Toxic causes	~3%

Work-up of new onset seizure:
1 Detailed history and physical. Particular attention should be given to possible secondary causes, especially as related to the list above. The semiology of the seizure event can give valuable clues. It is important, when possible, to interview

persons whom actually witnessed the event. Family history can also yield critical information. Careful exam should focus on any focal neurologic signs.

2 Electroencephalogram. Initially, a routine sleep/wake EEG should be ordered. It is common to observe a 'normal' recording over 30 minutes even in patients with known seizure disorders. Therefore, a routine interictal EEG may not demonstrate epileptiform activity and should not be interpreted as definitive in ruling out seizures. Sensitivity can be increased by: repeat exams, records obtained within 24 hours of an ictal event, or prolonged monitoring such as continuous telemetry.

3 Neuroimaging. MRI is the modality of choice and should include gadolinium contrast to assess infectious or neoplastic processes. A CT scan with and without contrast is acceptable only when MRI is not available or contraindicated.

Risk factors for recurrent seizures

- The decision to initiate anti-epileptic medication following a single seizure should take into account the likelihood of recurrence.
- Lifetime incidence of a single seizure in the general population is approximately 10%. This does not necessarily imply epilepsy requiring lifelong treatment.
- Good candidates for discontinuation of previously initiated anti-epileptic medical treatment include: seizures easily controlled with monotherapy, prior two-year seizure-free period, idiopathic seizure, normal EEG (2×), seizure onset in childhood, and normal neurological exam.
- The following list are features that should be considered risk factors for recurrent seizure.

1 EEG demonstrating epileptiform discharges
2 Abnormal neurological exam findings
3 History of neurological deficit from birth such as mental retardation or cerebral palsy
4 Age less than 16 years old
5 Seizure occurring during sleep
6 Status epilepticus or multiple seizures within 24 hours as the initial presentation
7 Partial seizures
8 Todd paralysis

Differential diagnosis of recurrent seizures

- Seizure recurrence should be divided into patients with a previous diagnosis who are currently treated and those individuals with a single previous seizure who are currently not treated.

- In patients with a single previous seizure, strong consideration should be given to initiating treatment, taking into account presumed etiology and risks for recurrent seizure (see recurrent risk document)
- Multiple physiologic, metabolic, and psychosocial factors may reduce seizure threshold in previously well-controlled patients

The following should be considered in evaluating recurrent seizures:
1 **Inadequate serum drug levels and patient compliance**
   - Check serum levels and also check for appropriate dose.
2 **Addition of other medications which may adversely influence anti-epileptic drug metabolism**
3 Ongoing infection
   - In patients with prior neurosurgical intervention, *CNS infection* must be ruled out.
   - Otherwise, CNS infection is fairly rare.
   - Epileptic patients with systemic infection/fever, may be more prone to break-through seizures at times of illness.
4 *Metabolic and/or electrolyte disturbances*
   - Hyponatremia, especially in patients on carbamazepine.
   - Hypocalcemia.
   - Hypoglycemia, especially in diabetics.
5 *Progression of previously documented disease, especially neoplastic processes*
6 *Alcohol or drug ingestion or withdrawal*
7 Heightened stress or anxiety
8 Sleep deprivation

Differential diagnosis of staring spells

- Characterized by fixed gaze of variable duration.
- Most commonly seen in the pediatric population.
- Usually benign in nature, though important to rule out seizure activity with careful history-taking and appropriate diagnostic testing.

1 **Daydreaming**
   - May be overcome by loud or startling noises.
   - No post-event confusion or lethargy.
   - Not associated with automatisms.
2 **Inattention**
   - As above.

3 **Hearing loss**
   - Concerning if staring cannot be interrupted by a variety of different sound sources.
   - Associated with developmental delay, especially concerning language.
   - Should be assessed with formal audiology.
   - Early identification and treatment is crucial, as loss of developmental milestones in language cannot typically be completely regained.
4 Absence seizure
   - Duration of seconds.
   - Automatisms are common.
   - Frequently associated with 3 Hz spike and wave on EEG.
5 Complex partial seizure
   - Duration seconds to minutes.
   - Automatisms are common.
   - Typically preceded by aura.
   - Post-ictal confusion and fatigue are common.

Differentiating absence from complex partial seizures

- These two seizure types do share some clinical overlap. However, the distinction is usually not difficult to make given adequate history-taking.
- Differentiating between these two seizure types is important, as their treatment, response to therapy, and prognosis is much different.

Clinical feature	Absence seizure	Complex partial seizure
Aura	None	Typically well-defined
Duration	Seconds	Seconds to minutes
Post-ictal state	Rare	Common
Automatisms	Common	Common
Age of onset	Usually childhood	Usually teens to early adult
Provoked by hyperventilation	Common	Uncommon
Interictal EEG	Generalized 3 Hz spike and wave	Normal or with focal spikes, sharp waves, or slowing

Episodic loss of consciousness

- Temporary loss of consciousness may be caused by a variety of neurological, medical, psychiatric, and non-medical etiologies.
- In most cases, clues to the proper diagnosis may be obtained by a careful history of the patient and observers.
- Utilizing history as a guide, work-up may include tests for metabolic derangements, cardiac function, and seizures.

1 **Syncope**
   - Work-up: ECG, careful cardiac exam, pulse, and blood pressure (lying, seated, standing), consider Holter monitor, echocardiogram.
   1.1 **Cardiac syncope**
      - Usually older patients, may occur with palpitations, chest pain.
      - Not necessarily postural, prodromal symptoms variable.
      1.1.1 *Ventricular tachycardia*
      1.1.2 *Bradyarrhythmias: sick sinus syndrome, bradyarrthmia, heart block, long QT syndrome*
      1.1.3 *Supraventricular tachycardia*
      1.1.4 *Outflow obstruction: aortic stenosis*
      1.1.5 *Reduced cardiac output: cardiomyopathy, myocardial infarction, cardiac tamponade*
   1.2 **Neurocardiogenic syncope**
      - History is very important; occurs in response to particular stimuli (see below).
      - Bradycardia during episode.
      1.2.1 **Vasovagal syncope**
         - Most common in adolescents and young adults.
         - Associated with heightened emotional state, prolonged fasting, prolonged standing, hot overcrowded areas, fatigue.
         - May occur with prodromal pallor, diaphoresis.
      1.2.2 **Reflex syncope:** cough, micturition, Valsalva, etc.
      1.2.3 Carotid sinus syncope: usually due to carotid atherosclerosis in older persons.
      1.2.4 Associated with trigeminal or glossopharyngeal neuralgia.
   1.3 Peripheral causes of syncope
      - May occur with prodromal pallor, diaphoresis.
      - Very often postural.
      - More common in older patients.
      1.3.1 Reduced vasomotor tone
         1.3.1.1 **Following prolonged recumbency or sitting**
         1.3.1.2 **Peripheral (autonomic) neuropathy**
            1.3.1.2.1 Diabetic neuropathy
            1.3.1.2.2 Amyloid neuropathy
            1.3.1.2.3 Shy-Drager: associated with Parkinsonism
         1.3.1.3 Medication-induced: L-dopa, antihypertensives, antidepressants, etc.
         1.3.1.4 Following sympathectomy.
         1.3.1.5 Following spinal cord injury.
      1.3.2 Hypovolemia
         1.3.2.1 Dehydration

          1.3.2.2 Medication-induced: diuretics

          1.3.2.3 *Blood loss*

          1.3.2.4 *Addison disease*

2 **Metabolic**

    2.1 **Hypoglycemia**

- Always check glucose, review medications (especially in diabetics), and assess for adequate PO intake.
- Commonly causes 'faintness', less often actual loss of unconsciousness.

    2.2 *Hypoxia*: assess oxygen saturation with pulse oximetry and arterial blood gas, exclude acute stroke and central venous thrombosis as etiology for global hypoxia, review gradient mismatch to evaluate perfusion vs. diffusion abnormalities.

    2.3 Hyperventilation-induced alkalosis: assess with arterial blood gases.

    2.4 Anemia

3 *Epileptic seizure*: refer to epilepsy differentials

- Work-up: careful history of event (particularly from witnesses); presence of risk factors (prior CNS infection or head trauma, prior seizure, family history), EEG, neuroimaging.

    3.1 Absence seizure

    3.2 Complex partial seizure.

    3.3 Post-ictal from an unwitnessed tonic-clonic seizure.

    3.4 Atonic or tonic seizure: associated with mental retardation, intractable seizures.

    3.5 Myoclonic seizure: may fall to ground; consciousness usually preserved.

4 *Elevated intracranial pressure*: rare cause of episodic symptoms

- Work-up: neuroimaging, look for papilledema.
- Associated with severe positional headaches.
- May experience drop attacks: sudden falls without loss of consciousness.

    4.1 *Third ventricle colloid cyst*

    4.2 *Aqueductal stenosis*

5 *Transient ischemic attack: vertebrobasilar insufficiency*

- Uncommon cause of isolated episodic loss of consciousness.
- May be associated with transient brainstem symptoms.

6 Confusional migraine: more often in younger persons; associated with confusion and headache

7 Breath-holding spell: common in children; history of precipitating event

8 Psychiatric

    8.1 Hysterical fainting

    8.2 Panic attack

- Symptoms include palpitations, chest pain, shortness of breath, fear.
- No consistent postural component.
- Presyncope is common, syncope rare. However, may lead to hyperventilation-induced syncope, above.

8.3 Pseudoseizure

- Most pseudoseizures occur in patients with true epileptic seizures also.
- Clinical characteristics that raise suspicion (but are NOT pathogno-monic) for pseudoseizures include alternating or asynchronous motor activity, pelvic thrusting, thrashing, prolonged motor episodes with apparently preserved consciousness, no post-ictal state following a pro-longed episode, lack of stereotypy, occurrence only in the presence of others, and precipitation by emotional factors.
- They are generally not associated with self-injury, severe falls, tongue-biting, or incontinence.
- Video-EEG telemetry is necessary in many cases to definitively diagnose.

Differentiating seizure from syncope

- Differentiating seizure from syncope is typically not difficult provided accurate descriptions of the 'spells' themselves. This is, however, an important distinction as the treatments are markedly different.
- Obtaining a description of the event from an eyewitness often provides the critical clues to allow differentiating these two phenomena.
- In some series, up to 50% of all syncopal episodes are cardiac in origin. Delaying the diagnosis may prevent appropriate cardiac care for the patient.

Clinical observation	Seizure	Syncope
Convulsions	Common	Rare
Injury	Common	Rare
Post-event confusion	Common	Rare
Urinary incontinence	Common	Rare
Tongue biting	Common	Rare
Duration of aura	Short	Usually longer
Aura	Somatosensory, visceral, psychic	Light-headed, dimmed vision, heart palpitations
Relationship to posture	No	Common

Metabolic etiologies of seizures

- Seizures arise as a common neurological complication of underlying metabolic disease.
- Suspicion should be particularly high in the ICU setting where seizures occur in as many as 1/3 of patients.
- Organ failure, especially renal, hepatic, cardiac, and pulmonary, are frequent causes of metabolic seizures.

- Initial work-up for metabolic derangements should include electrolyte disturbances, uremia, hyperammonemia, and hypoxia. Drug use should be excluded, especially cocaine and amphetamines, as well as alcohol withdrawal.
- Seizures may be generalized tonic-clonic, complex partial, or less commonly, simple motor in nature.

1 **Hypoglycemia**
  - Always assess glucose levels in the setting of a seizure, review medications, and evaluate for underlying diabetes.
2 **Hyponatremia**
  - Renal etiologies: diuretics, renal tubular acidosis, partial obstruction, salt wasting nephritis, SIADH.
  - Non-renal losses: adrenal insufficiency, water intoxication, hypothyroidism, gastrointestinal (hyperemesis, diarrhea).
3 Hypocalcemia
  - Remember to correct for low serum albumin.
  - Check circulating parathyroid hormone.
  - Common causes include:
    3.1 Hyperphosphatemia (renal failure, rhabdomyolysis)
    3.2 Hypovitaminosis D
    3.3 Pseudohypoparathyroidism
    3.4 Drugs/toxins: dilantin, phenobarbitol, citrated blood transfusions, protamine, colchicine, cis-platinum, gentamycin
4 Hypomagnesemia
  - Decreased intake: protein malnutrition, prolonged IV therapy.
  - Decreased absorption: sprue, short gut syndrome.
  - Excessive losses (body fluids): gastric suctioning, intestinal/biliary fistula, purgatives, colitis.
  - Excessive losses (urinary): diuretics, renal failure, chronic alcoholism, primary aldosterism, hypercalcemia, hyperthyroidism, renal tubular acidosis, resolving diabetic ketoacidosis.
  - Other: iatrogenic, pancreatitis, porphyria.
5 **Hepatic failure**: assess ALT, AST, alkaline phosphatase and INR (PT)
6 **Renal failure, uremia**: can result in electrolyte perturbations as well as uremia
7 Anoxia/hypoxia: stroke, near-drowning, cardiopulmonary collapse, carbon monoxide poisoning
8 **Drug/toxin-induced**
    8.1 Cocaine
    8.2 Amphetamine
    8.3 Alcohol-related

     8.4 Heavy metals: rare
9 Medication-induced: penicillins, cyclosporin, FK506; rarely carbamazepine, thorazine, haloperidol
10 Nonketotic hyperglycemia
11 Inborn errors of metabolism
     11.1 Porphyria: psychosis, constipation
     11.2 Pyridoxine deficiency
12 Thyroid storm: assess TSH, T3, free T4

Differentiating seizure from pseudoseizure

- The only reliable way to differentiate between an epileptic seizure and a pseudoseizure is with video/EEG telemetry during an actual event.
- Some general principles, though not without exception, are listed below.

Clinical symptom	Epileptic seizure	Psuedoseizure
Onset	Abrupt	Gradual
Duration	Self-limited and typically <3 minutes	Prolonged
Semiology	Usually stereotypic	Thrashing, head-banging, rolling side-to-side, pelvic thrusting
Course	Starts and ends with minimal fluctuation	Motor activity starts and stops repeatedly
Rhythmicity	Rhythmic and in-phase	Out-of-phase, arrhythmic, intermittent
Consciousness	Impaired with bilateral motor activity	Preserved with bilateral motor activity
Verbalization	Impaired with bilateral motor activity	Preserved with bilateral motor activity
Post-ictal confusion	Usually present	Usually absent
Suggestibility	Absent	Frequently present

Headaches

Approach to headache work-up

Essential elements of a headache work-up

- Benign headache syndromes are common and cause significant morbidity in the population.

- Work-up for headache consists primarily of thorough history-taking and a comprehensive neurological and physical exam. The goal is to rule out potentially serious etiologies and arrive at an accurate diagnosis for effective treatment.

Important elements of the history include:
1 Location of pain including migrating and/or radiating nature.
2 Description of the pain character (sharp, dull, throbbing, lancinating).
3 Duration of pain including onset, temporal nature, and seasonal/diurnal variations.
4 Severity of pain (frequently assessed on a scale from 1–10, though it is important to know whether it prevents work, normal activities, etc.).
5 Concurrent and recent medications, including the use patterns of over-the-counter analgesics.
6 Family history (migraine, seizures, psychiatric).
7 Associated symptoms or activities.
8 Precipitating, alleviating, and exacerbating features.
9 Past medical history.

Examination should consist of:
1 Complete neurological exam.
2 Blood pressure, temperature, and pulse rate.
3 Point tenderness, especially involving the temporal arteries, scalp, sinuses, musculature of the scalp, neck, and shoulders.
4 Evaluation for papilledema, retinal hemorrhage, optic disc sharpness, and retinal venous pulsations.
5 Detection of sensory asymmetry of the scalp.

Strong indications for imaging in headache

- Neuroimaging is not always necessary in the evaluation of headache.
- Neuroimaging has a low yield in patients with migraine headaches and a normal neurological examination.
- Neuroimaging has a low yield in chronic tension-type headache and normal neurological examination.
- In general, focality, new onset, or significant exacerbation of a previous headache pattern warrant neuroimaging.

1 Chronic or severe headache with onset after age 50 years (CT scan with/without contrast).
2 Sudden onset, especially when described as 'thunderclap' or 'worst headache of my life' (CT scan without contrast).
3 Accelerating pattern of intensity, severity, or chronicity of previously mild headache (CT scan with/without contrast).
4 New headache in patient with previous diagnosis of HIV or cancer (MRI with/without contrast).
5 Any headache which is concomitant with any focal neurological symptoms (MRI with/without contrast).
6 Persistent headache with failed management (CT with/without contrast).
7 Chronic headache with suspected sinusitis (CT scan).
8 Sudden onset of severe unilateral headache with suspected carotid or vertebral dissection and/or ipsilateral Horner syndrome (MRI/MRA).
9 New headache in patient older than 60 years. Sedimentation rate greater than 50 especially with temporal tenderness (MRI/MRA).

Acute headache (usually emergency or urgent care presentation)

- One of the most common complaints encountered by neurologists. However, there are only a few pathologies underlying headache that represent serious disease.
- Headaches may be primary or secondary.
  - Primary headaches have pain as the principle manifestation without known underlying disease.
  - Secondary headaches cause pain as a manifestation of an underlying disease process (hemorrhage, tumor, etc.).
- Some primary headache disorders, for example, migraine, are both acute (isolated exacerbations), and chronic (overall condition). However, it remains clinically useful to categorize headaches as acute versus chronic for the purpose of a diagnostic work-up and treatment plan.
- Patient descriptors such as 'worst', 'first', 'persistent', and 'different' may imply secondary headache and warrant immediate investigation, irrespective of chronicity.
- Evaluation should include onset, duration, severity, character, family and patient history, location, radiation, and associated symptoms such as visual disturbances, nausea, and emesis. Important clues may also lie in precipitating, exacerbating, and alleviating features, and diurnal/seasonal variations.

1 **Migraine headache**
  - Occurs in as many as 20% of females and 8% of males in the general population.
  - Either with aura (classic), neurological signs (complicated), or neither (common).
  - Clinical characteristics include nausea, vomiting, photophobia, phonophobia in conjunction with throbbing head pain that is uni- or bilateral. Precipitants include certain foods, odors, alcohol, hunger, and sleep deprivation.
  - Treatment is two-pronged: abortive therapy for acute attacks, and prophylactic therapy to prevent frequent attacks.
    - Triptans are the mainstay of abortive therapy. Other effective abortive treatments include ergotamines, midrin, intranasal lidocaine, oxygen, and opiates.
    - Prophylactic medications include tricyclic antidepressants, beta blockers, calcium channel blockers, or anticonvulsants such as valproic acid, topamax, carbamazepine, and gabapentin.

2 **Tension-type headache**
  - May include both episodic (acute) and chronic forms.
  - Typically bilateral with a non-throbbing character, usually worse as the day progresses and often exacerbated by psychosocial factors. Pain usually not exacerbated by Valsalva maneuver.
  - Treatment includes avoidance of precipitating etiologies, relaxation techniques, cranial/cervical massage, and over-the-counter NSAIDS.

3 **Sinus headache**
  - Frontal or maxillary pressure-like pain, uni- or bilateral in nature and associated with nasal congestion or rhinnorhea. Allergic persons have seasonal symptoms.
  - Percussion over the sinuses usually elicits tenderness.
  - CT imaging is indicated for confirmation.
  - Treatment: combination of analgesics, decongestants, and antibiotics.

4 *Subarachnoid hemorrhage*
  - Sudden onset, severe pancranial pain, and a complaint of the 'worst headache of my life'. May be accompanied by syncope, nausea, emesis, altered mental status, seizures, and focal neurologic signs.
  - Typical cause is aneurysmal or small vessel rupture in the hypertensive patient.
  - *Immediate diagnosis is imperative, and should be regarded as an emergency.*
  - Work-up is head CT scan. Even if negative, but clinical suspicion is high, a lumbar puncture (LP) should be performed. The presence of red cells out of proportion to white cells (>750:1) is highly suspicious.
  - If any of the above tests are suggestive of a subarachnoid hemorrhage, immediate neurosurgical consultation is indicated.

5 *Meningitis/encephalitis*
  - Usually subacute onset, associated fever, alteration in mental status, nausea, vomiting, stiff neck. Seizures can occur, particularly with encephalitis.

- Work-up must include an LP. Head CT scan is necessary if there is evidence of focal abnormality or elevated intracranial pressure.
- Positive CSF may show:
  - Elevated WBCs (mostly PMNs), few RBCs, low glucose, and elevated protein suggest bacterial meningitis.
  - Modestly elevated WBCs (mostly lymphs), many RBCs, variable glucose, and protein suggest HSV encephalitis.
  - Modestly elevated WBCs (mostly lymphs), few RBCs, normal glucose and protein are consistent with a picture of aseptic meningitis. This is usually a self-limited viral infection.
  - Extremely elevated WBCs (including blasts) and elevated protein is rare, but can be the presenting sign of acute leukemic meningitis.
- Antibiotics and antivirals should be administered immediately and not delayed while work-up is initiated.

6 *Temporal arteritis*
- Age is almost always >55 years. Pain is unilateral, localizes to the temporal area, and jaw claudication can occur.
- Physical exam frequently reveals tenderness at the temple, pulsations of the artery, and a tortuous arterial course.
- Work-up includes erythrocyte sedimentation rate. Temporal artery biopsy confirms diagnosis, but should not delay treatment in suspicious cases.
- Treatment with steroids. Due to potential involvement of the ophthalmic artery, failure to adequately treat may result in blindness.

7 *Other vascular headache*
  7.1 *Hypertensive headache*
  - Typically occurs in the setting of markedly elevated blood pressure (SBP > 220 mmHg) of acute onset. Altered mental status may occur.
  - Seen with certain drug ingestion or pheochromocytoma.
  - Parieto-occipital changes seen in CT imaging.
  7.2 *Arterial dissection*
  - Associated with neck pain. Carotid dissection may cause Horner syndrome.
  - Ischemic complications such as transient ischemic attacks and cerebral infarction may occur.
  7.3 *Sinus thrombosis*
  - Associated with encephalopathy, seizures.
  - May occur in pregnancy, hypercoagulable states, pericranial infections/mastoiditis, dehydration (particularly in children).
  7.4 *Other intracranial hemorrhage or ischemia*: intracerebral hemorrhage, subdural hemorrhage, cerebral infarction; usually with associated focal neurological signs.

     7.5 *Arteriovenous malformation*: focal deficits, seizures.

     7.6 Other vasculitides.

8 Post-traumatic/post-concussive headache
   - Most common symptom following closed head injury. May persist for days or weeks.
   - Can be associated with nausea, dizziness, impaired memory, inattention, cognitive slowing, visual complaints, sleep disturbance, irritability and is termed post-concussive syndrome.
   - Persistent/worsening symptoms, focal abnormalities, altered mental status, and seizures should prompt neuroimaging work-up, although intracranial pathology after mild head injury is very rare.

9 Cluster headache
   - More common among men than women. Typically has a cyclical, temporal nature, either seasonal or monthly (hence, it 'clusters').
   - Severe, abrupt on- and offset hemicranial/temple/retro-orbital pain lasting from 20 minutes to 2 hours, associated with autonomic features such as lacrimation, rhinnorhea, and conjunctival hyperemia.
   - Treatments include prophylaxis with verapamil, or abortive therapy with NSAIDS, triptans, ergotamines, intranasal lidocaine, or oxygen.

10 Situational headaches: cough, exertional, coital
   - Male-predominant, benign headache syndromes.
   - Transient severe headaches are provoked by coughing, exertion, sneezing, or even coitus. Subarachnoid hemorrhage is the main dangerous possibility in the differential diagnosis. Effort migraine may mimic exertional headaches.
   - Cough and exertional headache can be associated with Chiari malformation.
   - These headaches can be remarkably responsive to indomethacin.

11 Paroxysmal hemicrania
   - Nearly indistinguishable from cluster, except that they are more frequent (10–30/day) and typically of shorter duration (10–30 minutes).
   - Often without autonomic features found in cluster headache.
   - They are usually responsive to treatment with indomethacin.

12 Headache associated with neuralgia
   - Usually occur in the adult population.
   - Includes:
     - Trigeminal neuralgia (tic douloureux): unilateral, severe, lancinating pain in the distribution of cranial nerve V (usually V_2 or V_3).
     - Occipital neuralgia with similar symptoms in the occipital nerve distribution.
     - Glossopharyngeal neuralgia: pain in the auditory canal and tonsillar bed.
   - May be precipitated by minimal stimulation or dental malocclusion, and is not associated with sensory or motor deficits.

- Treatment includes anticonvulsants such as carbamazepine, phenytoin, gabapentin, and topamax. Refractory cases may require surgical referral.

13 *Brain tumor*: a rare cause of acute headache (see details under Chronic headache)
- Tumor headache can present acutely with *intratumoral hemorrhage, rupture of necrotic contents* into CSF spaces, or *positional obstruction* of CSF flow.
- Focal neurological deficits may be present; seizures can occur.
  - 13.1 *Colloid cyst*: not technically a neoplasm, but presents with severe positional headache and has been associated with sudden death, presumably due to ball-valve obstruction of CSF flow.

14 Post-lumbar puncture headache
- Postural headache worse when upright, due to persistent CSF leak.
- Treatment includes analgesics, caffeine, and occasionally, spinal blood patch.

15 Acute headaches associated with underlying medical conditions:
  - 15.1 Fever
  - 15.2 Carbon monoxide exposure
  - 15.3 Medication-induced
    - 15.3.1 Associated with high doses of anticonvulsants, beta-agonists, nitrates.
    - 15.3.2 Aseptic meningitis: intravenous immune globulin (IVIg).
    - 15.3.3 Analgesic rebound: see Chronic headache, below.
  - 15.4 Acute anemia
  - 15.5 Phenochromocytoma: associated with paroxysmal hypertension; very rare.

Chronic headache (usually clinic presentation)

- It is important to distinguish the time course of chronic headaches, as time course suggests different diagnoses.
  - Chronic recurrent: migraine, episodic tension headache, cluster
  - Chronic continuous or fluctuating: chronic tension-type headache, chronic daily headache, pseudotumor cerebri, sinusitis, TMJ, vasculitis
  - Chronic progressive: tumor, pseudotumor cerebri, subdural hematoma, AVM
- Worrisome features of chronic headaches include nocturnal awakening, focal neurological signs, seizures, persistent unilateral location, and progressive worsening in severity.
- Neuroimaging yield is low for chronic, unchanged headaches with a non-focal neurological exam.

Chronic recurrent headaches
- Characterized by pain-free periods punctuated by episodes of head pain.

1 **Migraine**
2 **Recurrent episodic tension-type headaches**
  A At least 10 previous headache episodes fulfilling criteria B and D listed below. Number of days with headache is <180/year or <15/month.
  B Headache lasting from 30 minutes to 7 days.
  C At least two of the following pain characteristics.
    i Pressing/tightening (nonpulsating) quality
    ii Mild or moderate intensity (may inhibit but not prohibit normal activity)
    iii Bilateral location
    iv No aggravation through climbing stairs or routine physical activity
  D Both of the following:
    i No nausea or emesis (anorexia may still occur)
    ii Photophobia and phonophobia are absent, or one but not both is present
  E At least one of the following:
    i History, physical, and neurologic exam do not suggest an alternative disorder
    ii History, physical, and neurologic exam do suggest an alternative disorder but it has been ruled out by the appropriate investigations
    iii An alternative disorder is present, but tension-type headache attacks do not occur for the first time in close temporal relation to the disorder
3 Cluster headaches
4 Situational headaches: exertional, cough, coital
5 Paroxysmal hemicrania
6 Headache associated with neuralgia
7 *Colloid cyst*: see Acute headache, above; danger due to intermittent ventricular obstruction.
8 Post-ictal headaches: not uncommon following a seizure in patients with epilepsy.
9 Pheochromocytoma: headache associated with paroxysmal hypertension, very rare.

Chronic constant, fluctuating, or progressive headaches
- Characterized by frequent or daily headache that is continuous, waxes and wanes or, more ominously, slowly progressive.

1 **Chronic tension-type headache (CTTH)**
  A Average headache frequency >15 days/month for more than 6 months and fulfilling criteria B and D.
  B At least two of the following pain characteristics:
    i Pressing/tightening quality
    ii Mild or moderate severity (may inhibit but not prevent activity)
    iii Bilateral location

    iv No aggravation caused by routine physical activity

  C Both of the following:

    i   No emesis

    ii No more than one of the following: nausea, photophobia, phonophobia

  D No evidence of underlying disease.

2 **Chronic (transformed) migraine (CM)**

  A Daily or almost daily (>15 days/month) head pain for >1 month.

  B Average headache duration >4 hours/day (if untreated).

  C At least one of the following:

    i   History of episodic migraine

    ii History of increasing headache frequency with decreasing severity of migrainous features over at least three months

    iii Headache at some time meets IHS criteria for migraine

  D Does not meet criteria for daily persistent headache or hemicrania continua.

  E No evidence for underlying disease.

3 Chronic daily headache (see Chronic daily headache, pp. 171–2).

4 *Vascular headaches*:

    4.1 *Chronic subdural hematoma*

    4.2 *Temporal arteritis*

    4.3 Other vasculitides

5 *Intracranial* and pericranial *infection*

    5.1 *Chronic meningitis*: usually associated with altered mentation, dementia, low grade fever.

    5.2 *Brain abscess*: focal neurological signs, seizures, fever.

    5.3 Sinusitis

    5.4 Dental abscess: pain referred to jaw, can cause throbbing headache.

6 Hemicrania continua

  A Headache present for >1 month.

  B Strictly unilateral.

  C All three of the following must be present:

    i   Continuous low level pain with periods of superimposed exacerbation

    ii Moderate severity, at least sometimes

    iii Lack of precipitants

  D Absolute response to indomethacin OR one of the following autonomic features associated with pain.

    i   Conjunctival injection

    ii Lacrimation

    iii Nasal congestion

    iv Rhinorrhea

    v   Ptosis

    vi Eyelid edema

  E No evidence of underlying disease.

7 Brain tumor (See chapter on Neuro-oncology for additional details)
  ◆ May be metastatic or primary in nature. High suspicion in patients with known disease, especially breast, lung, prostate, renal cell, and melanoma.
  ◆ Rare, but should be considered in a setting of progressively worsening headache with or without focal neurological deficit.
  ◆ More often a persistent, slowly worsening headache. May have features associated with increased intracranial pressure: worse headache at night, nocturnal awakening with headache, nausea, vomiting, blurry vision, diplopia.
  ◆ Work-up includes CT or, preferably MRI, both with and without contrast.
8 Pseudotumor cerebri
  ◆ Patient demographic is typically young, obese females.
  ◆ Headache frequently associated with visual changes, nausea, and dizziness. Papilledema may or may not be present.
  ◆ Imaging is normal, diagnosis based on clinical features as well as elevated opening pressure (>25cm) on lumbar puncture.
  ◆ Important to rule out venous sinus thrombosis, particularly in patients taking oral contraceptives who smoke.
  ◆ Visual changes/loss may be permanent if undiagnosed/untreated.
9 Low CSF pressure headache: similar to post-LP headache, but seen in some patients having valveless ventriculoperitoneal shunts.
10 Temporomandibular joint disorder
  ◆ Usually unilateral, severe, constant, aching, facial pain around the temporomandibular joint (TMJ). Often precipitated by chewing, with tenderness to palpation at the TMJ. Associated with bruxism or dental malocclusion.
  ◆ Dental referral is appropriate.
  ◆ Treatment is symptomatic and may include soft diet, muscle relaxants, and dental prosthesis. Joint replacement may be necessary.
11 Chronic headaches associated with underlying medical conditions.
     11.1 Cervical spine disorders
     11.2 Chronic lung disease: with hypercapnea
     11.3 Endocrine causes
          11.3.1 Hypothyroidism
          11.3.2 Cushing syndrome
     11.4 Medication-associated
          11.4.1 Corticosteroid withdrawal
          11.4.2 Chronic ergot ingestion
          11.4.3 Analgesic rebound
               ▫ Rare in general population (4%), but can be more than 50% presenting to specialized headache/pain clinics and centers.
               ▫ Associated with frequent analgesics/narcotic use (>15 days/ month).
               ▫ Can complicate treatment of any chronic headache.
     11.5 Pheochromocytoma – associated hypertension; very rare

Chronic daily headache (CDH)

- Defined by occurrence of greater than 15 episodes/month for at least 6 months.
- Pain is invariably bilateral and not exacerbated by routine physical activity.
- Etiology may be related to defective pain modulation mechanisms, abnormalities within brainstem central pain pathways, and abnormal excitation of peripheral pain pathways.
- Risk factors for CDH include:
  - Analgesic overuse
  - Stress
  - Head or cervical spine injury
  - Chronic snoring
  - Excessive caffeine intake
- For more details regarding specific diagnoses, see appropriate descriptions under Acute and Chronic headaches, above.

Primary CDH: duration >4 hours

1 **Chronic tension-type headache (CTTH; IHS classification)**
2 **Chronic (transformed) migraine (CM)**
3 New daily persistent headache (NDPH)
   A Average headache frequency >15 days/month for >1 month.
   B Average headache duration >4 hours/day (without treatment); frequently constant but may fluctuate.
   C No history of tension-type headache or migraine which increases in frequency and decreases in severity in association with new headache.
   D Acute onset (developing over <3 days) of constant unremitting headache.
   E Headache is constant in location.
   F Does not meet criteria for hemicrania continua.
   G No evidence of underlying disease.
4 Hemicrania continua

Primary CDH: duration <4 hours

1 **Cluster headache**
2 Chronic paroxysmal hemicrania
3 Short-lasting unilateral neuralgiform headache with conjunctival injection and tearing (SUNCT)
4 Hypnic headache
5 Idiopathic stabbing headache

Secondary CDH

1 **Post-traumatic headache**
2 **Cervical spine disorders**
3 *Headache associated with vascular disorders*
    3.1 *Arteriovenous malformation*
    3.2 *Chronic subdural hematoma*
    3.3 *Vasculitis*: including temporal arteritis
    3.4 *Dissection*: usually more acute and associated with neck pain +/– focal neurological signs
4 Intracranial infection: Epstein-Barr virus, HIV, etc.
5 Pseudotumor cerebri
6 Neoplasm
7 Sinusitis
8 Temporomandibular joint (TMJ) disorder
9 Analgesic rebound headache

Chapter 5
Neuropsychiatry and Dementia

Specific behavioral syndromes like aphasia, apraxia, etc. are covered in Chapter 2.

Approach to neurobehavioral evaluation

Neuropsychiatric interview

- Assessing the patient's general appearance is the first observation made in the neuropsychiatric examination. For example: a disheveled appearance reflecting a lack of self-care occurs in frontal lobe syndromes; a unilateral dressing disturbance occurs in hemispatial neglect.
- Disturbances of motor function are among the most revealing aspects of the neuropsychiatric examination. For example: 1) retarded depression is characterized by psychomotor slowing, long latencies of reply, and paucity of verbal output; 2) catatonic behavior with stereotypy and waxy flexibility can be seen in affective disorders.

Components of the neuropsychiatric interview and mental status examination
1 Interview:
- Appearance: well-groomed, disheveled
- Motor behavior: restless, akathisia, tremor, waxy flexibility
- Mood and affect: depressed, energized, cheerful, flat, blunted
- Verbal output: sparse, verbose, pressured
- Thought: circumstantial, flight of ideas, perseveration
- Perception: misperceptions, illusions, hallucinations
2 Mental status examination:
- Attention and concentration: digit span forward and backward
- Language: fluency, comprehension, reading, writing, repetition
- Memory: registration, immediate and delayed recall
- Construction: drawing objects
- Calculation skills: mathematics, word problems
- Abstraction: similarities, proverbs

- Insight and judgment: problem solving, hypothetical examples (what would you do if …?)
- Praxis: ability to perform complex motor tasks (brush teeth, comb hair, etc.)
- Frontal lobe system tasks: executive planning, Luria hand sequence
- Right-left orientation
- Finger identification

Clinical correlates of mental status impairment

- When testing mental status, remember there is a hierarchy of performance. If the patient is unable to perform a basic task, then detailed testing of higher functions will not necessarily reflect a specific localization-related deficit.
- Basic tasks include tasks of attention, language, and recognition. If a patient is unable to attend (such as in an acute confusional state/delirium), then deficits in memory or calculations, etc. should be interpreted with caution. Similarly, if a patient demonstrates a receptive aphasia, then failure to complete other tasks may not reflect additional deficits, but merely the inability to follow the examiner's commands.
- It is generally sensible to test basic functions first, and then modify the level of detail of the remainder of the mental status exam based on performance of these basic functions.

Test	Abnormal performance	Clinical correlates of poor performance
Attention		
Digit span	< 5 digits	Delirium Advanced dementia Conduction aphasia
'A' test: series of letters, patient identifies all 'A's	Errors of omission	Delirium Frontal lobe dysfunction
Serial subtraction	Erroneous subtraction	Delirium Dementia Acalculia, amnesia
Digit span backwards	< 4 digits	Delirium Dementia Frontal lobe syndrome
Reversed spelling	Slowing or failure	Delirium Dementia Frontal lobe syndrome

Continued

Test	Abnormal performance	Clinical correlates of poor performance
Memory		
Word list learning	Recall & recognition impaired	Amnesia with left hemispheric lesions Cortical dementia
Word list learning	Recall impaired, recognition intact	Frontal subcortical system dysfunction
Figure learning	Recall & recognition impaired	Amnesia with right hemispheric lesions
Figure learning	Recall impaired, recognition intact	Frontal subcortical system dysfunction
Remote recall	Variable: temporal gradient present	Amnesia
Remote recall	Impaired: no temporal gradient	Dementia
Language		
Spontaneous speech	Fluent aphasia	Posterior left hemispheric lesion
Spontaneous speech	Non-fluent aphasia	Anterior left hemispheric lesion
Comprehension	Impaired	Posterior left hemispheric lesion
Repetition	Impaired	Left perisylvian lesion
Naming	Impaired	Left or right hemispheric lesion Delirium Dementia
Writing	Agraphia	Left parietal lobe lesion
Reading	Alexia without agraphia	Left medial occipital lesion (and splenium?)
	Alexia with agraphia	Left parietal lobe lesion
Word list generation	Reduced	Anomia Left frontal lobe lesion Psychomotor retardation
Miscellaneous		
Calculation	Acalculia	Left inferior parietal lesion
Abstraction	Concrete	Dementia Frontal lobe syndrome
Judgment	Impaired	Dementia Frontal lobe syndrome
Motor programming	Perseveration	Lateral convexity of frontal lobes
Praxis	Apraxia	Left hemispheric lesion Corpus callosum

Dementia evaluation

- There is no single battery of laboratory tests that would adequately screen for all causes of dementia. In addition, many syndromes lack pathognomonic laboratory features that would allow such identification.
- Correct diagnosis of a dementing illness depends critically on the integration of clinical history, neurological, and general physical examinations, and mental status assessment as well as selected laboratory tests.
- Laboratory assessment of patients with suspected dementia is targeted to identify REVERSIBLE causes, with a core group of laboratory tests that should be performed on all demented patients for this purpose. Ancillary investigations are recommended when suspicion for a specific diagnosis is high.

1 **Core laboratory tests**
  - Complete blood count
  - Serum electrolytes, calcium, glucose, blood urea nitrogen, creatinine, liver function tests
  - Thyroid-stimulating hormone
  - Serum vitamin B_{12}
  - Structural imaging study
2 Ancillary investigations
  - Syphilis serology (RPR)
  - Sedimentation rate (ESR)
  - HIV testing
  - Chest X-ray
  - Urinalysis with 24-hour urine collection for heavy metals and toxicology screen
  - Neuropsychological testing
  - Apo-E genotyping, $A\beta_{42}$/tau CSF analysis
  - Electroencephalography
  - Single-photon emission computed tomography (SPECT)
  - Positron emission tomography (PET)

Note: apolipoprotein E genotyping is not useful in isolation from the clinical criteria of Alzheimer disease, but may increase the sensitivity of the diagnosis when patients do not have the Є-4 allele. Another biomarker for diagnosis of Alzheimer disease is the combined assessment of CSF amyloid $\beta_{(1-42)}$ protein ($A\beta_{42}$) and tau concentrations, which has a sensitivity of 85% and specificity of 87%.

Neuropsychiatry and behavioral neurology

Clinical signs and symptoms

Disorders of perception

- Abnormalities of perception may be classified according to modality (visual, auditory, touch, olfactory, and gustatory) and whether they represent positive or negative phenomena.
- Disorder of visual perception is the most common disorder of perception seen in clinical practice.

1 Positive phenomena
  - Hallucinations: formed or unformed distortions occurring without external stimulus
  - Illusions: distortions or misinterpretations of existing stimuli
  - Palinopsia: visual images that persist even when gaze direction changes
2 Negative phenomena
  - Unilateral neglect
  - Blindness
  - Achromatopsia (central color blindness)
  - Agnosia (inability to recognize)
  - Visual object agnosia
  - Prosopagnosia (agnosia for familiar faces)
  - Environmental agnosia (agnosia for familiar places)
  - Simultagnosia (inability to perceive multiple objects as a single entity at once)
  - Color agnosia

Memory disturbances

- For clinical purposes, memory disturbances can be divided into those that are short-lived (less than 24–48 hours) and those that are more prolonged.
- Alternatively, memory disturbances can be divided into stable and progressive.
- Amnesia refers to a specific clinical condition in which there is an impairment in the ability to learn new information *despite normal attention, preserved ability to recall remote information, and intact cognitive functions.*
- Amnesia should be distinguished from other causes of memory disturbances associated with lapses of consciousness including seizures, alcoholic blackouts, migraine, etc.

1 Transient episode of memory loss (< 48 hours)

   1.1 **Amnesia**

      ▪ **Transient global amnesia (TGA)** – (see below)

      ▪ **Psychogenic amnesia**

      ▪ **Post-traumatic amnesia**

   1.2 Memory lapses associated with alterations of consciousness

      ▪ Seizures

      ▪ Alcoholic blackouts

      ▪ Migraine

      ▪ Toxic-metabolic confusional states

      ▪ Benzodiazepine-induced amnesia

2 Prolonged period of memory loss (> 48 hours)

   2.1 Amnestic syndromes

      ▪ **Head trauma**

      ▪ *Wernicke-Korsakoff syndrome*

      ▪ *Herpes simplex encephalitis*

      ▪ Hippocampal infarction

      ▪ Basal forebrain lesions

   2.2 Dissociative states

      ▪ Fugues

      ▪ Multiple personality disorders

   2.3 Minimal cognitive impairment (MCI)

   2.4 Dementias

      ▪ **Alzheimer disease**

      ▪ Subcortical dementias

Transient global amnesia vs. psychogenic amnesia

- Psychogenic amnesia is most likely to be confused with transient global amnesia (TGA), especially in patients presenting with acute onset.
- However, there are several characteristics that aid in the differentiation of psychogenic amnesia from TGA.
- The most important clue is that TGA almost never includes a loss of personal identity, whereas it is one of the hallmarks in psychogenic amnesia.
- Psychogenic amnesia should also be distinguished from episodic disturbances of consciousness, such as those associated with complex partial seizures.
- The exact cause of TGA is still unclear. However, recent cerebral blood flow studies suggested diminished blood flow in the posterior hemispheric and inferior temporal regions.

Transient global amnesia	Psychogenic amnesia
A distinct clinical syndrome consisting of an acute period of amnesia lasting less than 24 hours	Hysterical conversion symptom in which patients suddenly forget their identity and life situations
Personal identity retained	**Personal identity lost**
Unable to learn new information	Ability to learn new information preserved
Amnesia not selective	Memory loss may be selective for specific information
Temporal gradient present, with relative preservation of remote memory beyond the period of retrograde amnesia	Temporal gradient absent
Depression and anxiety infrequent	Depression and anxiety common
Distressed by amnesia	Indifferent to amnesia
Common in older patients (5th to 7th decades)	Common in younger patients (teens–3rd decades)

Visual hallucinations

> • There are no etiology-specific or pathognomonic types of hallucinations, though features of visual hallucinations may facilitate identification of the clinical disorders from which they originate.

1 Lilliputian hallucinations
  - Vision of tiny humans and animal figures, named after the diminutive inhabitants of the Isle of Lilliput.
  - They are distinctive but appear to have little etiologic significance. They have been described in toxic/metabolic disorders, epilepsy, ocular diseases, affective disturbances, and schizophrenia.
2 Brobdingnagian hallucinations
  - Hallucinations of giants.
  - Have been reported in a small number of acute confusional state cases.
3 Autoscopy (heutoscopy)
  - Striking hallucinations in which one sees one's own image.
  - May suggest underlying organic brain disorders including epilepsy, tumor, trauma, subarachnoid hemorrhage, migraine, and infections. Also occurs with schizophrenia and depression.
4 'Psychedelic' hallucinations
  - Characterized by geometric forms, spirals, funnels, and chessboards that are most characteristic of the hallucinogenic drugs. However, can also occur with

sensory deprivation, and have been described in CNS disorders such as during recovery from acute viral encephalitis and with acute occipital lobe insults.

5 Palinopsia
   - A unique form of visual hallucination that involves the persistence or recurrence of visual images after the exciting stimulus has been removed. The images remain when the patient changes direction of gaze and may spontaneously recur.
   - Palinopsia can occur with lesions in either hemisphere, but is most common with acute damage to the posterior aspect of the non-dominant hemisphere.
   - It has also been reported as a possible side-effect of trazodone and LSD intoxication.

Auditory hallucinations

- Auditory hallucinations, unlike visual hallucinations, are more characteristic of idiopathic psychiatric disorders than of neurological or toxic metabolic disorders.
- An important exception to this observation is the common occurrence of auditory hallucinations in schizophrenia-like psychosis that may be associated with a variety of medical and neurological disorders.
- Unformed auditory hallucinations are called tinnitus, whereas formed hallucinations consist of melodies and occasionally voices.
- Deafness and auditory hallucinations appear to predispose to the development of paranoia in the elderly.
- Musical hallucination is a unique type of auditory hallucination and is most common with deafness. It can also be caused by central nervous processes, such as epilepsy, and can occur with depression and schizophrenia.

Etiologies of auditory hallucinations:
1 **Psychiatric disorders: the most common cause of auditory hallucinations**
   - Schizophrenia, occurs in 60–90% of patients
   - Depression
   - Mania
   - Post-traumatic stress disorder
2 Toxic metabolic disorders
   - Chronic alcoholic hallucinosis
   - Occurring as part of delirium?
3 Peripheral lesions
   - Deafness can be caused by the disease of middle ear, inner ear, and auditory nerve. This may produce both unformed and formed hallucinations.
4 CNS disorders
   - Temporal lobe epilepsy
   - Pontine lesions

Pharmacologic agents and toxins associated with hallucinations

- Among all medications, hallucinations commonly occur with four major groups: hallucinogens, anti-Parkinsonian medications, drugs associated with withdrawal syndromes, and a miscellaneous group.
- Any medications, when taken in excess, may produce an acute confusional state with concomitant hallucinations.

1 Hallucinogens
  - Lysergic acid diethylamide (LSD)
  - MDMA (ecstasy)
  - Ketamine
  - Abused inhalants, including ether, gasoline, glue, and nitrous oxide.
2 Antiparkinsonian medications: all anti-Parkinsonian medications have been reported to cause hallucinations.
  - Anticholinergic drugs
  - Levodopa
  - Dopamine agonists, including pramipexole, ropinirole, pergolide, and bromocriptine
  - Amantadine
  - Selegiline
  - Catechol-O-methyltransferase inhibitors (COMTI), including entacapone and tolcapone
3 Drugs associated with withdrawal syndromes
  - Barbiturates
  - Benzodiazepines
  - Chloral hydrate
  - Opiates
  - Ethyl alcohol
4 Miscellaneous
  - Cimetidine
  - Digoxin
  - Lithium
  - Antidepressants, e.g. imipramine
  - Corticosteroids
  - Propanolol
  - Disulfiram
  - Thyroxin
  - Amphetamines
  - Sympathomimetics

Neurological disorders and associated behavioral disorders

- Depression is a broad term that encompasses changes in mood as well as a complex clinical syndrome. It includes sadness, anhedonia, and impaired ability to experience pleasure.
- The interaction between depression and neurological diseases is complex. When depression precedes the onset of neurological disease, it is usually unclear whether the depression is the first manifestation or coincidentally preceded the onset of the brain syndrome.
- Depression itself can cause cognitive impairment, resulting in a dementia syndrome of depression or pseudodementia.
- In general, depression is under-recognized in neurological conditions and even when recognized, patients tend to be under-treated for depression.

Neurological conditions that have depression as a prominent feature

1 **Multiple sclerosis**
   - Up to 80% of patients with multiple sclerosis have depressive symptoms.
   - In addition, treatment with interferon ß-1b has been associated with new-onset depression.
2 Extrapyramidal diseases
   2.1 **Idiopathic Parkinson disease (PD)** and other Parkinsonian syndromes
      - Approximately 50% of PD patients will experience depressive episodes during the course of illness.
      - Risk factors include female gender with a past history of depression.
      - Depression in PD is associated with more impaired cognitive function, the presence of psychotic features, and greater disability.
      - Profiles of depression in PD include dysphoria, pessimism, and prominent somatic symptoms with less guilt and self-blame.
      - In other Parkinsonian syndromes, depression is observed in:
        - 20% of patients with progressive supranuclear palsy
        - 75% of patients with corticobasal ganglionic degeneration
        - 50% of patients with diffuse Lewy body disease
   2.2 **Huntington disease (HD)**
      - Approximately 40% of patients with HD have mood disorders.
      - The mood change in HD is not just a reaction to the illness, but reflects the underlying neuropsychiatric manifestation of the disease.
      - HD is also associated with a marked increased in suicide rate, up to 8 times greater among patients age 50–69 years old compared to a control group.

3 Primary degenerative dementias
  • **Alzheimer disease** (AlzD) and frontotemporal dementia
    ▪ Patients with cortical dementia tend to exhibit less severe depression than those with subcortical disorders.
    ▪ Approximately 40% of AlzD patients have depression.
4 Cerebrovascular disease
  • Up to 33% of stroke patients will experience depression.
  • Correlation between stroke location and risk of depression has been controversial.
  • Vascular depression is a rather new term, suggesting that the late-onset depression is related to silent cerebral infarction and subcortical white matter lesions.
5 Epilepsy
  • Depression in epilepsy patients may occur as part of a prodromal emotional change, part of an aura, part of an ictal manifestation, following seizures as part of the post-ictal state and lastly, may be an interictal manifestation.
  • Interictal depression is the most common type of psychopathology observed in epilepsy patients and is associated with complex partial seizures with left-sided foci.
  • Situational depression may also occur and can result from anticipation of seizures, reduced socialization, and decreased work productivity.
  • Interactions between anticonvulsants and antidepressants should always be considered in each patient. Monoamine oxidase inhibitors are least likely to exacerbate seizures.
6 Others
  • Traumatic brain injury
  • CNS infections
  • Cerebral neoplasms

Neurological causes of mania

• Mania is usually primary but may be secondary to other medical conditions.
• The most common associations are with lesions in the right hemisphere involving the orbitofrontal cortex, caudate nuclei, thalamus, and basotemporal area.

1 Right hemispheric lesions
  • In epilepsy, hypomania is usually seen peri-ictally, in the setting of clusters of right-sided temporal seizures.
  • Other causes have been reported, such as stroke, and traumatic brain injury.
2 Parkinson disease with dopaminergic therapy

3 Huntington disease
  ◆ Depression is more common than mania in HD.
4 Multiple sclerosis
5 Frontal lobe degeneration
6 Tertiary syphilis

Neurological conditions associated with psychosis

- Psychosis is defined as a loss of reality testing such that affected individuals cannot evaluate the accuracy of their perceptions or thoughts and draw incorrect inferences about external reality.
- A wide variety of neurological, toxic, and metabolic disorders cause secondary psychosis as their presenting manifestation, or as one aspect that emerges during the course of illness.
- The most common condition associated with psychosis is schizophrenia, followed by dementia of Alzheimer disease.

1 **Drug intoxication**
  ◆ Acute psychosis (including paranoia, agitation, and hallucinations) can result from intoxication, particularly with amphetamine, cocaine, phenylcyclidine (PCP), mescaline, LSD, and psilocybin.
2 Primary degenerative dementias
  ◆ Three common primary degenerative dementias associated with delusions are Alzheimer disease, diffuse Lewy body disease, and frontotemporal dementia.
  ◆ **40–70% of patients with Alzheimer disease manifest delusions, making it the most common cause of psychosis after schizophrenia**.
  ◆ Delusions in Alzheimer disease are usually simple, loosely held, and often transient. Typically, Alzheimer patients experience delusions of spousal infidelity, monetary theft, or uninvited strangers coming to the house.
3 **Extrapyramidal disorders**
  ◆ Psychosis is **more frequent in hyperkinetic diseases** than in patients with hypokinetic disorders. A good example is Huntington disease in which psychosis is one of the major manifestations. Others include Wilson disease, idiopathic basal ganglia calcification, and spinocerebellar degeneration.
  ◆ In hypokinetic disorders, psychosis is common in postencephalitic Parkinsonism (von Economo encephalitis) with delusions in up to 25% of cases. Psychosis is much less common in idiopathic Parkinson disease and usually occurs in the setting of a medication-induced effect.
4 **Central nervous system infections**
  ◆ Herpes simplex encephalitis preferentially involves the medial temporal lobes, inferior frontal areas, and cerebral cortices that are included in the limbic

system, and frequently presents with psychosis, delusions, and auditory hallucinations.

- Other common viral diseases with prominent psychoses include HIV and subacute sclerosing panencephalitis. Less common viral agents are mumps, measles, and infectious mononucleosis.
- Nonviral causes of infectious psychosis include malaria, syphilis, neurocysticercosis, and prion diseases.

5 Demyelinating diseases

- Multiple sclerosis is more commonly associated with depression than psychosis, though episodic psychosis is a well-recognized feature of patients with progressive demyelinating illness.
- Older individuals with new-onset psychosis and no identifiable cause have an increased number of white matter lesions on MRI compared to non-psychotic elderly individuals. However, it is controversial if ischemic white matter lesions on MRI play a role in late-onset psychosis.

6 Epilepsy

- Temporal lobe epilepsy is associated with a high prevalence of psychosis, especially if seizure activity originates from left-sided foci.
- Primary generalized epilepsy and complex partial seizures are also associated with psychosis.

7 Other causes

- Traumatic brain injury, especially if injury is to the left temporal region.
- Stroke and aneurysms
- Mitochondrial disorders
- Postanoxic encephalopathy
- Hydrocephalus

Neurological causes of episodic dyscontrol or violence

- No clear definition of episodic dyscontrol exists. It is sometimes referred to as intermittent explosive disorder.
- While some cases may be associated with brain lesions, milder degrees of this behavior may simply represent a person with a 'hot temper' or 'short fuse'. Intense outbursts of anger and violence may also be part of a borderline personality disorder.
- In simple terms, the more primitive or inappropriate the violence is, the more likely it is that a neuropathological substrate for the behavior change will be found.
- These patients are usually remorseful when they have calmed down.
- The relationship between epilepsy and violence remains controversial. It is unlikely that a seizure will manifest as a nonstereotypic violent act.

1 Orbitofrontal lesions
  - May manifest as a lack of impulse control, a 'short fuse', and violence that is typically triggered by a perceived threat or insult.
  - Examples include head injury and orbital groove meningioma.
2 Hypothalamic lesions
  - Associated with nonpurposeful rage attacks.
3 Mesial temporal lesions
  - Not necessarily associated with temporal lobe seizure.
4 Chronic confusional state/dementia
  - Associated with aggressive behaviors that are short-lived and nonpurposeful.
5 Epilepsy
  - Epilepsy patients may be violent as a consequence of peri-ictal confusion, but it is unlikely that seizure itself manifests as a violent act.

Common neurological disorders and associated behavioral disorders

- Various neurological disorders have distinct profiles of associated behavioral disturbances. These profiles reflect the different topography of brain dysfunction associated with each disease, and the dysfunction may reflect structural and neurochemical abnormalities.
- On the other hand, differences in symptom profiles exist within neuropsychiatric disturbances associated with different neurological disorders. For example, suicide is a common depressive symptom in epilepsy and Huntington disease, but rare in depressed patients with Parkinson disease. Psychotic depression is also common in epilepsy but rare in Parkinson disease.

Neurological disorders	Associated behavioral abnormalities
Alzheimer disease	Apathy Agitation Depression Irritability
Diffuse Lewy body disease	Hallucinations Delusions Depression
Frontotemporal dementia	Disinhibition Apathy
Vascular dementia	Depression Apathy

Continued

Neurological disorders	Associated behavioral abnormalities
Traumatic brain injury	Depression Disinhibition Apathy
Huntington disease	Depression Obsessive-compulsive disorders Irritability
Parkinson disease	Depression Anxiety Psychosis (associated with treatment)
Progressive supranuclear palsy	Apathy Disinhibition
Corticobasal ganglionic degeneration	Depression
Tourette syndrome	Obsessive-compulsive disorders
Multiple sclerosis	Depression Irritability Anxiety
Epilepsy	Depression Psychosis (depending on area involved)
HIV encephalopathy	Apathy

Substance abuse and neurological symptoms

- Substance abuse describes a maladaptive pattern characterized by:
  - recurrent use in spite of academic, social, or work problems,
  - use in situations in which changes in mental status may be dangerous, and
  - recurrent substance-related legal problems.

Substance	Clinical features
Amphetamine	Loquacity, hypervigilance, tachycardia, pupillary dilatation, moist mucous membranes
Cocaine	Euphoria with paranoia, psychosis, agitation, anxiety, hyperactivity, sympathetic stimulation including pupillary dilatation, visual and tactile hallucinations Serious complications include intracerebral hemorrhage, ischemic infarcts, seizures, and coronary events
Tricyclic antidepressants	Sedation, blurred vision, seizures, stupor, coma, hypotension, prolonged PR and QT intervals, cardiac arrthythmias, impotence, hyperhydriosis, anticholinergic side-effects

Substance	Clinical features
Opiates	Respiratory depression, stupor, coma, pupillary constriction, hypotension
Heroin withdrawal	Craving, anxiety, dysphoria, yawning, pupillary dilatation, rhinorrhea, restlessness, piloerection, muscle twitching
Phencyclidine (PCP)	Agitation, impulsiveness, hypertension, tachycardia, nystagmus, numbness, ataxia, dysarthria, hyperacusis, perceptual disorders, psychosis
Alcohol withdrawal (delirium tremens)	Coarse hand tremor, insomnia, anxiety, agitation, autonomic hyperactivity, confusion, tactile and visual hallucinations
Inhalants	Headaches, tremor, cerebellar findings, hearing loss, peripheral neuritis, muscle weakness (due to rhabdomyolysis)
LSD	Visual hallucinations, such as flashbacks, flashes of color and after images, persistence of trailing images when an object moves through the visual field
MDMA (ecstasy)	Disorientation, sensation of 'rush', euphoria, decreased appetite, bruxism, shortness of breath, cardiac arrhythmia
Anabolic steroids	Anxiety, irritability, acne, gynecomastia, muscle hypertrophy
Caffeine withdrawal	Withdrawal headache, anxiety

Neuro-ophthalmologic features of common neuropsychiatric disorders

- The neuro-ophthalmologic examination may contribute essential information to neuropsychiatric diagnoses.
- Neuro-ophthalmologic examination should include inspection, visual acuity, visual field testing, ocular motility, and fundoscopy in addition to the general neurological examination.

Diagnosis	Neuro-ophthalmic manifestations
Alzheimer disease	Inadequate visual exploration, 'visual grasp' Optic ataxia (as in Balint syndrome)
Frontotemporal dementia	Anti-saccade impairment
Diffuse Lewy body disease	Visual hallucinations
Parkinson disease	Poor convergence and upgaze Diminished blinking Visual hallucinations with dopaminergic therapy

Continued

Diagnosis	Neuro-ophthalmic manifestations
Progressive supranuclear palsy	Supranuclear gaze palsy with impairment of vertical gaze; early slowing of saccades, followed by loss of downgaze, upgaze, and horizontal gaze Supranuclear gaze palsy Anti-saccade impairment
Huntington disease	Supranuclear gaze palsy in advanced stage
Wilson disease	Blinking tics Sudden gaze tics
Corticobasal ganglionic degeneration	Kayser-Fleischer ring Cataracts
Tourette syndrome	Obsessional eye mutilation
Frontal lobe lesions	Acute: ipsilateral gaze deviation Chronic: contralateral gaze impersistence
Geniculocalcarine lesions	Homonymous hemianopia Release hallucinations
Midbrain lesions	Peduncular hallucinosis
Basilar bifurcation occlusion	Dreamlike state Visual hallucinations
Multiple sclerosis	Optic neuritis Internuclear ophthalmoplegia
Delirium	Visual hallucinations
Narcolepsy	Hypnagogic and hypnopompic hallucinations
Mass lesions	Papilledema Transient visual obscuration

Modified from Cummings, J.L., Mega, M.S. *Neuropsychiatry and Behavior Neuroscience*. 2003, Oxford University Press, Oxford.

Serotonin syndrome vs. neuroleptic malignant syndrome

- Serotonin is metabolized via monoamine oxidase (MAO-A), while dopamine is metabolized via MAO-B.
- In cases where patients are taking an MAO inhibitor, an SSRI, and a neuroleptic, distinguishing between the two diagnoses may not be possible.

Serotonin syndrome	Neuroleptic malignant syndrome
Occurs with the use of SSRIs	Occurs with the use of neuroleptics
Rigidity Altered mentation Tremors	Rigidity Altered mentation Tremors
Myoclonus	High fever High CPK level
Hydration with supportive treatment	Hydration Consider dopamine agonist, in addition to supportive measures
Usually resolves within several hours	Usually lasts days to weeks

Regional correlates of neuropsychiatric symptoms

- Various neuropsychiatric syndromes are associated with distinct patterns of anatomical involvement.
- Pathology in the frontal lobes, temporal lobes, caudate nucleus, globus pallidus, and subthalamic nucleus are implicated in many neuropsychiatric syndromes.
- The laterality of brain lesions influences the associated neuropsychiatric symptoms.
  - Secondary mania is associated with non-dominant hemispheric lesions.
  - Depression in the acute post-stroke period is associated with dominant hemispheric lesions

Neuropsychiatric symptoms	Regional pathology
Mania	Right inferomedial cortex Caudate nucleus Temporal-thalamic connections
Depression	Bilateral cerebral dysfunction Left caudate nucleus Left anterior frontal cortex Dorsolateral prefrontal cortex
Psychosis with first rank symptoms	Left temporal cortex
Psychosis with misidentification	Right hemisphere
Obsessive-compulsive disorders	Orbital or medial frontal cortex Globus pallidus Caudate nucleus

Continued

Neuropsychiatric symptoms	Regional pathology
Apathy	Anterior cingulate gyrus Nucleus accumbens Globus pallidus Thalamus
Disinhibition	Orbitofrontal cortex Hypothalamus
Paraphilia (sexual deviations)	Medial temporal cortex Hypothalamus Rostral brainstem
Akinetic mutism	Medial frontal cortex

Psychotic symptoms associated with focal brain abnormalities

- Secondary psychotic symptoms were categorized in DSM as psychoses associated with organic brain syndromes. The syndromes included in that category were dementias, delirium, and psychoses associated with other cerebral and systemic conditions.
- The differential diagnosis involves first establishing that the symptoms are in fact psychotic. For example, confabulation may be mistaken for delusions. Additionally, perceptual disturbances associated with focal cerebral pathology must be distinguished from hallucinations.

Psychotic symptoms	Site
First-rank symptoms • Thoughts spoken aloud • Third-person voices arguing • Delusions of control • Delusional perception • Thought withdrawal • Thought insertion • Thought broadcasting	Dominant temporal lobe
Complex delusions	Subcortical or limbic structures
Anton syndrome	Bilateral occipital lobe and optic tract
Anosognosia	Non-dominant parietal lobe
Misidentification syndromes • Capgras syndrome • Reduplicative paramnesia • Fregoli syndrome • Intermetamorphosis syndrome	Non-dominant or bilateral temporo-parietal-frontal lobes

Modified from Kaplan & Sadock's 'Study guide and self-examination review' in *Psychiatry*, 7th edition. 2003, Lippincott Williams & Wilkins.

Neuropsychological deficits associated with lateralized hemispheric damage

- Many functions are mediated by both the right and left cerebral hemispheres. Important qualitative differences between the two hemispheres can be demonstrated in the presence of lateralized brain injury.
- In most persons (regardless of handedness), the left hemisphere is dominant.
- Although language is the most obvious area that is largely controlled by the dominant hemisphere, this hemisphere is also considered to be primary for limb praxis.
- In contrast, the non-dominant hemisphere is thought to play a more important role in controlling visuospatial abilities and hemispatial attention, which are associated with the clinical presentations of constructional apraxia and neglect, respectively.

Dominant hemisphere	Non-dominant hemisphere
Aphasia	Visuospatial deficits
Right-left disorientation	Impaired visual perception
Finger agnosia	Neglect
Dysgraphia	Constructional apraxia (Gestalt)
Dyscalculia	Dressing apraxia
Limb apraxia	Anosognosia
Constructional apraxia (details)	

Dementia and delirium

DDx of dementia

- Dementia is a syndrome of acquired intellectual impairment characterized by persistent deficits in at least three of the following areas of mental activity: memory, language, visuospatial skills, personality/emotional state, and cognition (abstraction, mathematics, and judgment).
- Although Alzheimer disease (AlzD) is the leading cause of dementia, there are many potential causes of dementia. Among those with dementing diseases, at least half have pure AlzD or a mixture of AlzD and cerebrovascular disease, and about 15% have dementia with Lewy bodies.
- Its acquired nature distinguishes dementia from mental retardation and its persistence differentiates it from the delirium of acute confusional states.
- Approximately 5% of individuals over the age 65 are severely demented, and an additional 10–15% are mildly to moderately intellectually impaired. As the number of aged persons continues to increase, dementia will demand an increasing share of financial and other societal resources.

1 Primary dementia syndromes
   * **Alzheimer disease** (see Alzheimer disease)
   * **Vascular dementia**
   * Dementia with Lewy body disease
   * Frontotemporal dementia
2 Other neurodegenerative disorders
   * Parkinsonian syndrome with dementia (see Parkinsonism in Movement Disorders chapter)
      ▪ Idiopathic Parkinson disease
      ▪ Progressive supranuclear palsy
      ▪ Corticobasal ganglionic degeneration
   * Huntington disease (see Chorea in Movement Disorders)
3 Infections
   * HIV dementia: increasingly common as HIV-infected patients live longer
   * Neurosyphilis
   * Prion disease: Creutzfeldt-Jakob disease
   * Chronic meningitis (see Infection/Inflammatory chapter)
4 Paraneoplastic disorders (see Neuro-oncology chapter)
5 Toxic and metabolic causes
   * Vitamin B_{12} deficiency
   * Thyroid disorders
   * Chronic hypoxemia
   * Toxin exposure including manganese, lead, and mercury
6 Others
   * Traumatic dementia
   * Normal pressure hydrocephalus
   * Demyelinating disease with dementia, e.g. multiple sclerosis

Differentiating dementia and delirium

* Dementia and delirium are both the disorders of intellectual function that affect multiple cognitive domains.
* Attentional disturbance is the single most salient feature of delirium.
* It is crucial to distinguish delirium from dementia as the management of these two conditions is significantly different.
* *Dementia cannot be diagnosed until delirium resolves.* However, delirium and dementia can coexist in the same patient.
* Patients with dementia can easily become delirious with minor infections, fever, or electrolyte imbalance.

Features	Delirium	Dementia
Definition	The inability to sustain, direct, or appropriately shift attention.	An acquired persistent impairment in at least three of the following domains; language, memory, spatial skills, executive ability, and emotion
Onset	Acute or subacute	Chronic
Course	Fluctuating	Persistent
Duration	Limited	Chronic
Attention	**Impaired**	**Intact until advanced stage**
Speech	Slurred dysarthria	Dysarthria uncommon
Visual hallucinations	Common	Uncommon except in certain types of dementia
Tremor	Common	Uncommon
Myoclonus	Common	Uncommon except in certain types of dementia
EEG	Abnormal, e.g. triphasic waves	Mild changes, e.g. mild diffuse slowing

Table modified from Cummings J.L., Trimble M.R. *Concise Guide to Neuropsychiatry and Behavioral Neurology*. American Psychiatric Press, 1995.

Criteria for diagnosis of probable Alzheimer disease

- Premorbid diagnosis for these and other degenerative disorders is a 'probable' diagnosis.
- The diagnosis shifts to 'possible Alzheimer disease' if it is very early in its course, if another brain-based disorder is present but does not significantly contribute to the clinical picture, or if there is an atypical presentation.
- 'Definite' diagnosis requires a clinically probable diagnosis and autopsy or biopsy confirmation.

1 Dementia present
2 Onset between 40 and 90 years of age
3 Deficits in two or more cognitive areas
  - Memory
  - Language
  - Visuospatial skills
  - Personality or emotional state
  - Cognition
4 Progression of deficits > 6 months
5 Consciousness undisturbed

6 Absence of other potential etiology
(Modified from McKhann G., Drachman D., *et al.* Clinical diagnosis of Alzheimer disease: report of the NINCDS-ADRDA work group, Department of Health and Human Services Task Force on Alzheimer Disease. *Neurology* 1984; 34: 939–944.)

Infectious causes of dementia

- Dementias may be caused by viruses, bacterial encephalitis, or chronic meningitis.
- HIV-associated dementia is increasingly common, as HIV patients live longer with more effective antiretroviral therapy. Nearly 50% of patients with acquired immunodeficiency syndrome may suffer from dementia.

1 **HIV viral dementias**
   - Most HIV-associated dementia are of the subcortical type. Memory impairment is a retrieval type deficit. Additional symptoms: apathy and psychomotor slowing.
   - Motor symptoms are significant for poor coordination.
   - The presence of multinucleated giant cells in the central nervous system is the most specific finding in HIV infection and is a better correlate of the dementia than the extent of CSF viral load.
   - The best treatment for HIV dementia is effective control of systemic HIV replication and decreasing chronic macrophage activation.
2 Non-HIV viral/inflammatory dementias
   2.1 Progressive multifocal leukoencephalopathy (PML)
      - Slowly progressive papovavirus (JC and rarely SV40) infection occurring almost exclusively in patients with chronic lymphoproliferative, myeloproliferative, or granulomatous diseases.
      - Signs include gradual progression of focal neurological deficits and dementia.
   2.2 Subacute sclerosing panencephalitis (measles)
      - Usually in unvaccinated children; sometimes young adults.
      - Additional signs include myoclonus, ataxia, focal neurological signs.
      - Dx: elevated CSF measles antibodies; EEG may show 'burst-suppression' with bursts in synchrony with or independent of myoclonic jerks.
   2.3 Progressive rubella panencephalitis
      - Very rare; seen in children and young adults.
      - Progressive dementia and prominent ataxia. Later spasticity and retinopathy.
3 Bacterial and spirochetal causes of dementia
   3.1 **Syphilitic general paresis**

- Uncommon in Western countries, but still one of the most common causes of treatable dementia worldwide.
- General paresis typically manifests 15–30 years after the initial infection and is characterized by progressive intellectual impairment combined with psychosis. Facial and lingual tremors are common.
- Treponema pallidum organisms are abundant in the frontal cortex. Symptoms improve with penicillin treatment.

3.2 Chronic meningitis: caused by tuberculous, fungal, parasitic, and syphilitic infections (see Infection/Inflammatory chapter)

Rapidly progressive dementia

- Dementia is a syndrome of acquired intellectual impairment produced by brain dysfunction.
- AlzD has an insidious onset with a slowly progressive and chronic course lasting years. When the duration is acute or subacute, alternative diagnoses should be considered.
- The presence of movement disorders, abnormalities on motor examination, or gait disturbances should also raise other possible etiologies including infectious causes, paraneoplastic process, multisystem neurodegenerative diseases, or atypical presentation of common dementias.

1 **Treatable causes**
   - **Hashimoto encephalitis**
     - Usually younger age group.
     - Manifested by intermittent confusion, seizures, and cerebellar ataxia
     - Associated with elevated antithyroperoxidase and antithyroglobulin antibodies.
     - Treatable with intravenous steroids.

2 **Creutzfeldt-Jakob disease (CJD)**
   - Creutzfeldt-Jakob disease (CJD) is the most important and most common form of human prion diseases and should be considered in all patients who present with rapidly progressive dementia and myoclonus.
   - About 85% of cases of human prion disease occur sporadically as CJD (sporadic CJD or sCJD) with an equal incidence in men and women.
   - The etiology of sporadic CJD is unknown, although hypotheses include somatic human prion protein gene (PRNP) mutation, or the spontaneous conversion of the cellular prion protein (PrP^c) into an abnormal isoform. Homozygosity at a common coding polymorphism at codon 129 of PRNP encoding either methionine or valine predisposes to the development of sporadic and acquired CJD.

3 Rapidly progressive form of Alzheimer disease
   * May be difficult to differentiate clinically from CJD
   * Less frequent visual symptoms, cerebellar ataxia, myoclonus, and pyramidal signs
4 Dementia with Lewy bodies (DLB)
   * Associated with Parkinsonism.
   * Fluctuating cognition with pronounced variations in attention and alertness.
   * Recurrent visual hallucinations, which are typically well-formed and detailed.
5 Frontotemporal dementia
6 Cerebellar degeneration, especially with ataxic variant of sCJD
7 Paraneoplastic syndromes
8 Others
   * Anoxic brain damage
   * Postviral encephalitis
   * Subacute sclerosing panencephalitis

Creutzfeldt-Jakob disease: sporadic form versus variant

* CJD belongs to a family of prion diseases known as transmissible spongiform encephalopathy (TSE). These include scrapie in sheep and bovine spongiform encephalopathy (BSE) in cattle. Gerstmann-Sträussler-Scheinker disease (GSS), fatal familial insomnia (FFI), kuru, and most recently, variant CJD occur in humans.
* Prions are protein fragments devoid of nucleic acid that may self-polymerize and thus accumulate in the brain. Transmission occurs by ingestion of prion-containing tissue, but spontaneous (sporadic) genetic mutations also occur (sCJD). More recently, variant CJD (vCJD) in the UK and other European countries appears causally related to human exposure to BSE.
* All prion diseases have several features in common. They have incubation periods of months to years, and none evokes an inflammatory response.

Features	sCJD	vCJD
Age of onset	60–65 years	26 years
At presentation (in addition to rapidly progressive dementia)	Myoclonus, cortical blindness, pyramidal signs, akinetic mutism	Behavioral and psychiatric disturbances, cerebellar ataxia
Psychiatric symptoms	Late and less frequent	Early
Mean survival	4 months	13 months

Features	sCJD	vCJD
Neuroimaging findings	Abnormal signal in the basal ganglia, ribbon-like high signal intensity in the cerebral cortex on DWI	High T2W signal in the posterior thalamus bilaterally (Pulvinar)
EEG findings	Background slowing with periodic slow-wave complexes, often triphasic	Generally not helpful
CSF 14–3-3 protein	Elevated with varying sensitivity and specificity between 50–95%	Generally not helpful
PRNP analysis	No pathogenic mutations, many are codon 129 homozygotes	No PRNP mutations
Distribution of PrP^c in human tissues	Brain, spinal cord	Brain, eyes, tonsils, spinal cord, thymus, spleen, adrenal gland, lymph nodes, appendix, rectum

DDx of delirium or acute confusional state

- Delirium or acute confusional state is a condition of relatively abrupt onset and short duration whose major behavioral characteristic is **altered attention (the hallmark of delirium)**. Other behavioral abnormalities may coexist, including cognitive disturbances, hallucinations, and delusions.
- Delirium may be produced by a large number of metabolic, toxic, and intracranial conditions and should be considered a NEUROLOGICAL EMERGENCY.
- Delirium is particularly likely to occur in patients with pre-existing intellectual impairment and in the elderly.
- The prevalence of delirium in the hospitalized elderly is 10–40%, while 51% of postoperative patients develop delirium. Up to 80% of terminally ill patients will become delirious.
- The only definite criteria differentiating delirium from dementia is duration: delirium persists for hours or days, whereas dementia usually implies intellectual deficits over months or years.

Etiologies of delirium:

1 *Systemic conditions with toxic metabolic derangements*
   - **The most common cause of delirium.**
   - **Specific etiology is usually multifactorial as listed below.**
   - Most common metabolic conditions resulting in delirium include:
     - **Infections**

- **Dehydration**
- **Drug intoxication**
- **Nutritional deficiency**
- **Electrolyte abnormalities**
- **Cardiac and respiratory failure**
- **Hepatic encephalopathy**
- **Renal failure with uremia**
- Delirium can be caused by any medications with high concentration. However, particular medications include anticholinergics, analgesics, and anesthetics.

2 **Postoperative delirium**
- Very common, up to half of postoperative patients experience at least mild delirium.
- Delirium occurring immediately after surgery is usually due to anoxia or persistent medication effects, while delirium appearing later in the postoperative course is most likely to be a product of multiple factors including metabolic abnormalities, sleep deprivation, infections, and pain.

3 *Intracranial causes*
- *Meningitis/encephalitis* (see Chapter 7: Infectious/Inflammatory)
- *Hypertensive encephalopathy*
- *Cerebrovascular disease*, usually during acute phase
  - Thromboembolic
  - Vasculitic
- *Subdural hematoma*, history of head trauma may not be present – especially in the elderly.
- *Epilepsy*, manifested as post-ictal delirium. Delirium is uncommon during the ictal phase.
- *Head trauma*/concussion

4 Focal brain lesions: reported to cause delirium, although uncommon
- Right parietal lesions
- Bilateral medial occipitotemporal lesions

5 Others
- Underlying psychiatric disorders, precipitated by acute events
- Fever

(See also Chapter 2: Clinical Syndromes: Coma)

Common risk factors for delirium in elderly hospitalized patients
1 Age is a risk factor for hospital-associated delirium.
2 Underlying dementia
- Approximately 50% of hospitalized patients who develop delirium have underlying dementia and many have at least some cognitive impairment.
3 Associated toxic-metabolic conditions
- Dehydration, especially sodium disturbances (either hypo- or hypernatremia)
- Concomitant infection

Hydrocephalus and dementia

- Hydrocephalus refers to the presence of excessive CSF in the cranium, associated with ventricular enlargement and increased CSF within the ventricular cavities.
- Ventricular enlargement is a common finding in neuroimaging of the elderly. Difficulties often arise in determining if this dilatation represents hydrocephalus or hydrocephalus ex vacuo (see Neuroradiology chapter).
- Normal pressure hydrocephalus is a common cause of treatable dementia. Most patients present with apathy, inattention, poor memory, and impaired judgment. Associated gait impairment and urinary incontinence may or may not be present.
- In addition to clinical history and detailed examination, determination of the type of hydrocephalus is made by a combination of structural imaging, cisternography, and in some cases, a CSF flow study.

1 **Hydrocephalus ex vacuo**
  - The ventricular dilatation is a product of tissue loss manifested by enlarged cerebral sulci without any change in the dynamics of CSF flow.
2 Obstructive hydrocephalus
    2.1 Intraventricular blockade
      - Aqueductal stenosis
      - Ventricular mass
    2.2 Ventricular outlet foramina obstruction
      - Posterior fossa mass
      - Basilar meningitis
3 Communicating hydrocephalus (normal pressure hydrocephalus, NPH)
  - Idiopathic: most common cause of NPH
  - Post-hemorrhage, e.g. subarachnoid hemorrhage
  - Post-encephalitic process
  - Post-traumatic

Chapter 6
Movement Disorders

Movement disorders: an introduction

HYPOkinesias	HYPERkinesias
Akinesia/bradykinesia (**Parkinsonism**, 187)	**Essential tremor** (415)
Catatonia	**Tics, Tourette syndrome** (29–1052)
Psychomotor depression	Dystonia (33)
Freezing phenomenon	Hemifacial spasm (7.4–14.5)
Hypothyroid slowness	Ataxia (6)
Stiff muscles	Chorea (2–12)
	Others including akathisia, dyskinesia, hyperekplekia, jumpy stumps, moving toes, myokymia, myorhythmia, restless legs, and stereotypy

Numbers in parentheses indicate prevalence of disease per 100,000 in the general population.

Evaluation of a movement disorder

- The first question to be answered when seeing a patient suspected of having a movement disorder is whether or not involuntary movement is actually present.
- As a general rule, abnormal involuntary movements are exaggerated with anxiety and diminished during sleep.
- It is important to determine the nature of the involuntary movements, such as chorea, dystonia, myoclonus, and tremor.
- Features that one needs to consider during evaluation include rhythmicity, speed, duration, pattern, induction, complexity, and suppressibility

1 Rhythmic movements
  - Tremor
  - Myoclonus
  - Dystonic tremor
  - Tardive dyskinesias
  - Moving toes and fingers
2 Sustained movements
  - Dystonia
  - Stiff-person syndrome
3 Intermittent movements
  - Tics
  - Paroxysmal dyskinesias
4 Speed of movements
  - Myoclonus (faster) → chorea → athetosis (slower)
5 Suppressibility
  Tics (suppressible) → chorea → dystonia → tremor (hard to suppress)
6 Complex movements
  Tics (complex) → stereotypies → myoclonus → akathitic movements (simple)

(Ref: Fahn S., Greene P.E., Ford B., Bressman S.B. *Handbook of Movement Disorders.*)

Syndromes

Ataxia

Ataxia of acute or subacute onset

- Ataxia is an impairment of coordination in the absence of significant weakness.
- Acute ataxia (onset minutes/hours) is a NEUROLOGICAL EMERGENCY. A vascular lesion of the cerebellum (infarction, hemorrhage) must be considered. Other common causes of acute ataxia include drug/alcohol intoxication, post-concussive, and migraine.
- Subacute ataxia (hours/days) may be due to many causes. In addition to acute causes, infectious cerebellitis is common in children. Multiple sclerosis should be considered in young adults.

1 Ataxia of acute onset (minutes/hours):

   1.1 Suggests a ***vascular etiology; cerebellar hemorrhage, or infarction***

       • Suspect this particularly if hemiataxia or other brainstem signs.

       • **It is a neurological emergency.** Neuroimaging should be performed immediately.

   1.2 **Intoxication** with alcohol or drugs is perhaps the most common etiology of acute ataxia.

       • Ataxia due to intoxication is usually bilateral (not focal), more often involves truncal/gait ataxia, and altered mentation is also present.

       • May occur in children, too, as a result of accidental ingestion.

   1.3 Migraine: unsteadiness/dizziness can occur in typical migraines. In addition, the basilar migraine variant can present with cerebellar ataxia and brainstem signs; headache may not be prominent.

   1.4 Post-traumatic/post-concussive

2 Ataxia of subacute onset (hours/days):

   2.1 **Infectious causes: most common in children**

       • Viral cerebellitis/rhombencephalitis, especially in children 2–10 years old.

       • Usually pyrexia, limb/gait ataxia, and dysarthria develop in hours or days, with recovery over a period of weeks.

       • Postinfectious encephalomyelitis, especially related to varicella infection.

   2.2 **Intoxication**: see above

   2.3 Multiple sclerosis: consider this possibility especially in young adults.

       • Usually associated with other brainstem signs.

       • May have a history of relapse.

   2.4 Paraneoplastic syndromes

       • Related to neuroblastoma in children and lung carcinoma in adults.

       • Symptoms and signs include ataxia, vertigo, opsoclonus, and myoclonus.

   2.5 Others

       • Foramen magnum compression

       • Hydrocephalus

       • Labyrinthitis/vestibular neuritis: usually vertigo, nausea, and vomiting are more prominent symptoms than ataxia.

       • Miller-Fisher variant of Guillain-Barré syndrome: ophthalmoplegia, ataxia, areflexia.

       • Posterior fossa lesions: may be accompanied by signs/symptoms of increased intracranial pressure.

       • Post-concussion

Autosomal dominant spinocerebellar ataxias (SCA)

- The autosomal dominant spinocerebellar ataxias are a genetically heterogeneous group of neurodegenerative disorders, characterized by progressive motor incoordination.
- Patients usually have an affected parent or can trace the condition in family members in earlier generations who also have a similar onset of slowly progressive ataxia.
- The classification, established by the Human Genome Organization, assigns each form of SCA to a unique chromosomal locus by genetic linkage studies, designated by the symbol SCA, followed by a number.
- SCA3 is the most common recognized form of SCA in most populations, accounting for 21% of US patients with SCA.

1 Autosomal dominant ataxias caused by trinucleotide repeats and glutamine tracts

Disorder	Findings (besides ataxia; major findings in bold)	Age	Protein/gene/locus	Diagnosis
SCA1	**Hypermetric slow saccades**, pyramidal signs, neuropathy, **dysphagia**, optic atrophy	15–63	Ataxin-1 / SCA1 / 6p23	CAG repeats > 38 in SCA1 gene
SCA2	**Hypometric slow saccades, areflexia, ophthalmoplegia**	16–31	Ataxin-2 / SCA2 / 12q23–24.1	CAG repeats > 33 in SCA2 gene
SCA3 (Machado-Joseph)	Neuropathy, pyramidal signs, **dystonia**, nystagmus, **ophthalmoplegia**	5–65	Ataxin-3 / SCA3 / 14q21	CAG repeats > 55 in SCA3 gene
SCA6	**Gaze-evoked horizontal and vertical nystagmus, slow progression**	19–71	α-1A subunit of P/Q voltage-gated Ca channel / CACNA1A / 19p13	CAG repeats > 19 in CACNA1A gene
SCA7	**Abnormal color vision, central vision loss, retinal degeneration, macular dystrophy,** slow saccades	1–50	Ataxin-7 / SCA7 / 3p21.1-p12	CAG repeats > 40 in SCA7 gene

2 Autosomal dominant ataxias caused by noncoding nucleotide repeats

Disorder	Findings (besides ataxia; major findings in bold)	Age	Protein/gene/locus	Diagnosis
SCA8	Usually pure ataxia	15–66	SCA8 / 13q21	CTA/CTG repeats at SCA8 locus 101–345

Disorder	Findings (besides ataxia; major findings in bold)	Age	Protein/gene/ locus	Diagnosis
SCA10	**Generalized seizures**	10–49	E46L / SCA10 / 22q13	ATTCT repeats > 800 in SCA10 gene
SCA12	Tremor	8–55	Protein phosphatase 2A / 5q31–5q33	CAG repeats > 65 in SCA12 gene

3 Autosomal dominant ataxias with a defined genetic locus

Disorder	Findings (in addition to ataxia)	Age	Locus
SCA4	**Sensory loss, areflexia**	26–72	16q24-ter
SCA5	Pure ataxia, slow progression	10–68	11q
SCA11	Prominent nystagmus, almost pure ataxia	15–43	15q14–21.3
SCA13	**Mental retardation**	1–45	19p13.3–13.4
SCA14	**Myoclonus**	12–42	19q13.4-ter
SCA16	Prominent nystagmus, almost pure ataxia	20–66	8q22.1–24.1

Correlation between Harding clinical and genetic classification of ataxia

- Numerous classifications have been proposed to group different types of autosomal dominant cerebellar ataxias. The Harding clinical classification has gained wide acceptance by mainly dividing these ataxias into three distinct groups called ADCA type I, II, and III.
- Over the last several years, a new classification based on genetic loci of spinocerebellar ataxias has gained wide acceptance. These disorders are numbered according to their order of identification. However, this classification provides a long list and is difficult to apply in daily practice.
- Therefore, we have attempted to correlate the Harding classification with this genetic nomenclature. Both classifications are useful, and the correlation of both classifications should provide a better understanding of these important genetic causes of ataxia as well as better application in clinical neurology practice.

Harding classification	Genetic typing	Distinguishing features
ADCA I Ataxia with ophthalmoplegia, optic atrophy, dementia, or extrapyramidal features	SCA1	Nondescriptive spinocerebellar ataxia with neuropathy and pyramidal signs
	SCA2	Slow saccades, myoclonus, areflexia
	SCA3	Bulging eyes, fasciolingual fasciculations, extrapyramidal signs
	SCA4	Sensory neuropathy
	SCA12	Tremor, dementia
	Possibly DRPLA	Chorea, seizures, myoclonus
ADCA II Ataxia with pigmentary maculopathy with or without ophthalmoplegia or extrapyramidal features	SCA7	Macular degeneration
ADCAIII Relatively pure ataxia	SCA5	Slow course despite early onset
	SCA6	Very late onset, mild, apparently sporadic onset
	SCA8	Mild
	SCA10	Generalized complex partial seizures
	SCA11	Mild
	SCA13	Mental retardation
	SCA14	Occasional myoclonus

ADCA – autosomal dominant cerebellar ataxia, SCA – spinocerebellar ataxia. Note: ADCA IV (myoclonus and deafness) includes SCA14, DRPLA, mitochondrial disorders; ADCA V (essential tremor) includes SCA12 and SCA16; ADCA VI (episodic) includes EA1, EA2, EA3, EA4, and early SCA6.

Recessively inherited and X-linked ataxias

- About one half of patients with a hereditary ataxia have a recessively inherited condition.
- The two most common and important conditions are ataxia telangiectasia (AT) and Friedreich ataxia (FRDA)

1 **Ataxic telangiectasia (AT)**
  - **Most common form of infantile-onset cerebellar ataxia.**
  - It is a systemic condition resulting from defective DNA repair.
  - In classic form, progressive gait unsteadiness begins in the 2nd year of life, soon after learning to walk. Slurred speech and poor hand coordination follow.

Gaze apraxia and extremely slow saccades are also present. Some have choreoathetosis.

- Associated with recurrent sinopulmonary infections, cutaneous telangiectasia, and a higher frequency of lymphoreticular malignancy.

2 **Friedreich ataxia (FRDA)**

- **Most common hereditary ataxia; approximately one half of all cases.**
- The diagnosis is confirmed by finding a GAA repeat expansion in the frataxin gene, associated with 66 to more than 1700 repeats.
- Age of onset is usually 2–25 years, with progressive gait unsteadiness, posterior column signs, dysarthria, optic atrophy, and sensory neuropathy.
- Common non-neurological manifestations include cardiomyopathy (the most frequent cause of death), kyphoscoliosis, and diabetes mellitus.
- Variants of FRDA include late-onset Friedreich ataxia (LOFA), Friedreich ataxia with retained reflexes (FARR), and Acadian form of Friedreich ataxia.

3 Ataxia with isolated vitamin E deficiency (AVED)

- A very rare form of autosomal recessive ataxia; clinically similar to FRDA.
- Patients usually present < 20 years of age with progressive gait ataxia and dysarthria. Diffuse muscle weakness, retinopathy, and dystonia may occur.
- Diagnosis is confirmed by severely reduced or absent vitamin E level.
- Underlying pathogenesis is caused by defective α-MTP, a cytosolic liver protein.

4 Others causes of non-dominant ataxias: individually rare

- Abetalipoproteinemia, hypobetalipoproteinemia
- Aminoacidopathy: Hartnup disease, maple syrup urine disease, many others
- Autosomal recessive spastic ataxia of Charlevoix-Saguenay
- Baltic myoclonus (Unverricht-Lundborg): progressive myoclonus and ataxia

Chorea

- Chorea refers to an irregular, nonrhythmic, rapid, unsustained involuntary movement that flows from one part of the body to another.
- It is differentiated from other types of movement disorders by its unpredictable quality and its unpatterned direction, timing, and distribution.
- One of the characteristic features is motor impersistence (or negative chorea). A common example is dropping objects.
- Many of the causes of chorea are apparent from the history. The most common cause of chorea in adults is Huntington disease, whereas infections and cardiac surgery constitute the most common causes in children.

1 Primary chorea:

  1.1 **Huntington disease**

- The most common cause of chorea in adults.
- A trinucleotide repeat disorder (CAG) of chromosome 4 that causes the production of an abnormal protein, called huntingtin.
- There is an inverse correlation between repeat length and age of onset.

  1.2 Other causes of hereditary chorea

- Benign hereditary chorea
- Neuroacanthocytosis

2 Secondary chorea:

  2.1 **Infections**

    2.1.1 Sydenham chorea

- A common cause in childhood.
- Neurological complication of group A streptococcal infection.
- May occur as a part of manifestations of rheumatic fever.
- Acute onset clinical syndrome that involves chorea, dysarthria, weakness, and behavior changes.
- Self-limited illness with a good prognosis for recovery.

    2.1.2 Other infectious causes

- Bacterial and TB meningitis
- Encephalitis
- HIV infection

  2.2 Drug-induced chorea

- Drugs known to cause chorea include neuroleptics, dopamine agonists, levodopa, lithium, cocaine, and anticonvulsants.
- Chorea does not always remit with the discontinuation of the offending drug.
- **Tardive dyskinesia** is a term used when the chorea occurs after use of dopamine blocking agents for more than three months.

  2.3 **Post-cardiac surgery** (in children)

- Up to 10–18% of children with congenital heart disease, post-bypass
- Typically resolves in weeks/months
- Often associated with some cognitive disturbance

  2.4 Immune-mediated chorea

- 4% of patients with systemic lupus have chorea during exacerbation.
- Associated with antiphospholipid syndrome.

  2.5 Others

- Structural lesions of the striatum have been reported to cause chorea.
- Toxins, such as carbon monoxide
- Multiple sclerosis
- Anoxic encephalopathy
- Chorea gravidarum
- Birth control pills

Inherited neurological disorders with prominent chorea

- Orofacial dyskinesias and choreiform movements can be prominent manifestations of inherited diseases of the central nervous system.
- Chorea is characterized as primary, when idiopathic or genetic in origin, or secondary, when related to infectious, immunological, or other medical causes
- Most of these diseases are very rare, with the exception of Huntington chorea.
- Huntington disease is a choreic prototypic disorder and is probably the most common inherited movement disorder.

1 **Huntington disease (HD)**
   - An autosomal dominant neurodegenerative disorder, caused by an expansion of an unstable trinucleotide repeat near the telomere of chromosome 4.
   - Clinical features include involuntary movements of mainly chorea, psychiatric disturbances, and cognitive decline.
2 Benign hereditary chorea
   - A distinct disease of early onset, nonprogressive uncomplicated chorea
3 Neuroacanthocytosis
   - A rare multisystem degenerative disorder of unknown etiology that is featured clinically by the presence of deformed erythrocytes with spicules known as acanthocytes and abnormal involuntary movements.
4 Dentatorubralpallidoluysian atrophy (DRPLA)
   - A trinucleotide repeat polyglutamine disorder with the gene defect localized to chromosome 12. It is inherited in an autosomal dominant fashion, and clinical features include chorea, myoclonus, ataxia, epilepsy, and cognitive decline.
5 Wilson disease
   - A systemic disorder of copper metabolism that is transmitted as an autosomal recessive trait with an abnormal gene mapped to chromosome 13q.
6 Others: very rare disorders, for example;
   - Paroxysmal choreoathetosis
   - Familial chorea-ataxia-myoclonus syndrome
   - Pantothenate kinase-associated neurodegeneration (PKAN or Hallervorden-Spatz syndrome)

Distinguishing features between Huntington disease and benign hereditary chorea

Features	Huntington disease (HD)	Benign hereditary chorea (BHC)
1) Age of onset	Approximately 40 years	Early childhood
2) Genetics	Unstable CAG repeats on chromosome 4	Mutation in TITF-1 gene on chromosome 14q
3) Natural history	Relentlessly progressive with mean duration of 17 years	Non-progressive with normal life expectancy
4) Motor impersistence	Characteristically present	None
5) Neuropsychiatric features	Depression with tendency to suicide, agitation, aggression, global cognitive impairment	None
6) Eye movement	Fixational instability, slowing of saccades, increased saccadic latency	Normal
7) MRI findings	Caudate atrophy, generalized cerebral atrophy	Normal

Drug-induced chorea

- Chorea may result from exposure to a variety of drugs.
- Certain drugs seem to require pre-existing basal ganglia dysfunction to induce chorea, such as contraceptive pills, levodopa, and dopamine agonists.
- Some other drugs, however, appear to be capable of inducing chorea to anyone exposed, for example, dopamine antagonists.
- The most prevalent types of drug-induced chorea result from treatment of elderly patients with dopamine antagonists, or of PD patients with levodopa.

	Neuroleptic-induced chorea	Levodopa-induced chorea in PD
Age of onset	Elderly > young	Young > elderly
Sex	Female > male	Female = male
Prevalence	10% after treatment	50% after 3–5 years of treatment
Characteristics	Buccolinguomasticatory movements, asymmetric in the limbs	Asymmetric, worse in the more severely Parkinsonian limbs
Pathophysiology	Unknown, possibly related to chemical denervation of striatal neurons	Unknown, possibly related to denervation hypersensitivity of dopamine receptors
Treatment	Discontinuation of neuroleptics, reserpine, tetrabenazine	Reduction of levodopa use, amantadine

Chorea in the elderly

- Although Huntington disease (HD) usually begins in early to mid-adulthood, it may also begin in childhood (Westphal variant) or after age 50 (late-onset HD).
- Late-onset HD accounts for approximately 25% of all HD cases, half of which do not present until after age 60.
- Late-onset HD is a potential diagnostic pitfall. The family history may be unknown, hidden, or misleading. In addition, patients usually have a slower disabling course, more subtle chorea, predominant gait disorder, dysphagia, or dysarthria.
- Most cases of chorea in the elderly are medication-induced or due to structural lesions, for example, in the subthalamic nucleus.

1 **Medication-induced**
   - Dopaminergics, e.g. in Parkinson disease patients on chronic levodopa treatment
   - Antidopaminergics, most commonly neuroleptics (tardive syndromes)
   - Amphetamines
   - Anticonvulsants
2 **Vascular**
   - Infarction of subthalamic nucleus may result in acute hemichorea or hemiballism.
3 Senile chorea
   - Unclear identity. Some authorities do not believe that this condition exists.
   - It is important to rule out late-onset HD and tardive syndrome.
   - Buccolingual chorea may be seen in the edentulous elderly.
4 Metabolic derangements
   - Hypo or hypernatremia
   - Hypo or hyperglycemia
   - Hyperthyroidism
   - Hypo or hyperparathyroidism
   - Polycythemia vera
5 Degenerative conditions
   - Late-onset HD
   - Dentatorubralpallidoluysian atrophy (DRPLA)
6 Others
   - Lupus or antiphospholipid antibody syndromes
   - Syphilis

Dystonia

- Dystonia is defined as a syndrome of sustained muscle contractions, frequently causing twisting, repetitive movements or abnormal postures.
- Important features of dystonia include sustained contractions, consistent directional or patterned character (predictable), and exacerbation during voluntary movements.
- A characteristic and unique feature of dystonia is the presence of sensory tricks (that is, tactile stimulus to a particular body part may alleviate the dystonia).
- Dystonia can be classified by age of onset, body region(s) affected, and etiology.

1 Primary dystonia (not associated with any laboratory abnormalities)
- Most childhood-onset dystonia begins with a leg or arm, and then spreads to other limbs and trunk. It is due to mutations in a gene located on chromosome 9q34 and classified as **DYT1 or Oppenheim dystonia.**
- Adult-onset primary dystonia usually starts in the neck, cranial muscles, or arm and progression is limited to adjacent muscles. Generalization and leg involvement are rare.

2 Secondary dystonia
  - 2.1 **Dystonia associated with environmental-exogenous factors** (80% of secondary dystonia)
    - 2.1.1 Tardive dystonia
      - □ The most common cause of secondary dystonia.
      - □ Usually secondary to dopamine receptor blockers.
    - 2.1.2 Perinatal cerebral anoxia (15%)
      - □ Onset can be delayed for years.
    - 2.1.3 *Focal lesions*
      - □ Hemidystonia can occur secondary to structural lesions (hemorrhage, tumor, or infarction) in the basal ganglia, usually the putamen.
  - 2.2 Inherited secondary dystonia
    - Dopa-responsive dystonia: DYT5, GTP cyclohydrolase 1
    - Dystonia-myoclonus syndrome
    - Ataxia telangiectasia
  - 2.3 Dystonia as a manifestation of neurodegenerative diseases (2–3% of secondary causes)
    - Idiopathic Parkinson disease
    - Parkinson-plus syndrome
    - Spinocerebellar ataxias 1–8
    - Huntington disease
  - 2.4 Psychogenic dystonia (< 5%)

Dopa-responsive dystonia (DRD) and important DDx

- Diagnostic errors as well as delayed diagnosis of DRD are frequent because knowledge of the disease is still limited, and also because there are many atypical presentations.
- Common misdiagnoses include spastic paraparesis, paraplegia, or diplegia due to hyperreflexia, extensor toes, and localization of disturbances in the lower limbs.
- Absence of history of perinatal distress or MRI abnormalities, or the presence of mild dystonic rigid features, full term birth, and/or diurnal worsening should suggest DRD. Dystonic cerebral palsy should be diagnosed cautiously in these settings.
- A dopa test is indicated even when the diagnosis of DRD is in the slightest doubt.

Features	DRD	Childhood-onset ITD	Childhood-onset PD	Dystonic cerebral palsy
Age at onset	0–12 years	Less common, <6 years	< 8 years	Infancy
Family history	Often	Maybe	Often	No
Perinatal distress	No	No	No	Yes
Initial signs or symptoms	Arm/leg dystonia	Foot dystonia, gait disorder	Bradykinesia, rigidity, resting tremor	Hypotonia
Later signs or symptoms	Axial dystonia rare, resting tremor late	Axial dystonia and resting tremor rare	Axial dystonia (65%)	Focal or axial dystonia, choreoathetosis
Diurnal worsening	Prominent	Sometimes	No	No
Hyperreflexia	Common	No	No	Yes, especially early
Levodopa responsiveness	Excellent at low doses	Partial response	Excellent at low to moderate doses	No

ITD – idiopathic torsion dystonia, PD – Parkinson disease.

Iatrogenic movement disorders

- The administration of drugs having antagonistic effects on striatal dopamine receptors is frequently associated with the development of different types of movement disorders.
- These disorders are most often seen in psychiatric patients undergoing neuroleptic treatment.
- The clinical presentation and time of onset of movement disorders resulting from the use of offending drugs are quite variable.
- Tardive syndromes often run a persistent fluctuating course despite cessation of therapy. Symptoms can become permanent and irreversible.

Dopamine antagonist-induced movement disorders

1 Acute onset

   1.1 Acute dystonic reaction

- Usually evident soon after the initiation of neuroleptic therapy (90% within 5 days of therapy), ranging from brief jerks to prolonged muscle spasms involving the craniocervical region.
- This reaction is often associated with psychiatric manifestations.
- Laryngeal muscles can be involved, resulting in respiratory difficulties.
- Risk factors include young male (<30 years old), high neuroleptic dosage, potency of the drug involved and familial predisposition.
- Treatment includes parenteral administration of anticholinergics and antihistamines.

   1.2 Acute akathisia

- Very common, very early and dose-related side-effect of neuroleptics.
- Usually self-limited upon discontinuation of neuroleptics.

2 Subacute onset

   2.1 Parkinsonism

   2.2 *Neuroleptic-induced malignant syndrome*

- Characterized by fever (may be low-grade or high), muscle rigidity, movement disorders, autonomic instability, and mental status changes.
- Usually occurs within the first two weeks of initiating dopamine receptor antagonists.
- Although rare (0.2%), it has rapid onset with severe medical complications (50%) and a high mortality rate (20%).

3 Chronic onset

   3.1 **Tardive syndromes**

- Refers to persistent, sometimes irreversible, abnormal involuntary movements appearing over the course of prolonged neuroleptic treatment.

- Tardive syndromes can reproduce almost the entire spectrum of known abnormal involuntary movements of the hyperkinetic type: tardive stereotypy, tardive dystonia, tardive tourettism, tardive tremor, tardive myoclonus, tardive akathisia.
- Buccolinguomasticatory syndrome is the most common form of tardive syndrome in clinical practice, especially in elderly subjects.

Tardive dyskinesia: risk factors

- Tardive dyskinesia is an involuntary movement disorder that occurs with long-term neuroleptic use, usually after 1 year of treatment.
- Patients may have buccolinguomasticatory movements and athetoid movements of the arms, legs, and trunk.
- The main treatment is the withdrawal of the offending agent. The symptoms usually remit in 40% of patients after discontinuation.
- Numerous medications have been used to treat this condition; reserpine is usually considered to be the most effective. Other agents include atypical antispychotics, clonazepam, valproate, baclofen, and diltiazem.

Common risk factors for developing tardive dyskinesia include:
1 **Increasing age**
2 Female sex
3 Neuroleptic dose
4 Cumulative duration of neuroleptic exposure
5 Presence of dementia

Tardive syndromes: phenomenology

- The American Psychiatric Association Task Force requires 3 months of exposure to a dopamine receptor blocking agent (DRBA) for diagnosis of tardive syndromes, although tardive syndromes can occur in individuals 60 years of age or older after only 1 month of exposure to a DRBA.
- There are several phenomenologically distinct types of tardive syndromes that are historically referred to as tardive dyskinesia (TD). However, the term TD is used to refer to a specific subtype, characterized by oro-buccal-lingual dyskinesias.
- Among all tardive syndromes, tardive dyskinesia (TD) is the most common form.
- There are other types of tardive syndromes in addition to those described in the list below, including tardive myoclonus, tardive tremor, and tardive tourettism. It remains unclear if tardive Parkinsonism truly exists.

1 **Tardive dyskinesia (TD)**
   1.1 Definition: TD that presents with rapid, repetitive, stereotypic movements involving oral, buccal, and lingual areas
   1.2 Epidemiology: **most common of all tardive syndromes**. Annual incidence: 5% in the young and 12% in the elderly. In general, 20% of patients on neuroleptics are affected by TD.
   1.3 Differential:
      ▪ Spontaneous buccal-lingual dyskinesia of the elderly
      ▪ Edentulous dyskinesia
      ▪ Hereditary choreas (e.g. HD)
      ▪ SLE, vasculitides
      ▪ Wilson disease
   1.4 Treatment: mild TD – reducing the neuroleptic dose, switching to atypical agent, or discontinuing antipsychotic treatment.
2 Tardive dystonia
   2.1 Definition: tardive syndrome that presents with co-contraction of agonist and antagonist muscles, resulting in twisting, abnormal posture and turning.
   2.2 Epidemiology: prevalence 2–20%, more common in younger men. DRBA exposure may be shorter for tardive dystonia, compared to TD.
   2.3 Differential:
      ▪ Idiopathic torsion dystonia
      ▪ Meige syndrome
      ▪ Oromandibular dystonia
      ▪ Wilson disease
   2.4 Treatment: same as TD.
3 Tardive akathisia
   3.1 Definition: tardive syndrome that is characterized by a feeling of inner restlessness/jitteriness, often objectively manifest by semipurposeful movements.
   3.2 Epidemiology: usually accompanied by other tardive syndromes. Exact incidence is unclear, between 20–40% of DRBA-treated patients with schizophrenia. Mean DRBA exposure of 4.5 years with mean age of onset of 58 years.
   3.3 Differential:
      ▪ Restless leg syndrome
      ▪ Anxiety/hyperactivity disorder
      ▪ Stereotypy
      ▪ Drug-induced, e.g. levodopa, dopamine agonists
   3.4 Treatment: same as TD.
4 Withdrawal emergent syndrome

4.1 Definition: a benign tardive syndrome occurring mainly in children who were abruptly withdrawn from their chronic neuroleptic therapy. Movements are choreic, random, and involve mainly the limbs, trunk, and neck.

4.2 Treatment: the movements usually last for weeks, but DRBAs can be reinstituted for immediate suppression or withdrawn gradually.

Tardive syndromes: DDx

- Tardive syndromes are a group of disorders characterized by predominantly late-onset and sometimes persistent abnormal involuntary movements (or a sensation of restlessness) caused by exposure to a dopamine receptor blocking agent (DRBA) within 6 months of the onset of symptoms and persisting for at least 1 month after stopping the offending drug.
- Common DRBAs include traditional neuroleptics, drugs for nausea (metoclopramide and prochlorperazine), and depression (amoxapine).
- Age has been the most consistent risk factor for TD. Higher incidence and lower remission rates are noted in older patients, especially among women.
- The only way to prevent these syndromes is to avoid the etiologic agents.

The diagnosis of a tardive syndrome can be easy in most cases and should be based on a complete neuropsychiatric history and examination. However, the diagnosis can be challenging in older patients with a history of dementia.

Conditions that may mimic tardive syndromes include:

1 **Benign conditions in the elderly**
   1.1 Spontaneous buccal-lingual dyskinesias of the elderly
   1.2 Edentulous dyskinesia

2 **Hereditary choreas**
   2.1 Huntington disease (HD)
       ■ TD primarily involves the tongue, lips, and jaw causing twisting, protrusion, lip smacking, and puckering. The stereotypic pattern is in contrast to the dyskinesias seen in HD, where movements are random and unpredictable.
   2.2 Benign hereditary chorea
   2.3 Wilson disease

3 Medical conditions
   3.1 Hyperthyroidism
   3.2 Systemic lupus erythematosus or other vasculitides
   3.3 Polycythemia vera
   3.4 Sydenham chorea

4 Non-DRBAs that can cause dyskinesias (exact mechanism unclear)
   ◆ Levodopa

- Amphetamines
- Cocaine
- Cimetidine
- Cinnarizine
- Antihistamines
- Phenytoin
- Lithium

Myoclonus

- Myoclonus is defined as sudden, brief, jerky, and shock-like involuntary movements involving the face, trunk, and extremities.
- Most myoclonic jerks are caused by abrupt muscle contractions ('**positive myoclonus**'), but abrupt movements are also caused by sudden cessation of muscle contraction associated with a silent period on EMG ('**negative myoclonus' or asterixis**).
- The diagnostic approach to myoclonus is first to identify the site of origin (cortical vs. subcortical vs. brainstem vs. spinal) and then establish the cause.
- Myoclonus may be physiologic, such as hiccups and sleep jerks.

Localizations and etiologies:
1 **Cortical myoclonus**
   - Most commonly encountered.
   - Cortical myoclonus is seen in a variety of diseases but the most common and important underlying etiology is generalized epilepsy.
      - 1.1 Progressive myoclonic epilepsy
         - Has various diseases as the underlying cause; mostly hereditary.
         - 1.1.1 Progressive myoclonic epilepsy of unknown etiology
         - 1.1.2 Progressive myoclonic ataxia
      - 1.2 Juvenile myoclonic epilepsy
      - 1.3 **Postanoxic myoclonus** (Lance-Adams syndrome)
         - Most common cause of myoclonus in the intensive care unit setting.
      - 1.4 Others
         - Creutzfeldt-Jakob disease
         - Corticobasal ganglionic degeneration
         - Rett syndrome
2 Subcortical myoclonus
   - Myoclonus from brainstem origin may present as exaggerated startle reflex or hyperekplexia, brainstem reticular myoclonus, or palatal myoclonus syndrome.
3 Spinal myoclonus
   - Spinal segmental myoclonus can occur secondary to focal spinal cord pathology.

- Propiospinal myoclonus produces generalized axial jerks.

4 Peripheral myoclonus

- Myoclonus can occur secondary to peripheral lesions in the spinal roots, plexus, or nerve. An example is hemifacial spasm.

Parkinsonism

- Parkinsonism is applied to neurological syndromes in which patients exhibit some combination of resting tremor, rigidity, bradykinesia, and loss of postural reflexes.
- Parkinson disease (PD) is the most common form of Parkinsonism (77%), with an incidence of 200 per 100,000 in the general population.
- One of the major problems when seeing patients with Parkinsonism is to distinguish PD from its clinical imitators.
- Before diagnosing patients with PD or other neurodegenerative disorders, it is important to exclude any treatable and reversible causes, such as drug-induced or structural lesions.

1 **Idiopathic Parkinson disease (77%)**
2 **Parkinson-plus syndromes (12%)**
    2.1 Multiple system atrophy (MSA): autonomic instability
    2.2 Corticobasal ganglionic degeneration (CBGD): alien hand syndrome
    2.3 Progressive supranuclear palsy (PSP): slow and restricted vertical saccades
    2.4 Diffuse Lewy body disease (DLB): prominent visual hallucinations
3 **Drug-induced Parkinsonism (5%)**: common drugs include
    3.1 Dopamine receptor blockers
        ▪ Neuroleptics
        ▪ Antiemetics
    3.2 Dopamine depletors; reserpine, tetrabenazine
    3.3 Calcium channel blockers
4 Other neurodegenerative conditions
- Alzheimer disease
- Pick disease
- Motor neuron disease-Parkinsonism
5 Toxic, metabolic, and infectious causes
- Toxins: carbon monoxide, manganese, methanol, cyanide, disulfiram
- Metabolic: hepatolenticular degeneration, Wilson disease, hypocalcemic Parkinsonism, post-anoxic Parkinsonism
- Infectious causes: fungal, toxoplasmosis, HIV, post-encephalitic Parkinsonism (1960+)

6 *Structural lesions (rare causes of Parkinsonism but should be excluded in suspected cases)*
   - Normal pressure hydrocephalus
   - Communicating hydrocephalus
   - Subdural hematoma
7 Others
   - Vascular Parkinsonism
   - Other neurodegenerative conditions, such as PKAN, Huntington disease, Neuroacanthocytosis
   - Familial conditions such as SCA1, 2, 3, 12, FTD with Parkinsonism

Tremor in Parkinson disease vs. essential tremor

- 3–6 Hz resting tremor with pill-rolling is typical.
- Besides resting tremor, up to 40% of PD patients have postural and/or action tremor, which can occur in isolation or together with resting tremor.
- The differential diagnosis of tremor in PD and classical essential tremor (ET) can be difficult, especially in the early stage of the condition.
- It has been estimated that 20% of patients with ET are misdiagnosed for PD and vice versa.

Features	Parkinsonian tremor	Essential tremor
Tremor	At rest, increases with walking. Decreases with posture holding or action	Posture holding or action
Frequency	3–6 Hz	5–12 Hz
Distribution	Asymmetric	Symmetric
Body parts	Hands and legs	Hands, head, voice
Writing	Micrographia	Tremulous
Course	Progressive	Stable or slowly progressive
Family history	Less common	Often
Other neurological signs	Bradykinesia, rigidity, loss of postural reflexes	None
Substances that improve tremor	Levodopa, anticholinergics	Alcohol, propanolol, primidone
Surgical treatment	Patients usually have other Parkinsonian features, requiring subthalamic nucleus or internal globus pallidus deep brain stimulation (DBS)	Thalamic VIM DBS or thalamotomy

Young-onset Parkinson disease: DDx

- Young-onset Parkinson disease (YOPD) is arbitrarily defined as that which produces initial symptoms between the ages of 21 and 39, inclusive.
- In contrast to juvenile Parkinsonism, which is a heterogeneous group of clinicopathologic entities presenting before age 21, YOPD appears to be the same nosologic entity as older-onset PD.
- YOPD comprises approximately 5% of referral populations in Western countries and about 10% in Japan.
- In general, YOPD tends to have more gradual progression of Parkinsonian signs and symptoms, earlier appearance of levodopa-induced dyskinesias and levodopa-dose-related motor fluctuations and frequent presence of dystonia as an early presenting sign.
- The most important differential diagnosis in patients presenting with Parkinsonian signs before the age of 40 is Wilson disease. The absence of Kayser-Fleischer rings or of a positive family history must not deter one from obtaining screening blood tests including ceruloplasmin and copper levels.

Some differences between young-onset PD and older-onset PD are provided in the table below.

Features	YOPD	Older-onset (typical) PD
Age of onset	21–39 years	After 40 years
Annual incidence	0.15/100,000	1.5/100,000 (60–64 years)
Dystonia at onset	15–50%	Very rare
Disease progression	Slower	Faster
Motor complications after 3 years of levodopa treatment:		
• Dyskinesia	72%	28%
• Dose-related fluctuations	64%	28%
Dementia	Less common	More common

Ref: Golbe LI. Young-onset Parkinson disease. A clinical review. *Neurology* 1991; 41: 168–173.

Surgical treatment of Parkinson disease

- There are three types of approaches to surgery for Parkinson disease (PD):
  - ablative surgery,
  - deep brain stimulation (DBS), and
  - restorative therapies, including intracerebral cell transplantation or growth factor infusion.

- Currently, there are three surgical targets for ablative surgery and DBS:
  - the globus pallidus interna (GPi),
  - the subthalamic nucleus (STN), and
  - the motor thalamus (Vim).
- Surgical destruction of portions of the GPi is called pallidotomy, and destruction of the motor thalamus is called thalamotomy.
- Deep brain stimulation is gaining popularity over ablative procedures and is increasingly considered as the surgical procedure of choice in PD. The mechanism of DBS is not exactly known but may be related to activation of inhibitory presynaptic axons, depolarization blockade, block of ion channels, synaptic exhaustion, or jamming. At present, it is still unclear which target between GPi and STN is preferable for DBS, although STN is considered by many experts to be the 'favorite'.

DBS surgery: advantages and disadvantages over ablative procedures

Advantages	Disadvantages
Reversible	Expensive
Adjustable setting	Requires expertise and training
Less tissue is destroyed	Available only in major medical centers
Does not exclude patients from future therapies	Time consuming for both physicians and patients for programming and frequent visits
Benefits are easy to document objectively	Hardware problems can occur as well as infections

DBS Surgery: Choice of surgical target

Surgical target	Potential benefits	Possible side-effects
Nucleus ventralis intermedius thalami (Vim)	• Effective on tremor • No improvement on rigidity, bradykinesia • Adjustment of stimulator parameters and medication simple • Potentially useful in older patients with a monosymptomatic tremor at rest or tremor-dominant PD with little rigidity and akinesia	• Risk of dysarthria, balance problems with bilateral procedures

Surgical target	Potential benefits	Possible side-effects
Globus pallidus interna (GPi)	• Effective on all cardinal symptoms of PD • Significant reduction of dyskinesia • Few therapy-related side-effects • Postoperative adjustment of stimulator parameters and medication simple and less time consuming	• Larger energy consumption • No benefits of dose reduction of dopaminergic therapy
Subthalamic nucleus (STN)	• Effective on all cardinal symptoms of PD • Significant reduction of dopaminergic medications postoperatively • Significant reduction of dyskinesias • Low energy consumption	• Risks of psychiatric and neurobehavior side-effects • Adjustment of stimulator parameters and medication more complex and time consuming

Paroxysmal movement disorders

- Paroxysmal movement disorders are the most common movement abnormalities encountered by pediatric neurologists.
- The list of this differential is extensive, although it is useful to categorize it by first identifying the type of movement disorders.
- Although it is often difficult to witness the movements in person, it is often useful to see and identify the movement, possibly by video recording, as the history and description can be vague and inconclusive.

1 **Tic disorder: the most common type of paroxysmal movement disorder**
   - Refers to brief, intermittent movements (motor tics) or sounds (phonic tics).
   - Tics can be simple (involving only one group of muscle), complex, part of Tourette syndrome, or caused by neuroleptic exposure (tardive tourettism).
2 Paroxysmal choreoathetosis or dystonia
   - Heterogeneous group of disorders that present with sudden abnormal involuntary movements out of a background normal behavior. May have a dominant familial component or be sporadic.
   - Abnormal movements can be complex, including a combination of dystonia, chorea, athetosis, and ballistic. The condition is often mistakenly labeled psychogenic.
   - Commonly used classification identifies four variants:
     - Parosymal kinesogenic dyskinesia (PKD)
     - Paroxysmal nonkinesogenic dyskinesia (PNKD)

- Paroxysmal exertional-induced dyskinesia (PED)
- Paroxysmal hypnogenic dyskinesia (PHD)

3 Startle (hyperekplexia)
- A startle response is a brief motor response, usually a jerk, elicited by an unexpected auditory, or less commonly tactile or vestibular, stimulus.
- A normal startle response usually involves the upper half of the body and habituates, while startle syndrome usually elicits greater movement amplitudes, is more widely distributed and habituates poorly.
- In startle syndromes, the startle is usually followed by another movement abnormality, like tonic spasm, or is associated with nocturnal myoclonic jerks.

4 Stereotypy
- A repetitive nonfunctioning motor behavior, that is monotonous in fashion without apparent conscious control, despite a normal level of consciousness.
- Stereotypy can be distinguished from tics by easy suppressibility without the tension buildup that often accompanies suppression of a tic.

5 Ataxia
- Episodic ataxia is rare, caused by a point mutation in the voltage-gated potassium channel gene KCNA1.
- A second, milder type is associated with a mutation in the voltage-gated calcium channel gene CACNL1A4.
- Clinically, it is characterized by attacks of ataxia and dysarthria (less often dystonia or chorea) lasting for seconds to minutes, provoked by movements or startles.

Psychogenic movement disorders

- Neurologic dysfunction of psychogenic origin has been reported to occur in 1–9% of all neurological diagnoses. Abnormal movements or motor disorders are among the most frequent symptoms.
- The presence of a psychiatric disorder does not prove that the movement disorder is psychogenic.
- The diagnosis of psychogenic movement disorders should be a diagnosis of exclusion and is best made by a neurologist familiar with movement disorders.

When this diagnosis is considered, the correct psychiatric diagnosis may fall under the categories listed in the DSM-IV. The following psychiatric disorders can be associated with psychogenic movement disorders:

1 Somatoform disorders
2 Malingering
3 Depression
4 Anxiety

5 Histrionic personality disorder (very rare)

Clinical features that are suggestive of psychogenic movement disorders include:
1 Acute onset
2 Static course
3 Inconsistent character of movements
4 Movement increases with attention
5 Movement decreases with distraction
6 Responsive to placebo
7 Remission with psychotherapy
8 Diagnosed psychopathology

Tics

- Tics refer to spontaneous, purposeless, simple, and complex movements or vocalizations that abruptly interrupt normal motor activity.
- Often associated with an urge to make the movement: sensory tics.
- Temporarily suppressible (myoclonus is not).
- Cease during sleep.
- Associated with obsessive-compulsive disorder.
- Rarely associated with brain lesions.

1 Idiopathic: most likely these represent a diagnostic continuum
   1.1 **Transient tic disorder**
      - Most common, affecting up to 15% of children
      - Boys especially affected
      - Involves motor or vocal tics but not both
      - Lasts more than 1 but less than 12 months
      - Onset before 21 years old
   1.2 Chronic motor or vocal tic disorder
      - Same as above except for duration of more than 12 months.
   1.3 **Gilles de la Tourette syndrome**
      - Multiple motor tics and at least one vocal tic
      - Onset before 21 years old
2 Secondary
   2.1 Tics as components of specific neurodegenerative disease
      - Huntington disease
      - Neuroacanthocytosis
   2.2 Tics in association with neurodevelopmental disorders
      - Learning disability
      - Autism
      - Schizophrenia

2.3 Medication-induced tics
- Amphetamine, cocaine
- Levodopa
- Neuroleptics (tardive tourettism)
- Carbamazepine, phenytoin

2.4 Tics following acute brain injury (rare)
- Stroke (case report of caudate infarct)
- Encephalitis lethargica (called 'klazomania')
- Sydenham chorea

2.5 PANDAS (pediatric autoimmune neuropsychiatric diseases associated with streptococcal infection)
- Associated with:
  □ onset between 3 and 12 years
  □ obsessive-compulsive disorder
  □ abrupt onset or abrupt worsening of symptoms
  □ onset/exacerbation temporally associated with group A beta hemolytic streptococcal infection
  □ neurological abnormalities, including choreoathetosis and/or tics

Tics: characteristics and differentiation from other movement disorders

- Tics are repetitive, stereotyped, involuntary, sudden, inopportune, non-propositional, and irresistible movements involving skeletal and pharyngo-laryngeal muscles. The latter are responsible for emission of sounds or noises.
- The involuntary nature is not absolutely clear as patients can exert some control over the movements. Moreover, they are 'urged' to do it as a compulsive action.
- The voluntary suppression of tics generates an unpleasant feeling that is resolved with the execution of the tics. Frequent tics can produce pain.
- Tics can be divided into simple motor, complex motor, and phonic tics. The association with multiple motor and phonic tics before the age of 21 is required for the diagnosis of Tourette syndrome.

Unique features of tics include:
1 Patients can partially control them (temporarily suppressible).
2 Tics may increase with stress or anxiety.
3 Tics do not generally interfere with voluntary activities, for example, they do not alter handwriting.
4 Tics predominate facial muscles, trunk, and proximal parts of the limbs. The further from the face, the rarer the involvement.

5 Tics generally do not persist during sleep.
6 Clinical course of tics usually fluctuates in severity, and the majority of tics tend to improve in adulthood.

Tremor

- A rhythmic oscillation of a body part produced by alternating or synchronous contraction of opposing muscles.
- Tremors can be classified on the basis of clinical appearance, distribution, and/or etiology. The following two main categories are described: at rest and with action.
- Tremors can be physiological. The most common cause of rest tremor is Parkinsonian tremor, while essential tremor is the most common cause of action tremor. 40% of patients with Parkinson disease may also have postural tremor.

1 Rest tremor
 - Tremor which is present when a limb is fully supported against gravity and the relevant muscles are not voluntarily activated.
 - The amplitude of tremor increases during mental and sometimes motor activation.
 - Usually 3–6 Hz tremor occurring at rest, suppressed by posture-holding or action.
 - The classical tremor of **Parkinson disease** is a tremor at rest, but it tends to recur when the limbs are outstretched.
2 Action tremor
 - Tremor occurring during any voluntary muscle contraction. Types include the following:
   2.1 Postural tremor
    - Tremor apparent during the voluntary maintenance of a particular posture, which is opposed by the force of gravity.
    - Examples include **exaggerated physiological tremor, essential tremor**, and midbrain or rubral tremor.
   2.2 Intention tremor
    - Action tremor that increases towards the end of goal-directed movement.
    - Suggests a clinical localization to the cerebellum or its outflow tracts.
   2.3 Kinetic tremor
    - A tremor that occurs during any voluntary movements. Kinetic tremor can occur in non-goal-directed and goal-directed movements.
    - Example includes dystonic tremor, **essential tremor**.
   2.4 Task-specific tremor

- Tremor which occurs only during the performance of highly skilled activities such as writing, playing musical instruments, etc.
- Examples include variants of essential tremor, such as primary writing tremor, isolated voice tremor.
2.5 Isometric tremor
  - Tremor which occurs when a voluntary muscle contraction is opposed by rigid stationary object.

Specific clinical differentials

Dopa-responsive movement disorders

- Although the mechanism of hypokinetic-rigid syndrome is thought to be secondary to defective dopaminergic activity, not all cases will respond to the administration of levodopa or dopamine agonists.
- Patients with idiopathic Parkinson disease have a remarkable response to dopaminergic medications. In other conditions of hypokinetic-rigid syndromes, the degree of responsiveness varies.
- Dopaminergic medications should be considered in all cases with hypokinetic-rigid syndrome to assess the responsiveness. Levodopa should always be given with peripheral decarboxylase inhibitor (carbidopa or benserazide).

1 Conditions with an excellent response to dopaminergic medications
  1.1 **Idiopathic Parkinson disease**
  - Levodopa is the most effective treatment.
  - Most patients with PD have a remarkable response to levodopa. This effect is commonly used to determine if patients have PD.
  1.2 **Dopa-responsive dystonia** (hereditary progressive dystonia with diurnal fluctuations or Segawa disease)
  - Characterized by dystonia, Parkinsonism, hyperreflexia, and a good response to low doses of levodopa.
  - The dystonia is usually better in the morning and increases during the day.
  - The onset is usually within the first 12 years of life (Median age is 4.5 years).
  - The first symptoms are insidious, with fatigability, clumsiness of gait, and dystonic posture of one foot.
2 Conditions with a partial response to dopaminergic medications
  2.1 **Parkinson-plus syndromes**
  - Multisystem atrophy (MSA): 40% have a partial response to levodopa.

- Corticobasal ganglionic degeneration (CBGD), progressive supranuclear palsy (PSP): 10–20% with minimal response.

2.2 Machado-Joseph disease or spinocerebellar ataxia type 3 (SCA3)
  - Autosomal dominant disorder with variable clinical expression.
  - Clinically, it is characterized by cerebellar and progressive external ophthalmoplegia, spasticity, and late peripheral neuropathy.

2.3 Other very rare disorders
  - Rapid-onset dystonia Parkinsonism
  - X-linked dystonia Parkinsonism
  - Hydrocephalic Parkinsonism

Involuntary forceful eye closure

- Involuntary, inappropriate, forceful eye closure is termed blepharospasm.
- The most common presentation is essential blepharospasm, which is a form of adult-onset focal dystonia. It typically affects both eyes symmetrically and begins insidiously in the 5th to 7th decade of life.

1 **Essential blepharospasm**
  - **The most common cause of involuntary forceful eye closure.**
  - A form of adult-onset focal dystonia.
  - Almost always bilateral.
  - Meige syndrome: blepharospasm associated with oromandibular, laryngeal, and cervical dystonia.
  - Prodromal symptoms including photophobia and ocular discomfort are common.

2 Secondary blepharospasm
  - Blepharospasm can be a feature of ocular diseases, such as corneal abrasion.
  - Blepharospasm is seen in about 25% of patients with neurodegenerative conditions; for example, progressive supranuclear palsy (PSP), generalized dystonia, and idiopathic Parkinson disease.

3 Apraxia of eyelid opening
  - Sometimes called atypical blepharospasm or akinetic blepharospasm.
  - Characterized by excessive eyelid closure, due to failure to activate the levator palpebrae muscle.
  - A useful clue to differentiate from blepharospasm is that the lower eyelid tends to be elevated in blepharospasm.

4 Motor tics
  - Frequently present as increased blink rate or forceful blinking and even persistent blepharospasm.

5 Psychogenic causes
  - Psychogenic blepharospasm is unusual.

Primary neurological conditions associated with several types of movement disorders (mixed movement disorders)

- In some disorders, several types of movement disorders may coexist and none is characteristic. Therefore, early diagnosis is often difficult in these conditions.
- Wilson disease is the most common condition of this group. Wilson disease should be considered in all cases under the age of 40 with any types of movement disorders. Clinical presentation can be quite variable.
- In these conditions, any type of movement disorder, can occur, although dystonia tends to be the most common.

1 **Wilson disease** (familial progressive hepatolenticular degeneration)
   - Caused by abnormal deposition of copper in the liver, brain, cornea, and other tissues.
   - Autosomal recessive inheritance with the gene mapped to chromosome 13. The basic defect is of P-type ATPase involved in the cellular transport of copper.
   - Neurological manifestations usually appear after the age of 10 with the dystonic form being the most common. Others include pseudo-sclerotic form, rigid-akinetic form, and choreic form. About one-third of patients present for fairly long periods with mental deterioration and psychiatric problems.
2 Pantothenate kinase associated neurodegeneration (PKAN or Hallervorden-Spatz syndrome)
   - Characterized clinically by a progressive movement disorder, usually with dystonia or Parkinsonism, associated with dementia and pyramidal tract signs.
   - The most specific pathological finding includes dysmyelination and deposition of iron-staining pigments in the pallidum and the substantia nigra pars reticulate.
   - Main clinical feature depends upon age of onset: early onset – delay in walking; juvenile onset – dystonia; late onset – hypokinetic rigid syndrome.
3 Machado-Joseph disease or spinocerebellar ataxia type 3 (SCA3)
   - Autosomal dominant disorder with variable clinical expression.
   - Clinically, it is characterized by cerebellar, progressive external ophthalmoplegia, spasticity, and late peripheral neuropathy.
4 Dentatorubralpallidoluysian atrophy (DRPLA)
   - Autosomal dominant disorder associated with unstable expansion of CAG trinucleotide on chromosome 12p.
   - Alternative diagnoses include: mitochondrial encephalopathies, cerebellar ataxias, and Huntington disease (HD). The most common misdiagnosis is HD.
   - As a rule, DRPLA should be considered in families initially diagnosed as having HD when this has been excluded.
5 Familial progressive encephalopathy with calcification of the basal ganglia

♦ Autosomal recessive disorder with presominant dystonia, spasticity, acquired microcephaly, and abnormal ocular movements in the first year of life.

Recurrent facial twitches

- Recurrent facial twitches normally involve muscles innervated by the facial nerve.
- They are typically unilateral and the lesion localization tends to be peripheral, involving different parts of the facial nerve or muscles supplied by its nerve.
- Associated facial weakness is a common finding.

1 **Hemifacial spasm**
   - ♦ **The most common cause of recurrent facial twitches**.
   - ♦ Hemifacial spasm is peripherally induced and is not a form of focal dystonia as commonly misinterpreted.
   - ♦ As its name states, it is almost always unilateral.
   - ♦ Typically, it is more common in women and it starts in the orbicularis oculi, spreading slowly to other muscles over months or years. Eye closure and mouth retraction are the most commonly encountered movements.
   - ♦ Mild lower motor neuron facial weakness with a slightly closed palpebral fissure is characteristic and nearly always diagnostic. There are no other associated cranial nerve signs.
2 Essential blepharospasm
   - ♦ Typically bilateral and involves only the peri-orbital areas.
3 Focal seizures
   - ♦ Less frequent for seizure activity to localize only in the face, but this can occur; for example, epilepsia partialis continua.
4 Facial myokymia
   - ♦ Characterized by subtle, continuous, ripple-like quivering, usually over small areas of the face
5 Facial tics
   - ♦ Usually not limited to one side of the face.
6 Bell palsy with aberrant regeneration and synkinesia
   - ♦ There is usually a clear history of lower motor neuron facial weakness before the appearance of facial twitching.

Restless legs syndrome: causes

- Restless legs syndrome (RLS) is one of the most common movement disorders, with a prevalence of approximately 4%.

- The fundamental problem of RLS is a complex sensory-motor disorder, predominantly involving the legs.
- The International RLS Study Group has published major (minimal) criteria for the diagnosis of RLS and these include a desire to move the limbs, usually associated with paresthesia or dysesthesia, motor restlessness, worsening of symptoms or exclusive presence at rest, and worsening of symptoms in the evening or night.
- The physiological mechanism for RLS is unknown, although dopaminergic theory has gained the most popular support. The onset of disease is usually in middle-aged and elderly subjects. The course is usually chronic and progressive. Iron deficiency anemia is the most important provocative factor for RLS in which treating iron deficiency often improves RLS symptoms or patients' response to other RLS medications.
- The most important involuntary movements are periodic limb movements during sleep (PLMS), occurring in at least 80% of patients with RLS.

1 Idiopathic
2 Secondary causes
  2.1 Neurological disorders
  - **Polyneuropathy**, especially associated with diabetes mellitus
  - Parkinson disease
  - Lumbosacral radiculopathies
  - Amyotrophic lateral sclerosis
  - Multiple sclerosis
  - Myelopathies
  2.2 Medical conditions
  - **Anemia**, especially iron and folate deficiency anemia
  - **Uremia**
  - **Diabetes mellitus**
  - Rheumatoid arthritis
  - Peripheral vascular disease
  - Hypothyroidism
  - Gastrectomy
  2.3 Medications
  - **Caffeine**
  - **Withdrawal from sedatives or narcotics**
  - Neuroleptics
  - Lithium

Restless legs syndrome vs. akathisia

- Many conditions can mimic restless legs syndrome, although the most important and difficult condition to differentiate from RLS is akathisia. The main motor component of both conditions is restlessness.
- Others mimics include: painful leg and moving toes, myokymia, painful nocturnal leg cramps, hypnic jerks, muscular pain-fasciculation syndrome, causalgia-dystonia syndrome.

Features	Restless legs syndrome	Akathisia
Definition	Clinical diagnosis with the criteria, established by international RLS Study Group	Inner restlessness, fidgetiness with jittery feeling, or generalized restlessness
Occurs as a side-effect from neuroleptics	Less common	More common
Disease course	Chronic and progressive	Can be acute, chronic, or tardive
Character of restlessness	Tossing, turning in bed, floor pacing, leg stretching, leg flexion, foot rubbing	Swaying, rocking movements, crossing, uncrossing the legs, shifting body positions, inability to sit still, resembling mild chorea
Day/night	Worsening of symptoms in the evening or at night	Mostly during the day
Stress/rest	Worsening of symptoms or exclusively present at rest	Worsening with anxiety or stress
Distribution	Focal	More generalized
Family history	30–50%	No relevant family history
Abnormal sensation	Commonly described as creeping, crawling, cramping, and itching	Less common
Myoclonic jerks (associated)	Common	Uncommon
Treatment	Dopaminergic therapy	Anticholinergics, beta-adrenergic agonists

Sleep-associated movements and disorders: classification

- Movement disorders specialists tend to see patients with various involuntary movements that occur during the daytime, while sleep specialists are often consulted by patients with paroxysmal involuntary movements that occur during sleep at night. These daytime and night-time movement disorders are quite distinct from each other.

> • Movement disorders during sleep can be physiological. Pathological motor activity during sleep also includes motor parasomnias and nocturnal seizures, in addition to involuntary movement disorders.
> • Most involuntary movement disorders occur during the daytime and disappear during sleep. However, certain types of movement disorders can persist in sleep and their presence in sleep provides an important clue in differential diagnosis.

1 Physiological motor activity during sleep
   • Postural shifts, body and limb movements during sleep
   • Physiological fragmentary myoclonus
   • Hypnic jerks
   • Hypnagogic imagery
2 Pathological motor activity during sleep
   2.1 **Periodic limb movements in sleep (PLMS)**
      ▪ Characterized by periodically recurring stereotyped limb movements that occur during NREM sleep (stage I and II), most commonly, patients dorsiflex ankles or flex knees or hips every 20–40 seconds.
      ▪ PLMS is noted in at least 80% of cases of restless legs syndrome (RLS), while RLS is seen in 30% of cases of PLMS.
      ▪ PLMS can occur as an isolated condition, called periodic limb movement disorder (PLMD), or may be associated with other conditions, including Parkinson disease, neuropathies, general medical conditions, and medications, such as tricyclic antidepressants or levodopa.
   2.2 Involuntary movement disorders
      ▪ Always persisting during sleep:
         ▫ Palatal myoclonus or palatal tremor
      ▪ Frequently persisting during sleep:
         ▫ Hemifacial spasm
         ▫ Spinal or propriospinal myoclonus
         ▫ Hyperekplexia or exaggerated startle syndrome
      ▪ Sometimes persisting during sleep, usually in advanced cases:
         ▫ Tremor, chorea, dystonia, hemiballism
   2.3 **Motor parasomnias**
      ▪ Parasomnias are defined as abnormal movements or behaviors that intrude into sleep intermittently or episodically during the night without disturbing sleep architecture.
      ▪ Different categories include:
         ▫ Sleep-wake transition disorder
         ▫ NREM sleep parasomnias

□ REM sleep parasomnias
□ Diffuse parasomnias
2.4 Nocturnal seizures, examples include
- Tonic seizure
- Benign rolandic seizure
- Autosomal dominant nocturnal frontal lobe seizure
2.5 Drug-induced nocturnal dyskinesias
- Levodopa-induced myoclonus
- Tricyclic antidepressants
- Lithium
2.6 Others
- Sleep-related panic attacks
- Nocturnal jerks and body movements in obstructive sleep apnea
- Excessive fragmentary myoclonus
- Dissociative disorders

Torticollis: causes and mimics

- Torticollis, meaning twisted neck, is a physical sign, not a diagnosis.
- The most common cause of torticollis is idiopathic cervical dystonia. However, several disorders can mimic this condition.
- Nearly two-thirds of patients with cervical dystonia have bony degenerative change apparent on cervical spine X-rays, but there is no clear relationship between symptoms and the X-ray.

1 **Idiopathic cervical dystonia**
- The most frequent form of idiopathic focal dystonia and the most common neurological condition for which botulinum toxin treatment is indicated.
- The average age of onset is in the 40s, with over 75% of patients developing cervical dystonia between the ages of 30 and 60 years.
- Most adult-onset idiopathic cervical dystonia will stabilize without progression to segmental or generalized dystonia. This is in contrast to young-onset focal dystonia, which tends to become generalized.
2 Secondary cervical dystonia
- Approximately 8% of cervical dystonia patients suffer from cervical dystonia as parts of neurodegenerative diseases.
- Neck injury may precede the development of cervical dystonia in 15% of patients, even when there is no fracture.
- It is possible that local trauma triggers cervical dystonia in some genetically susceptible people.
3 Drug-induced cervical dystonia

- Cervical dystonia may occur following the treatment with some medications, for example: metoclopramide and other neuroleptics.
- 8% of patients with tardive dystonia have torticollis, with elderly women being the most susceptible.

4 Psychogenic cervical dystonia
- Although cervical dystonia was considered psychogenic in the first part of the last century, psychogenic dystonia is rare and should only be diagnosed with caution.
- Clues suggesting psychogenic etiology are:
  - Abrupt onset
  - Accompanying bizarre movements
  - Great variation in clinical presentation
  - Obvious psychiatric illness

Writer's cramp and its mimics

- Writer's cramp is a form of task-specific dystonia in which there is intense muscle co-contraction that locks the wrist and fingers, twisting them into abnormal postures and interfering with handwriting.
- Although the patient complains of a cramping sensation in the hands, severe pain is an uncommon feature and suggests an alternative diagnosis, such as nerve or nerve root entrapment.
- Sometimes, it can be very difficult to differentiate it from primary writing tremor, a condition in which writing is the only task that brings on tremor. Some believe that primary writing tremor is also a form of focal task-specific dystonia.
- Some patients with writer's cramp have a sensory trick that improves writing, such as lightly touching the hand or forearm with the other hand.

1 Focal nerve entrapment
- For example, carpal tunnel syndrome, ulnar neuropathy, or thoracic outlet syndrome.
- Physical findings of mononeuropathy or weakness of affected nerves suggest this alternative diagnosis.
- Usually accompanied by intense pain, uncommon in writer's cramp.

2 Systemic neurological conditions
- Multiple sclerosis can present with focal hand cramps.
- Patients with Parkinson disease can present with focal limb dystonia; however, it is usually a complication of levodopa treatment.

3 Soft-tissue disorders
- For example, tendonitis, epicondylitis
- These conditions can be coincidental or appear to be secondary to the muscle spasms and dystonic postures.

Chapter 7

Infectious, Inflammatory, and Demyelinating Disorders

Neurological infectious disorders

Signs and syndromes

Aseptic meningitis vs. acute encephalitis

- Aseptic meningitis is an inflammatory reaction in the subarachnoid space. Most cases are acute, benign, and self-limited. Viral etiology is common.
- Acute encephalitis is an inflammatory reaction of the brain parenchyma. Viral etiology is common, although encephalitis can be due to bacteria, parasites, fungi, protozoa, etc.
- Most acute encephalitides are viral infections and may involve the entire brain or be confined to focal areas. As the meninges are often involved, the term meningoencephalitis may be appropriate in most cases.
- In most cases, the clinical features of either syndrome are so nonspecific that diagnosis of the precise virus causing the infection is seldom possible without laboratory determination.
- Distinguishing between the two syndromes is useful because the natural course of aseptic meningitis typically is benign, while patients with acute encephalitis may be severely ill.

Symptom/sign	Aseptic meningitis	Acute encephalitis
Headache	Common	Common
Fever	Common	Common
Nuchal rigidity	Common	Common
Photophobia	Common	Common
Nausea/vomiting	May occur	May occur
Focal neurological signs	Absent	May be present
Seizures	Absent	May occur
Spasticity	Absent	May occur
Altered mental status	Rare	Common
Nystagmus, ocular palsies	Rare	May occur

Encephalitis vs. encephalopathy

- A common differential diagnosis when neurologists are asked to see the patient with stupor and coma is whether the patient has encephalitis or encephalopathy from various causes.
- Encephalitis implies brain inflammation, while encephalopathy refers to disturbance of brain function from different causes, commonly toxic-metabolic in origin.
- Recognition of the difference between encephalitis and encephalopathy is clinically important as the evaluation and treatment can be different.

Features	Encephalitis	Encephalopathy
History	Abrupt or subacute onset	Usually subacute or chronic
Fever	Present	Often absent
Headache	Present	Often absent
Attention, orientation	Fluctuates	Impaired
Focal neurological signs	Can be present	Usually none
Seizures	Common	Less common
Underlying general condition	Less common	Usually have underlying medical condition, e.g. renal or hepatic failure
Medication-induced	Less common	Common
Diagnostic testing		
Leukocytosis	Common	Less common, usually none
EEG	May show focal abnormalities	Usually demonstrates generalized slowing
Neuroimaging	May show focal lesions or leptomeningeal enhancement	Usually normal

Meningismus (neck stiffness) with fever and headache

- Symptoms may range from relatively mild to severe.
- Symptoms may be preceded by an antecedent illness.
- May be accompanied by focal neurological deficits, altered mental status, seizures, photophobia, nausea, or emesis.

1 **Viral meningitis**
   - Accounts for as much as 70% of community cases of meningitis.
   - LP results usually characterized as aseptic.
   - *Herpes encephalitis*: symptoms include seizures and behavioral changes with typical MRI findings and EEG changes. High mortality and morbidity if untreated.

2 *Bacterial meningitis*
  * LP is typically diagnostic.
  * Treatment should be initiated immediately.
  * Kernig and Brudzinski signs frequently present.
3 *Subdural empyema*
  * Often with focal neurological signs.
  * Often with focal seizures.
4 *Brain abscess*
  * Focal neurological signs frequently progressive in nature.
  * Often patient lacks obvious signs of systemic infection.
  * May present with signs of elevated intracranial pressure.
5 *Subarachnoid hemorrhage*
  * Meningismus, headache, altered mental status. Fever is variable.
  * Noncontrast CT scan is diagnostic. If high suspicion and CT negative, then carry out LP.
6 *Neuroleptic malignant syndrome*
  * Altered mental status, fever/hyperthermia, rigidity.
  * Associated with phenothiazine/neuroleptic use.
  * Monitor for rhabdomyolysis, myoglobinuria.
7 Tuberculosis meningitis
  * Patients with HIV infection or chronic alcohol abuse at higher risk.
  * Basilar meningitis.
  * Often with isolated cranial nerve abnormalities.

Exposures/risk factors associated with central nervous system infections

* The history of exposures and risk factors may be helpful in narrowing the possibilities of causative agents in central nervous system infections.
* The prevalence of a particular exposure in certain geographic areas where the patient lives is also important.
* Travel, exposure to animals or their waste, insect bites, ingestion of certain foods are all important aspects of the history to ascertain when a CNS infection is suspected.

Exposures/risk factor	Possible causative agents
Accidental or surgical trauma	• Staphylococcal brain abscess
Contact with infected patients	• Neisseria meningitidis
	• Hemophilus influenza meningitis
	• HIV infection
	• Syphilis
	• Tuberculosis

Exposures/risk factor	Possible causative agents
Deer, deer ticks	• Lyme disease
Mexico, South America, and Africa	• Cysticercosis
	• Amebic abscess
	• Malaria
	• Tuberculosis
	• Measles
	• Mumps
	• Rubella
Montana, Long Island, Virginia, Tennessee, and ticks	• Rocky mountain spotted fever
Mosquitoes	• Arbovirus encephalitis
	• Malaria
	• West Nile virus encephalitis
Ohio, Mississippi River valleys	• Histoplasmosis
	• Blastomycosis
Pork, uncooked or undercooked	• Trichinosis
Rabbit, squirrel hunting	• Tularemia
Southwestern United States	• Coccidioidomycosis
Swimming in ponds or lakes	• Amebic meningoencephalitis
Ticks, inhalation of dusts and handling of materials infected by causative organisms	• Coxiella burnettii (Q fever)
Tsetse fly in Africa, Central and South America	• Trypanosomiasis
Unpasteurized dairy products	• Brucellosis
Urine-contaminated soil or water (urine of rats, dogs, swine, and cattle)	• Leptospirosis

Geographic and seasonal incidence in United States	Encephalitis
Eastern US in early autumn	Eastern equine encephalitis
West of Mississippi	Western equine encephalitis
Nationwide in US, especially along the Mississippi River in August through October	St. Louis encephalitis
Florida, Southern half of US	Venezuelan equine encephalitis
Northern Midwest and Northeastern states in US	California virus encephalitis

Disorders by pathogen

Botulism

- Clostridium botulinum is a Gram-positive anaerobic rod typically found in water and soil.
- Clinical botulism is a flaccid paralysis, caused by neurotoxins of Clostridium botulinum. Other clinical manifestations include blurred vision, mydriasis, diplopia, ptosis, bulbar weakness, GI dysfunction, and loss of sweating. Botulism, unrecognized, can lead to respiratory failure and death.

- There are five types of clinical botulism. All forms have similar signs and symptoms but vary in the source of toxin.
- The toxin acts by binding to autonomic and motor nerve terminals. Then the toxin reduces the number of quanta of acetylcholine released by a nerve stimulus. Recovery from the toxin involves sprouting of nerve terminals, which form new synapses.

1 **Infantile botulism**
- The most common form of botulism.
- Almost all cases are under 1 year of age (90% are less than 6 months).
- It is assumed that infants consume spores that germinate in the gut, forming organisms that produce toxin in the large intestine.
- The combination of an infant who develops constipation, then feeding and respiratory difficulties, and later weakness of the neck and limbs, should raise the diagnosis of infantile botulism.
- The treatment is largely supportive, particularly respiratory management, as respiratory arrest occurs in 30% of patients. Antitoxin has been shown to accelerate recovery and reduce hospital stay if administered promptly.

2 **Food-borne (classic) botulism**
- Food-borne botulism is different from infantile botulism in that a source of toxin is present, and more than 50% of cases occur in outbreaks, with type A toxin being the most common.
- The common sources of type A and B toxins are home-canned food, baked potatoes in aluminum foil, and cheese sauce.
- Most patients are between 30 and 40 years old, with descending paralysis associated with respiratory failure being common presentations.
- Treatment is mainly supportive, with particular attention to respiratory support.

3 Wound botulism
- Once thought to be rare, wound botulism has increased in recent years, associated with drug injections, resulting in skin abscess, and intranasal cocaine administration causing sinusitis. 75% of cases are due to toxin type A.
- The combination of a wound and a descending paralysis should suggest this diagnosis. Circulating toxin in the serum is found in 46% of patients and the organism is cultured from the wound in 50–60% of cases.
- The treatment is focused on supportive measures and local wound care. Some studies suggest that the use of antitoxin may shorten the hospital stay and reduce mortality and morbidity.
- The most sensitive test for wound botulism is repetitive nerve stimulation showing an incremental response.

4 Inhalational botulism
  - Resulting from accidental or intentional aerosolization while attempting to use it as a weapon or to defend against it.
5 Iatrogenic botulism
  - Botulinum toxin injection may cause side-effects of local or generalized weakness.

Fungal infections

- Increasing frequency worldwide, fungal infections occur in a setting of intravenous drug abuse, immunosuppressant drugs, HIV, cancer, invasive CNS procedures, and use of broad-spectrum antibiotics.
- Characteristic fungal infections are largely dictated by host immune status.
- Fungal meningitis may present subacutely/chronically with nausea, vomiting, meningismus, seizures, and cranial nerve palsies. On the other hand, it often presents indolently, with vague symptoms such as headache with/without fever and a nonspecific deterioration in functional status.
- CSF studies demonstrate lymphocytic pleocytosis, elevated protein, and low/normal glucose.
- Fungal infections may also present as large, space occupying abscesses with focal neurological signs and characteristic neuroimaging findings.
- Other fungal syndromes include epidural cord compression via direct invasion from vertebral infection and acute syndromes such as stroke (vascular invasion) and rhinocerebral syndrome (from fungal sinusitis with direct extension into the surrounding soft tissues causing tissue necrosis).

Overall incidence of fungal infections

Species	Incidence per million per year
Candida species	73
Cryptococcus neoformans	66
Coccidioides immitis	15
Aspergillus species	12
Histoplasma capsulatum	7
Zygomycetes species	2

Fungal infections by pathogen
I Fungal pathogens in immunocompetent patients
  1 **Cryptococcus neoformans**
     - Infection via inhalation.

- Mild antecedent pulmonary symptoms followed by meningitis, altered mental status, increased intracranial pressure, and meningocerebral symptoms.

2   Coccidioides immitis
  - Infection via inhalation.
  - Usually benign and self-limited.
  - 1% incidence of disseminated disease, which may include headache, fever, altered mentation and behavior, cranial nerve palsies, nausea, and emesis.
  - Meningismus uncommon.

3   Histoplasma capsulatum
  - Infection via inhalation.
  - Typically benign and self-limited.
  - Rarely may disseminate and cause CNS disease via basilar meningitis, focal cerebritis, and granulomas.

II Fungal pathogens in immunocompromised patients

1   **Candida albicans**
  - Ubiquitous organism.
  - Disseminated candidiasis may involve brain parenchyma, meninges, and eyes.
  - CNS pathogenesis includes microabscesses, vasculitis with small vessel infarcts, and microvascular thromboses from pseudohyphae.

2   **Cryptococcus neoformans**

3   **Blastomyces dermatiditis**
  - Infection via inhalation.
  - 40% of AIDS patients with infection will develop CNS involvement.
  - CNS manifestations include intracranial or spinal abscesses or meningitis.

4   *Zygomycetes rhizopus (Mucor)*
  - Usually occurs in poorly-controlled diabetics.
  - CNS manifestations include ischemic lesions from vascular invasion, orbital cellulitis, rhinocerebral syndrome.
  - Internal carotid artery and cavernous sinus thromboses common.
  - Zygomycosis with acute necrotizing tissue reaction and surrounding vessel thrombosis.
  - >50% overall mortality in rhinocerebral mucormycosis.

5   *Aspergillus fumgatus*
  - Seen in patients with chronic sinusitis.
  - CNS involvement typically via direct extension or embolization.
  - CNS manifestations include cerebral vascular occlusions.
  - May give rise to rhinocerebral syndrome.
  - Brain abscess and cranial nerve compression in immunocompetent patients.

Neurological manifestations of HIV

- Neurological presentations in HIV infection can be attributed to:
  1. Direct HIV infection
  2. Secondary opportunistic infections
  3. Neoplasms
  4. Disorders of uncertain origins
  5. Neurological complications secondary to therapy
- HIV infects the CNS early in the course of disease and before the appearance of any clinical manifestations of neurological involvement.
- HIV can be recovered from CSF at all stages of viral infection and independent of clinically apparent degree of immunosuppression.
- Neurological manifestations differ markedly based on the stage of the infection.

1 Due to primary HIV infection
  - **Aseptic meningitis**
  - **AIDS dementia complex**
  - Vacuolar myelopathy
  - Demyelinating polyneuropathy
2 Secondary infections (opportunistic infections)
  2.1 Secondary viral infections
  - **Papovavirus (PML)**
  - Herpes simplex virus
  - Cytomegalovirus
  - Varicella zoster virus
  2.2 Secondary non-viral infections
  - **Toxoplasmosis**
  - **Cryptococcosis**
  - Candidiasis
  - Mycobacterium, like M. tuberculosis, M. kansasii, M. avium-intracellulare
  - Norcardiasis
  - Aspergillosis
3 Neoplasms
  - Primary CNS lymphoma
  - Metastatic Kaposi sarcoma
  - Metastatic systemic lymphoma
4 Vascular diseases
  - Cerebral infarction
  - Cerebral hemorrhage
  - Cerebral vasculitis

5 Complications to systemic therapy
  ◆ Encephalopathy
  ◆ Neuropathy

Neurocysticercosis: active vs. inactive presentations

- Neurocysticercosis is a common neurological disorder seen in many developing countries and is increasingly recognized in non-endemic areas. **Cysticercosis is the most common parasite in the CNS.**
- Cysticercus is the encysted larva of the cestode, Taenia solium. The life cycle of Taenia solium starts in the intestine of carriers. Ingestion of contaminated food will induce cysticercosis in humans or pigs as intermediate hosts. Consumption of undercooked pork containing cysticerci will complete the cycle.
- The most common form of cysticercosis in man is neurocysticercosis, with an incidence of up to 3.6% of the general population in endemic areas. Muscle cysticercosis is rarely diagnosed.
- The classification of neurocysticercosis presentations into active and inactive forms is based on the results of radiological and CSF studies. Indications for and expected results from drug therapy depend on the form of neurocysticercosis, with the best response in parenchymal cysticerci.

I Active neurocysticercosis
  1 **Arachnoiditis**
    ◆ Most frequent form of active cysticercosis (48%).
    ◆ Prominent inflammation in the subarachnoid space and positive immune reaction in the CSF.
    ◆ Common clinical presentations include headache, vertigo, cranial nerve dysfunction.
    ◆ 50% of patients with this form develop hydrocephalus.
    ◆ Poor prognosis.
  2 Hydrocephalus secondary to meningeal inflammation
    ◆ Usually as a complication of arachnoiditis.
    ◆ **Hydrocephalus must always be treated by a shunt before drug therapy.**
  3 Parenchymal cysts
    ◆ Commonly presents with partial seizures.
    ◆ Can cause significant edema resulting in mass effects and intracranial hypertension.
  4 Vasculitis
    ◆ As a complication of meningeal and parenchymal neurocysticercosis resulting in infarctions of small arterioles.
  5 Intraventricular cysts

- ◆ Can cause obstructive hydrocephalus and Brun syndrome (valvular obstruction of the fourth ventricle).
6   Spinal cysts
II Inactive cysticercosis
1   **Parenchymal calcifications**
- ◆ Most frequent form of inactive cysticercosis (57%).
- ◆ The most common presentation is simple or complex partial seizure.
2   Hydrocephalus secondary to meningeal fibrosis

Prion disease

- Diseases characterized by progressive dementia, insomnia, agitation, memory loss, imaging, and EEG abnormalities.
- All are uniformly fatal with differences in the rapidity of disease progression.
- All are accompanied by varying neurological deficits.
- Treatment is supportive.

1   **Creutzfeldt-Jakob disease**
- ◆ $1/10^6$ sporadic cases, 15% familial.
- ◆ Characterized by paranoia, early dementia, pyramidal and extrapyramidal signs, seizures, and myoclonus.
- ◆ 90% 1-year mortality.
2   Gerstmann-Sträussler-Scheinker disease
- ◆ Autosomal dominant transmission.
- ◆ Characterized by euphoria, pyramidal signs, and supranuclear gaze palsy.
- ◆ Slowly progressive over 2–10 years.
3   Fatal familial insomnia
- ◆ Autosomal dominant transmission.
- ◆ Characterized by agitation, ataxia, dysarthria, and autonomic dysfunction.
4   Kuru
- ◆ Transmitted primarily through cannibalistic practices first described in the Fores tribe of New Guinea.
- ◆ Characterized by euphoria and loss of facial muscle control.
- ◆ Progression over months to years.

Spirochete infections

- Important neurological pathogens due to under-recognition and incomplete treatment.
- Characterized by multiphasic/relapsing disease and multifocal neurological sequelae.
- Effective treatments exist, making proper diagnosis critical.

1 *Syphilis*
   - Caused by Treponema pallidun.
   - Multiphasic illness characterized by primary (local chancre), secondary (disseminated with rash), and tertiary (diffuse inflammation and neurological deficits) stages.
   - Neurological signs are protean and may include dementia, apathy, dysarthria, myoclonus, tremor, tabes dorsalis, Argyll-Robertson pupils, seizures, and hyperreflexia.

2 Lyme disease
   - Caused by Borrelia burgdorferi which is transmitted via a tick bite.
   - Systemic illness involving neurological, rheumatological, dermatological, and cardiac manifestations.
   - Typically heralded by a non-painful rash (erythema chronicum migrans) at the bite site.
   - Neurological manifestations include meningitis/encephalomyelitis, cranial nerve abnormalities, radiculoneuritis, optic neuritis, and mononeuritis multiplex.

3 Leptospirosis
   - Caused by Leptospira interrogans.
   - Worldwide zoonotic illness transmitted via contact with urine of infected animals, typically rodents.
   - Biphasic illness characterized initially by fever, myalgia, headache, and GI symptoms.
   - Secondary phase starts approximately one week after initial symptoms and typically involves more severe systemic illness and may include meningitis, meningoencephalitis, and uveitis.

Viral encephalitis

- Estimated at over 20,000 cases is the US every year, 70% of aseptic meningitis is viral.
- Characterized by fever, headache, and altered mentation.
- Severe infections may include seizures, focal neurological deficits, signs of elevated intracranial pressure, stupor, and coma.
- Detailed history should include recent travel, exposure to animals, and insect bites.
- Care is typically supportive, except in the case of herpes simplex I, when intravenous acyclovir is indicated ASAP.
- Must be distinguished from bacterial meningitis, brain abscess, subdural empyema, atypical fungal and parasitic infections, and toxic metabolic encephalopathies.

1 *Herpes simplex*
   - HSV-1 in adults, HSV-2 in neonates.
   - Early personality and behavioral changes.
   - Primarily a temporal lobe encephalitis, frequently with MRI correlation. Neonatal form is diffuse.
   - EEG may show temporal periodic lateralizing epileptiform discharges.
   - Acyclovir treatment should be instituted immediately on suspicion.
   - CSF is PCR positive.

2 **Arboviruses**
   - Include Eastern equine, Western equine, St. Louis, and West Nile.
   - Transmitted by mosquito or tick bites.
   - Most cases seen during summer months.
   - Treatment is supportive.

3 **Enteroviruses**
   - Include coxsackie, polio, and echovirus.
   - Often characterized by focal encephalitis.
   - Seen in epidemics of gastrointestinal illness.
   - Seen in summer and early fall.
   - Polio rarely seen in US due to active vaccination programs.
   - Treatment is supportive.

4 Varicella zoster
   - Usually a benign self-limited disease.
   - Post-infectious encephalomyelitis seen in immunocompromised patients and approximately 1/2,500 healthy children.
   - Immunization now available.
   - Treatment may include acyclovir.
   - Reactivation of latent virus from dorsal root ganglia causes herpes zoster (shingles).

5 Rabies
   - Nearly 100% mortality following onset of encephalitis.
   - Almost always transmitted via the bite of an infected animal (dog, raccoon, bat).
   - Long incubation period of weeks to several months.
   - Prodrome characterized by headache, fever, parasthesias, and pain at inoculation site.
   - Acute neurological phase accompanied by agitation, hallucinations, autonomic instability, and seizures.
   - Post-exposure treatment involves administration of rabies vaccine and antirabies immunoglobulin.

Meningoencephalitis

Bacterial meningitis pathogens by age and host

- Incidence approximately 4–10 per 100,000 per year.
- Offending organisms vary as a function of immune status and patient age.
- Mortality as high as 20%.
- Symptoms include headache, fever, malaise, meningismus, emesis, and photophobia.
- Seizures in up 40% of cases.
- Focal neurological signs less common but possible.

1 Immunocompetent hosts
  a <3 months
- *Escherichia coli* (other Gram-negative rods) ~50–60%
- *Group B streptococcus* ~30%
- *Listeria monocytogenes* ~2–10%

  b 3 months to 18 years
- *Haemophilus influenza* ~50%; now reduced due to routine immunization
- *Neisseria meningitidis* ~30%
- *Streptococcus pneumoniae* ~20%

  c 18 to 50 years
- *Streptococcus pneumoniae* ~50%
- *Neisseria meningitidis* ~25%
- *Staphlycoccus aureus* ~15%

  d >50 years
- *Streptococcus pneumoniae*
- *Listeria monocytogenes*
- *Gram-negative bacilli*

2 Immunocompromised hosts
- *Listeria monocytogenes*
- *Gram-negative bacilli*

3 Head trauma or neurosurgical intervention
- *Staphlycoccus aureus*
- *Gram-negative bacilli*
- *Streptococcus pneumoniae*

Chronic meningitis

- Characterized by low-grade headache and fever in the presence of meningismus and abnormal CSF.

- 'Chronic' designation implies persistence for 1 month or greater, though many patients will have adequate work-up prior to this timeline.
- Most cases are caused by infections, inflammatory conditions, or neoplasms.
- Infectious etiologies are often seen in immunocompromised individuals.
- In this setting, many of the potential etiologies should be investigated, as the specific diagnosis can be elusive without extensive evaluation. Hence, a large number of potential etiologies are listed in **bold** below.

1 Infectious etiologies
- **Fungal meningitis**: associated with immunodeficiency states
  - **Candidiasis**
  - **Cryptoccocus neoformans**
  - **Aspergillus**
    - Lung involvement
  - Coccidiodes immitis
    - Endemic to southwestern US
  - Histoplasma capsulatum
    - Endemic to midwest, Ohio Valley
    - Oral lesions, hepatosplenomegaly
  - Sporotrichosis: rare fungus
- **Bacterial/mycobacterial/spirochete meningitis**
  - **Partially treated bacterial meningitis**
  - **Tuberculosis**: Mycobacterium tuberculosis
  - **Lyme disease**: Borrelia burgdorferi
    - History of tick bite, visit to endemic area
    - History of 'bullseye' rash (erythema chronicum migrans)
    - Associated facial palsy, other cranial neuropathies
  - **Neurosyphilis**: Treponema pallidum
  - Brucellosis: unpasteurized dairy products
  - Leptospirosis
    - Exposure to urine of infected animals
    - Associated hepatomegaly, hepatitis
- **Viral meningitis**
  - **HIV**
  - **CMV**: associated chorioretinitis
  - LCMV: lymphocytic choriomeningitis virus
    - Exposure to rodents
    - Associated with orchitis, leukopenia, thrombocytopenia
  - Echovirus: associated with agammaglobulinemia, dermatomyositis
  - Mumps

- No vaccination
- Associated parotitis, orchitis, oophoritis
  - Acanthamoeba
  - Angiostrongylus cantonensis
    - Nematode endemic to SE Asia/Pacific
    - Ingestion of raw fish/seafood
  - Cysticercosis: Taenia solium
    - Calcified lesions on head CT scan, hydrocephalus
    - Endemic to southwestern US, Mexico
2 Non-infectious etiologies
  - Autoimmune conditions
    - **Behçet disease**
      - Recurrent oral and genital ulcers
      - Uveitis and other ocular symptoms (90%); arthritis (50%)
    - **Sarcoidosis**
      - Associated facial palsy, other cranial neuropathies
      - Lung, lymph node, bones, skin, muscle, ocular involvement
    - Systemic lupus erythematosus
  - Chronic benign lymphocytic meningitis
  - CNS angitis
    - Progressive encephalopathy, may have stroke symptoms
    - Angiography not very sensitive; biopsy is best
  - Uveomeningoencephalitis (Vogt-Koyanagi-Harada syndrome)
  - **Neoplasm**: diagnostic yield increases with multiple CSF cytology samples
    - Leukemia
    - Lymphoma
    - Leptomeningeal carcinomatous metastases – breast, lung, melanoma
3 Drugs
  - NSAIDS
  - Intravenous immune globulin
  - Sulfa, other antibiotics

Chronic meningitis: diagnostic tests

- Signs and symptoms include, but are not limited to, headache, fever, chills, focal neurological signs, and meningismus.
- Parasitic and fungal infections account for most chronic forms of meningitis.

Listed below are readily available diagnostic tests helpful when considering chronic meningitis in the differential.

Organism/diagnosis	Non-CNS/serum tests	CNS/CSF tests
Cryptoccocus	Antigen (+ serum & CSF = 94%) Urine, sputum, blood cultures	Smear: India ink stain (60%) Antigen (85%), [95%] Culture (75%)
Syphilis	FTA-ABS (fluorescent treponemal antibody-absorption)	VDRL
M. tuberculosis	Sputum: AFB culture (14–50%)	Smear: AFB visible (10–22%) Culture (38–88%) PCR (27–85%), [95%]
Coccidioides	Antibody	Smear: spherules visible occ. Antibody (55–95%) Culture (33–50%)
Histoplasmosis	Antibody (60–90%) Antigen (+ urine, blood, or CSF = 61%) Blood culture	Antibody Antigen (+ urine, blood, or CSF = 61%) Culture (27–65%)
Borrelia (Lyme)	Antibody (75%)	Antibody PCR (25–38%), [95%]
Cysticercosis	Antibody (50%)	Antibody (84%)
Candida		Smear: yeast visible (33%) Culture usually diagnostic
Brucella	Antibody	Antibody
Sporotrichosis		Antibody
Sarcoidosis	Angiotensin converting enzyme elevated (66%), CXR/chest CT/biopsy (67%)	Angiotensin converting enzyme elevated
Granulomatous angiitis	Angiography (27–65%)	Brain biopsy (71%)
Leptomeningeal carcinomatosis	Cancer screening (CXR, CBC, skin exam, mammogram, etc.)	Cytology (1 tap 42%; multiple taps 74%) Beta-glucuronidase?

(Sensitivity; % of true positives that test positive.) [Specificity; % of true negatives that test negative.]

Drug-induced meningitis

- A large number of drugs have been implicated in aseptic meningitis. The mechanism is uncertain, although it may be related to cellular immune hypersensitivity.

- The signs and symptoms of drug-induced meningitis usually start a few hours or weeks after ingestion. Symptoms and signs are typical of meningitis, including headache, photophobia, and meningismus. In addition, patients can develop facial edema, pruritus, and low-grade fever.
- The CSF studies often show pleocytosis (varies from 10–10,000 cells/mm³) with mostly PMNs or mononuclear cells as well as relatively increased eosinophils. CSF protein is usually elevated (up to 500 mg/dl).
- Drug-induced meningitis should be considered in all cases with acute or recurrent meningitis.

1 **Nonsteroidal anti-inflammatory agents (NSAIDS)**
   - The most common drug
   - Examples include ibuprofen, sulindac, and naproxen
2 **Trimethoprim-sulfamethoxazole**
3 **Intravenous immunoglobulins**
4 Antibiotics
   - Penicillin
   - Isoniazid
5 Others
   - Cytosine arabinoside
   - Azathioprine
   - Carbamazepine
   - Phenazopyridine
   - Monoclonal antibodies

Eosinophilic meningitis

- Defined by the presence of eosinophils in the CSF of patients with clinical meningitis.
- Characteristic etiologies include helminthic and protozoan parasites.
- Non-infectious causes may include malignancies, drugs, and dye reactions.

1 **Infectious etiologies**
   - **Angiostrongylus cantonensis**
     - #1 worldwide
     - Endemic to SE Asia and Pacific
     - Exposure to raw fish or seafood
   - Gnathostoma spinigerum
   - Baylisascaris procyonis

- Naegleria fowleri
- Acanthamoeba species
- Entamoeba histolytica
- Trichinella spiralis
- Cysticercosis: Taenia solium
- Coccidioidomycosis: 30% have >10 Eos/mm^3

2 Non-infectious etiologies
  - Neoplastic processes
    - Leukemia
    - Lymphoma
  - Drug reactions
    - Antibiotics
    - NSAIDS
  - Myelography dye

Recurrent meningitis

- Recurrent meningitis implies discrete episodes of abnormal clinical and CSF findings interspersed with asymptomatic periods and normal CSF profiles.
- Multiple etiologies include infections and inflammatory conditions.
- Infectious causes include undertreated bacterial, viral, and fungal etiologies.
- Recurrent bacterial meningitis may be due to undertreated infections, atypical pathogens, parameningeal abscess, CSF leak, or impaired immunity (B-cell).

1 **Infectious etiologies including:**
  - **Partially treated meningitis**
  - **Parameningeal infection with recurrent seeding of meninges: sinusitis, mastoiditis, osteomyelitis, brain abscess**
    - *Bacterial*: Borrelia burgdoferi, Streptococcus pneumoniae, Haemophilus influenza, Neisseria meningitidis, Mycobacterium tuberculosis
    - *Fungal*: Cryptoccocus neoformans, Coccidiodes immitis, Blastomyces dermatitides
    - *Parasitic*: Cysticercosis, Toxoplasma gondii
  - **Viral**
    - HIV
    - HSV-1
    - HSV-2
    - Epstein-Barr (EBV)

2 Inflammatory conditions
  - Rheumatologic conditions

- Systemic lupus erythematosus
- Polyarteritis nodosa
- Behçet disease
  - Mollaret meningitis: CSF shows 'Mollaret cells', actually monocytes
    - Most common in young adults; symptoms remit in 2–5 days.
    - Possibly associated with herpes virus infection (HSV, EBV)
  - Sarcoidosis
3 **Structural conditions**
  - Dermoid/epidermoid cyst with CSF leakage
  - Craniopharyngioma with CSF leakage
  - Myelomeningocele
  - Petrous fistula
  - Post-traumatic
4 Drugs (with rechallenge)
  - NSAIDS
  - Antibiotics, sulfa
  - Intravenous immune globulin

Brain abscess by location, organism, and other risk factors

- The location of brain abscesses reflects the prominence of spread from contiguous primary sites of infection.
- Symptoms include fever, chills, malaise, nausea, and emesis.
- 50–70% of patients with abscesses complain of headache.
- 33% of patients with abscesses will have a seizure prior to diagnosis.
- Patients with prior instrumentation, traumatic skull injury, or neurosurgical intervention are particularly vulnerable, with the location typically at or around the site of compromise.

1 Abscess location
  - **Frontal lobe**
  - **Frontoparietal region**
  - Parietal lobe
  - Cerebellum
  - Occipital lobe
2 Organisms
  - **Streptoccoccal species (50–70% of all cases)**; 30–60% of mixed cases
    - Aerobic, anaerobic, and microaerophilic
    - S. milleri group (anginosus, constellatus, intermedius)
  - **Anaerobic bacteria (40–100% of cases**, with proper culture techniques)
    - Bacteroides and Prevotella (20–40%)

- **Gram-negative enteric bacilli** (23–33%)
  - E. coli
  - Klebsiella
  - Pseudomonas
  - Proteus, Enterobacter
- Staphylococcal species (10–25%)
- Common organisms for meningitis but rarely form abscess (<1%)
  - H. influenza
  - Strept. pneumoniae
  - Listeria monocytogenes
- Rare organisms for meningitis but relatively high likelihood of abscess
  - Facultative Gram-negatives: Citrobacter, Proteus, Serratia, Enterobacter
- Other rare organisms
  - Nocardia
  - M. tuberculosis, other mycobacteria
  - Fungal abscesses: generally associated with immunosuppressed state
    - Candida, Aspergillus, Mucormycosis, Cryptococcus, Coccidioides, Histoplasma, Blastomyces
  - Parasitic abscesses: more common in developing countries
    - Toxoplasma gondii, Cysticercosis (Taenia solium), Trypanosoma cruzi, Entamoeba histolytica, Schistosoma
- Negative culture (0–43%): usually due to prior treatment with antibiotics

3 Common causes of brain abscesses by risk factor
- **Sinusitis (15%)**
  - Staphylococcus aureus
  - Streptococcus
  - Bacteroides
  - Haemophilus
- **Unknown (25%)**: no identifiable risk factor
  - Staphylococcus aureus
  - Streptococcus
  - Bacteroides
- Otitis or mastoiditis
  - Gram-negative bacilli
  - Streptococcus
  - Bacteroides
- Dental infections
  - Streptococcus
  - Mixed flora (Bacteroides, Fusobacterium, Prevotella)
- Pulmonary infections
  - Streptococcus
  - Nocardia

- Mixed flora (Bacteroides, Fusobacterium, Actinomyces, Prevotella)
- Penetrating head trauma or post-neurosurgical
  - Staphylococcus aureus
  - Streptococcus
- Endocarditis
  - Streptococcus
  - Staphylococcus aureus
- Immunodeficiency states (chemotherapy, transplantation, HIV infection)
  - Toxoplasmosis
  - Nocardia
  - Aspergillus
  - Candida
  - Cryptococcus
  - M. tuberculosis

Neurological inflammatory and demyelinating disorders

Central nervous system

CNS demyelination

- Classified as demyelinating, when a disease process affects myelin integrity, or dysmyelinating, when the disease is a biochemical disorder affecting myelin formation.
- Neurological manifestations are multiple and affect motor, sensory, autonomic, visual, and cerebellar systems.
- Upper motor neuron signs predominate.
- Neuroimaging is critical in diagnostic work-up.

1 Inflammatory/immune disorders
  - **Multiple sclerosis (MS)**
    - Female:male (2:1), usual onset age 20–40 years, more common in Northern hemisphere.
    - Multiple presentations: diagnosis made by neurological lesions separated in space and time.
    - Lesions are oval, periventricular; active lesions may enhance with contrast.
  - **Optic neuritis**: demyelination of optic nerves, may be initial presentation of MS.
  - **Acute disseminated encephalomyelitis**
    - Monophasic illness, associated with recent infection or vaccination.

- More common in children, but can occur in adults.
- Paraneoplastic encephalomyelopathies
- Rheumatoid arthritis
- Systemic lupus erythematosus
- Behçet disease
- Sjögren disease

2 Infectious diseases
- **HIV:** diffuse, patchy, bilateral white matter signals abnormalities
- Progressive multifocal leukoencephalopathy (JC virus)
  - Associated with HIV, transplantation, immunodeficiency states.
  - Multifocal demyelinating lesions, usually parietal or occipital.
- Lyme disease
- Neurosyphilis
- Human T-cell lymphotropic virus type I

3 Granulomatous disease
- Sarcoidosis
- Wegener granulomatosis
- Lymphoid granulomatosis

4 Myelin disorders
- Metachromatic leukodystrophy (AR)
  - Onset in infancy or childhood, associated peripheral neuropathy.
  - Diffusely affects white matter, U-fibers are spared.
- Adrenoleukodystrophy/adrenomyeloneuropathy
  - Usually XL inheritance. Neonatal form very rare, AR inheritance.
  - Elevated serum very long chain fatty acids.
  - Progresses occipital to frontal, involves splenium. N-acetylaspartate (NAA) may be decreased, choline and lactate increased on MR spectroscopy (MRS).
- Krabbe globoid leukodystrophy (AR)
  - Onset in infancy, opisthotonic posturing.
  - Elevated CSF protein, slowed peripheral nerve conduction velocity.
- Alexander disease
  - Associated macrocephaly, childhood onset.
  - Progresses from frontal to occipital, U-fibers initially spared.
- Canavan disease (AR)
  - Associated macrocephaly, onset in infancy.
  - Deficiency of N-acetylaspartylase results in increased NAA on MRS.

5 Toxic/metabolic disorders
- B_{12} deficiency.
- Central pontine myelinolysis: associated with abrupt sodium shifts, associated with alcoholism, sepsis, burns, malignancies.
- Carbon monoxide

- Radiation-induced myelinolysis
- Medication-induced leukoencephalopathy
  - Cyclosporin, tacrolimus: typically occipital, may involve gray matter, too.
  - Methotrexate: usually in conjunction with radiation.
- Posterior reversible encephalopathy syndrome (PRES)
  - Associated with hypertension, renal failure, immunosuppressants (steroids).
  - Bilateral, parietal, and occipital lesions in gray and white matter.

Clinical features suggestive of multiple sclerosis

- Several presenting symptoms are common features amongst MS patients.
- Clinical features should be considered to differentiate between MS or other forms of demyelinating disease.

Common PRESENTING symptoms and signs in MS	Percentage
Motor weakness	10–40%
Sensory impairment/paresthesias	13–40%
Optic neuritis	14–29%
Diplopia	8–18%
Ataxia	2–18%
Genitourinary dysfunction	0–13%
Vertigo	2–9%

Common CHRONIC symptoms and signs in MS	Percentage
Motor weakness/spasticity	65–100%
Hyperreflexia/Babinski sign	62–98%
Fatigue/pain	59–85%
Bowel/bladder dysfunction	39–93%
Impaired vibration/proprioception	48–82%
Tremor	36–81%
Ataxia	37–78%
Nystagmus	54–73%
Impaired pain/temperature/touch	16–72%
Dysarthria	29–62%
Visual symptoms	27–55%
Sexual dysfunction	33–59%

Clinical feature	Suggestive of MS	Less suggestive of MS
Age of onset	15–50 years	<10 or >60 years
Course	Relapsing-remitting	Steady progression
Symptoms	Optic neuritis, internuclear ophthalmoplegia	Dementia, early focal cognitive deficits
Environment	Worse with elevated body temperature	Unrelated

Classification of multiple sclerosis (MS)

- Devised by Lublin and Reingold (1996) to describe the pattern and course of the illness.
- Disease progression, age-of-onset, gender, and prognosis are somewhat characteristic for each category.

1 Relapsing-remitting (RRMS)
   - Characterized by exacerbations with clear remission and minimal/no residual sequelae, no disease progression between relapses.
   - Female predominance
   - Typically earlier onset
   - Best prognosis
2 Primary-progressive (PPMS)
   - Characterized by chronic disease progression from onset with occasional plateau periods.
   - Myelopathy common
   - Sex ratio 1:1
   - Later age onset
   - Poor prognosis
3 Secondary-progressive (SPMS)
   - Characterized by initial relapsing-remitting course with gradual progression of disease with or without relapses.
   - >50% of initial RRMS patients develop this form 10 years following onset.
4 Progressive-relapsing (PRMS)
   - Characterized as initially progressive disease with subsequent acute relapses with or without full recovery.
   - Unusual form

Acute demyelination

- A diverse set of conditions resulting from a variety of pathologic mechanisms including inflammatory, infectious, autoimmune, and metabolic syndromes.
- Pathologically linked by common features:
   - Destruction of myelin sheaths
   - Relative sparing of other nerve tissue
   - Inflammatory cell infiltration
   - White matter lesions
   - Relative lack of secondary (Wallerian) degeneration

- Clinically diverse, typically corresponding to lesion location and extent.
- Symptoms may be upper motor neuron, sensory, autonomic, and cognitive.
- Demyelinating syndromes may involve either spinal nerve roots, the CNS, or both.
- Designation of acute implies clinical pathology in days. However, in some cases the clinical entity may actually present as acute or chronic.

1 **Multiple sclerosis (MS)**
   - Relapsing-remitting MS
   - Marburg variant
2 **Optic neuritis**
   - A common initial presentation of multiple sclerosis.
3 *Transverse myelitis*
   - A common initial presentation of multiple sclerosis with pathology confined to the spinal cord.
   - May also be due to a variety of other etiologies (see differential on transverse myelitis).
4 *Acute inflammatory demyelinating polyradiculopathy (AIDP)*
   - Guillian-Barré syndrome
   - Miller-Fisher syndrome (ophthalmoplegia, ataxia, and areflexia)
5 Acute disseminated encephalomyelitis (ADEM)
   - Inflammatory demyelination of the brain and/or spinal cord.
   - Associated with recent vaccination or infection.
6 Central pontine myelinolysis
   - Seen in chronic alcoholism, rapid correction·of hyponatremia, and extreme serum hyperosmolality.
7 Cerebellitis
   - Isolated ataxia most frequently seen with varicella infections.
8 Acute necrotizing hemorrhagic encephalomyelitis (Weston Hurst disease)
   - Considered a hyperacute form of ADEM.
   - Associated with antecedent upper respiratory tract infection.

Chronic and recurrent demyelination

- Classification as chronic implies progression over months to years, though an acute phase may be present.
- Classification as recurrent implies repeated acute clinical symptoms, though this may be superimposed on chronic progressive decline.
- Myelin pathology due to inborn errors of metabolism is more accurately characterized as *dys*myelination.
- See acute demyelination gray-box discussion for additional details.

1 **Multiple sclerosis (MS)**
- Primary progressive MS
- Secondarily progressive MS
- Neuromyelitis optica (Devic disease)
  - Affects optic nerves and spinal cord.
- Recurrent optic neuropathy

2 **Chronic inflammatory demyelinating polyradiculopathy (CIDP)**

3 Progressive multifocal leukoencephalitis
- Seen most often, though not exclusively, in immunosuppressed patients.
- Caused by oligodrendrocytic infection by opportunistic papovavirus (JC or SV-40 strains).

4 HIV
- CIDP variant

5 Subacute combined degeneration
- B_{12} deficiency
- Intrinsic factor deficiency
- Nitrous oxide inhalation.

6 Carbon monoxide poisoning
- Diffuse, subcortical leukoencephalopathy occurring several weeks after acute intoxication

7 Adrenoleukodystrophy

8 Globoid cell leukodystrophy (Krabbe disease)

9 Metachromatic leukodystrophy

10 Marchiafava-Bignami disease
- Selective demyelination of the central corpus callosum seen in association with alcoholism and nutritional deficiency.

Peripheral

Inflammatory disorders causing neuropathies

- Peripheral and cranial nerves are commonly affected in systemic inflammatory disorders.
- Neurological manifestations may arise after a long course of disease, or may be the presenting feature of systemic disease.
- Neuropathies may occur as a part of the primary disease process or secondarily as a result of other organ system involvement.

1 **Systemic lupus erythematosus**
- Presumed pathology arises from immune-mediated vasculitis.
- CNS more frequently involved than PNS
- Chronic axonal sensory polyneuropathy is most common PNS manifestation.

2 **Rheumatoid arthritis**
  - Common disorder affecting 2–5% of the general population.
  - Peripheral neuropathies occur in up 10% of patients.
  - Neuropathies can be compressive secondary to inflammation and fibrosis, or symmetric, sensory, distal polyneuropathy, mononeuropathy/mononeuropathy multiplex, and fulminant sensorimotor polyneuropathy due to vasculitis or vascular occlusion.

3 *Vasculitis*
  - Spectrum of disorders characterized by inflammation of blood vessels and resultant luminal occlusion with downstream tissue ischemia.
  - Peripheral nerve involvement is common.
  - Broadly characterized as systemic necrotizing vasculitis, hypersensitivity vasculitis, giant cell arteritis, or localized vasculitis.

4 Sarcoidosis
  - Multisystem granulomatous disorder.
  - 5% of patients have neurological manifestations.
  - Cranial neuropathies are the most common neurological manifestation (73%).
  - Additional neurological manifestations include: multiple motor/sensory mononeuropathies, polyradiculoneuropathies, cauda equina syndrome, and symmetric sensorimotor neuropathy.

5 Amyloidosis
  - Multisystem disorder characterized by extracellular deposition of β-pleated sheet fibrillar proteins.
  - Usually presents after age 40, men affected 2:1 over women.
  - Peripheral neuropathy present in 10–35% of patients.
  - Clinical symptoms include painful dysesthesias with decrement in spinothalamic modalities, carpal tunnel syndrome, and dysautonomia.

6 Systemic sclerosis
  - Connective tissue disease characterized by excessive collagen deposition.
  - Neurological complications include myopathies but are uncommon.

Inflammatory demyelinating polyradiculopathies

- Acquired, immune-mediated, demyelinating diseases characterized primarily by their clinical course as chronic or acute.
- Acute forms, with maximal deficits occurring within 4 weeks of illness, are classified as Guillain-Barré syndromes.
- Disease with chronic progression or multiple relapses is classified as chronic inflammatory demyelinating polyradiculopathy (CIDP).

1 **Guillain-Barré syndrome**
 ◆ Annual incidence is approximately 1.8/100,000
 ◆ Antecedent illness reported in 2/3 of patients
 ◆ Presentation includes parasthesias, sensory symptoms, and weakness
 ◆ Weakness distal and symmetric, with ascending progression
 ◆ Hypo/areflexia invariably present
 ◆ Dysautonomia common
 ◆ Syndromes
  ▪ *Acute inflammatory demyelinating polyradiculopathy (AIDP)*
  ▪ Acute motor axonal neuropathy
  ▪ Acute motor/sensory axonal neuropathy
  ▪ Miller-Fisher syndrome
   ▫ Ophthalmoplegia and ataxia predominate
   ▫ Associated with α-GQ1b antibodies
2 Chronic inflammatory demyelinating polyradiculopathy (CIDP)
 ◆ Similar features with motor predominance and chronic progression or relapsing/remitting course

Inflammatory myopathies

- Characterized by disease of muscle in which inflammatory cells are a prominent feature.
- Hallmark features include generalized myalgias and muscle weakness.
- Electrodiagnostic studies are helpful in establishing diagnosis.
- Deep tendon reflexes are typically preserved out of proportion to weakness.
- Etiology is poorly understood.
- Treatment includes steroids and immunosuppressants.

Signs/symptoms	Childhood dermatomyositis	Adult dermatomyositis	Polymyositis	Inclusion body myositis
Pattern of weakness	Proximal dysphagia	Proximal dysphagia	Proximal dysphagia	Proximal distal dysphagia
Presence of myalgia	>50%	<25%	<10%	Rare
Skin involvement	Periorbital edema, rash	Periorbital edema, rash	None	None
Joint involvement	Contractures	Contractures	Rare	None
Other systems involved	Rare	Heart, lung	Heart, lung	None
Other characteristics			Onset typically after age 20	Male predominance, onset typically after age 50

Chapter 8
Peripheral Neurology

General approach

Neuropathy vs. myopathy vs. ALS

- Careful physical examination of the patient with weakness will quickly suggest whether the pattern is neuropathic, myopathic, or consistent with ALS (amyotrophic lateral sclerosis; motor neuron disease).
- Six items to examine clinically include: atrophy, distribution of weakness, fasciculations, sensory loss, deep tendon reflexes, and plantar response.

Physical findings

Signs	Neuropathy	Myopathy	ALS
Atrophy	Yes	Yes	Yes
Distribution of weakness	Distal	Proximal	Distal, bulbar
Fasciculations	Yes	No	Yes
Sensory loss	Yes	No	No
Reflexes	Hypoactive	Maybe hypo	Hyperactive
Babinski sign	No	No	Yes

Diagnostic tests

Tests	Neuropathy	Myopathy	ALS
Nerve conduction	Slow	Normal	Normal
Electromyography	Fibrillations, large motor units	Small motor units	Giant motor units
CSF protein	May be elevated	Normal	Normal
Muscle enzymes	Normal	Often elevated	May be elevated
Muscle biopsy	Group atrophy	Degeneration of muscle fibers	Group atrophy

Peripheral neuropathy: distribution of findings

- The temporal evolution of the neuropathy is diagnostically helpful and directs the acuity of investigations and management.
- Physicians should define the time from onset to nadir or from onset to the current state as being acute (days to weeks), subacute (6 weeks to 6 months), or chronic (6 months to years).
- The clinical course should also be described as being monophasic, progressive, or relapsing-remitting.
- The temporal differentials below presume that the cause of sensorimotor dysfunction has been determined to be neuropathic. For predominantly motor impairment, it is important to consider non-neuropathic processes such as acute central lesions, disorders of the neuromuscular junction, and myopathies.

Focal	Multifocal (asymmetric)	Diffuse (symmetric)
Mononeuropathy	Multiple mononeuropathy (Mononeuritis multiplex)	Polyneuropathy
Monoradiculopathy		Dorsal root ganglionopathy
Plexopathy	Polyradiculopathy	Motor neuronopathy
	Motor neuropathy	
	Motor neuronopathy	

Peripheral neuropathy: temporal profile

- Peripheral nerve disorders are characterized as being focal, multifocal (asymmetric), or diffuse (symmetric).
- Most acquired neuropathies evolve symmetrically, initially with sensory disturbances in the feet that gradually ascend, referred to as a length-dependent or dying-back neuropathy.
- Neuropathy that begins in one leg or hand usually indicates an asymmetric disorder.

- Multifocal neuropathies may have characteristic distributions, for example temperature-dependent distribution in lepromatous neuropathy. Pure or predominant sensory neuropathy is unlikely to be multifocal in distribution.

Acute

Axonal	Demyelinating
Alcohol	**GBS**
Vasculitis	**HIV-AIDP**
Acute axonal neuropathy	Diphtheria
Toxins (thallium, arsenic, etc.)	

Subacute/chronic

Axonal	Demyelinating
Diabetes	**CIDP**
Uremia	**Monoclonal gammopathy**
Alcohol	**Hereditary** (CMT, etc)
Vitamin deficiency	Hypothyroidism
HIV	Diabetes
Medications	Medications
Gastric surgery	
Hypothyroidism	
Connective tissue disease (SLE, Sjögren, etc.)	
Paraneoplastic	
Toxins (arsenic, etc.)	

Primarily motor involvement

- Rapidly progressive weakness is a relatively common neurological presentation.
- Primary motor neuropathies will present with muscle weakness and minimal, if any, sensory loss or impairment. However, non-neuropathic processes such as myopathies, neuromuscular junction disorders, and even acute central lesions must be considered.
- Deep tendon reflexes are often diminished or absent.
- Differential diagnosis can be divided into acute (hours/days) or chronic (weeks/months) duration of symptoms.
- Neuropathic weakness tends to be more distal. Weakness due to myopathy or neuromuscular junction disorders is more proximal.

Rapidly progressive weakness

Features	Botulism	GBS	MFS	MG	Tick paralysis
Weakness	Descending, fatigable	Ascending	Ascending	Fatigable	Ascending
Reflexes	Depressed in 50%	Areflexia or depressed	Areflexia or depressed	Normal	Areflexia or depressed
Ataxia	Maybe	No	Yes	No	Maybe
Ophthalmo-plegia	Yes	No	Yes	Yes and variable	No
Pupils	Fixed, sluggish response	Normal	Normal	Normal	Normal
Paresthesia or pain	No	Yes	Some	No	No
Autonomic dysfunction	Yes	Some	Some	No	No
CSF protein	Normal	Increased	Increased	Normal	Normal
Neuro-physiology	Normal NCV, small MAP, unchanged on rep. stim.	Slow or no potentiation of MAP with rep. stim.	Slow or no potentiation of MAP with rep. stim.	Decrement of MAP on rep. stim.	Small MAP, absence or prolonged latencies
Tensilon test	Weakly positive	Negative	Negative	Positive	Negative
Serum antibodies	Clostridium botulinum	Antiganglioside antibody	Antiganglioside antibody	Antiacetylcholine receptor antibody	None

GBS – Guillain-Barré syndrome, MFS – Miller-Fisher syndrome, MG – myasthenia gravis, NCV – nerve conduction velocity, MAP – motor action potential.

Acute weakness with minimal sensory symptoms

- Acute myelopathy, neuromuscular junction disorders, periodic paralysis, and other acute myopathies may mimic acute motor neuropathy.
- The greatest concern with ACUTE WEAKNESS is the progression to respiratory failure. Vital capacity must be monitored and artificial ventilation initiated if necessary.
- Many causes of acute motor weakness are treatable, so many less common causes are still important to consider.

1 ***Guillain-Barré syndrome (GBS)/acute inflammatory demyelinating polyneuropathy (AIDP)***
   - Worldwide incidence (0.4–1.7/100,000), often preceded by viral illness.
   - Ascending symmetric paralysis with minimal sensory symptoms. Hypotonia, hypo/areflexia, autonomic disturbances. May progress to respiratory failure. Facial diplegia and ophthalmoplegia variants.
   - CSF: increased protein, acellular. Nerve conductions slowed.
   - Respiratory support if needed. Treatment includes plasma exchange or intravenous immunoglobulin.
   - An acute axonal form of GBS has been described.
   - Clinically mimicked by polyneuropathy/neuritis associated with AIDS, infectious mononucleosis. or viral hepatitis.
2 *Acute myelopathy* (can present with areflexia and para- or quadriparesis)
3 *Neuromuscular disease*
   3.1 *Myasthenia gravis*
      - Clinical characteristics: fluctuating weakness, muscle fatigability, ocular/cranial nerve muscles affected, then neck and limbs.
      - Myasthenic 'crisis' with respiration and oropharyngeal muscle weakness; precipitated by intercurrent illness, surgery, or occurs spontaneously.
      - EMG: decremental response to repetitive stimulation; increased jitter.
   3.2 **Drug-induced**: aminoglycoside and polypeptide antibiotics; possibly worse with concomitant renal failure and steroid use.
      - Most severe: neomycin, colistin > moderate: kanamycin, gentamicin, streptomycin, tobramycin, amikacin > negligible effects: tetracycline, erthyomycin, vancomycin, clindamycin
4 *Poliomyelitis*: incidence (0.01/100,000), very rare
   - Fever, headache, abdominal pain, paralysis (usually asymmetric), meningismus. Bulbar variant.
   - CSF: aseptic meningitis. Increased WBCs, protein.
5 *Botulism*
   - Food poisoning due to toxin released by *Clostridium botulinum.*
   - Initial symptoms: blurred vision, unreactive pupils, ptosis, diplopia, ophthalmoplegia, bulbar paralysis. Followed by respiratory failure and weakness of limbs and trunk. Constipation.
   - Treat with trivalent botulinum antiserum.
6 *Diphtheria*
   - Due to toxin produced by *Corynebacterium diphtheriae.*
   - Inflammatory pharyngitis. Cardiac and neurological involvement in 20%.
   - 1–2 weeks: palatal paralysis, cranial neuropathies, ciliary paralysis, blurred vision; however, external ophthalmoplegia rare.

- 5–8 weeks: sensorimotor polyneuropathy, may be GBS-like.
- Acutely, treatment with antitoxin. No effective treatment for neuropathy.

7 *Myopathy*

7.1 *Periodic paralysis*: familial, weakness may lead to respiratory failure.
- Hypokalemic. Attacks may be precipitated by cold, ingestion of food. Associated with thyrotoxicosis, GI loss, renal loss.
- Hyperkalemic. Attack precipitated by cold or high potassium.

7.2 Acute polymyositis (see Chronic weakness, p. 276).

7.3 Acute steroid-induced myopathy.

8 *Porphyric polyneuropathy (acute intermittent porphyria)*

- Autosomal dominant inheritance. Attacks triggered by many drugs.
- Abdominal pain, psychosis (delirium), seizures, predominantly motor polyneuropathy. Respiratory failure can occur. Autonomic symptoms.
- Urine porphobilinogen elevated (turns dark when standing).

9 Other viral: other enteroviruses, West Nile virus.

10 Acute uremic polyneuropathy: can mimic GBS/AIDP
- Associated with end-stage renal failure and diabetes.

11 Acute toxic motor polyneuropathy
- Triorthocresylphosphate, other organophosphates, thallium salts.
- Less often: arsenic polyneuropathy, eosinophilia-myalgia syndrome due to contaminated L-tryptophan.

12 *Tick paralysis*
- Toxin produced by feeding tick. History of outdoor activity, insect bites. More often in children.
- Ascending paralysis that may progress to bulbar and respiratory weakness.
- Search for and remove tick.

13 Vasculitic: systemic lupus erythematosis, polyarteritis nodosa.

14 Paraneoplastic (occult carcinoma, Hodgkin)

15 Alcoholism
- May present with subacute axonal motor neuropathy

Plasmapheresis vs. intravenous immunoglobulins

- Both plasmapheresis (or plasma exchange) and intravenous immunoglobulin (IVIg) are effective treatment in various neuromuscular disorders. Both treatments have been shown to be equally effective in the treatment of Guillain-Barré syndrome.
- In addition to the underlying disorder and patient's general condition, the decision to choose either plasmapheresis or IVIg also depends on potential side-effects. Most commonly, both treatments are administered to patients who are critically ill in the intensive care setting, with IVIg being better tolerated by patients with impaired hemodynamics.

- Common indications for plasmapheresis or IVIg include:
  - Guillain-Barré syndrome
  - Myasthenia gravis (during attack or crisis)
  - Lambert-Eaton myasthenic syndrome
  - Chronic inflammatory demyelinating polyneuropathy (CIDP)
  - Some inflammatory myopathies
  - Paraneoplastic syndromes

Features	Plasmapheresis	Intravenous immunoglobulin
Dose	40–50 ml/kg of plasma is removed, replacing the plasma with albumin or saline. A series of 3–6 exchanges on a daily or alternate-day regime is often administered	2 g/kg, divided into 2–5 daily infusions
Side-effects	**Flu-like illness** (most common, particularly in patients with reduced immunoglobulin levels) Hemodynamic instability • Cardiac arrthymias • Orthostatic hypotension • Autonomic dysfunction Venous access complications • Bleeding • Thrombophlebitis • Line infections • Pneumothorax Coagulopathy • Prolonged PT • Prolonged PTT • Thrombocytopenia Electrolyte imbalance • Hypocalcemia • Hypomagnesemia	**Flu-like illness** (most common) Vascular-like headache Atrial and venous thrombosis Pulmonary embolism Hypertensive encephalopathy Leukopenia Worsening renal failure Electrolyte imbalance • Hypocalcemia • Hyponatremia IgA anaphylaxis (serum IgA measurement is required before therapy) Cerebral symptoms • Delirium • Cortical blindness • Seizures Retinal necrosis Hepatitis C (rare)

PT – prothrombin time, PTT – partial thromboplastin time.

Chronic weakness with minimal sensory symptoms

- Neuromuscular disease, myopathy, and motor neuron disease can present with LOWER MOTOR NEURON signs and mimic chronic motor neuropathy.
- Examination findings consistent with chronic motor disorders include atrophy, fasciculations, and reduced reflexes. Spontaneous fasciculations tend to be more prominent in chronic neuropathies or motor neuron disease than in myopathies or neuromuscular junction disorders.

- Most of these disorders are sensorimotor in nature, but can present with predominantly motor findings.
- Excluded from this differential are causes of chronic weakness with primarily UPPER MOTOR NEURON signs, such as cervical spondylosis, MS, tropical spastic paraparesis, and vitamin B_{12} deficiency.

1 **Chronic inflammatory demyelinating polyneuropathy (CIDP)**
   - Chronic or relapsing sensorimotor neuropathy. Motor signs tend to predominate.
   - CSF: may show increased protein (less than AIDP), no cells.
   - NCV shows segmental demyelination.
2 Motor neuron disease
   2.1 **Amyotrophic lateral sclerosis**
      - Clinical characteristics: involves both upper and lower motor neuron degeneration, progressive weakness, atrophy, fasciculations, hyperreflexia, and upgoing toes.
      - Bulbar signs and symptoms common.
   2.2 **Post-polio syndrome**: delayed progressive weakness years/decades after acute poliomyelitis.
   2.3 Spinal muscular atrophy: more so in children and adolescents.
3 *Neuromuscular disorders*
   3.1 *Myasthenia gravis* (see Acute weakness, p. 273)
   3.2 Lambert-Eaton syndrome
      - Clinical characteristics: proximal weakness, reduced/absent reflexes.
      - EMG shows incremental response to repetitive stimulation.
      - Associated with small cell lung cancer 60% of the time.
4 *Myopathy*
   4.1 Polymyositis
      - Inflammatory myopathy associated with collagen vascular disease, occult malignancy, infections, medications, endocrine disorders, and metabolic conditions.
      - Progresses over weeks. Somewhat responsive to immunosuppressants.
   4.2 Drug-induced
   4.3 Acute steroid-induced myopathy: days to weeks after high dose steroids
   4.4 Muscular dystrophy: children, adolescents, young adults
5 Multifocal motor neuropathy
   - Onset tends to be in young adults.
   - Clinical characteristics: upper extremity > lower weakness, asymmetric.
   - Responds to immunosuppressive therapy (IVIg, cyclophosphamide).

6 Toxins
   6.1 Lead: focal weakness of hand/wrist extensors
   6.2 Dapsone: dose-related motor neuropathy
7 HIV-associated motor neuropathy: can mimic CIDP
8 Paraproteinemia (multiple myeloma, osteosclerotic myeloma, MGUS – mono-clonal gammopathy of uncertain significance, POEMS syndrome – polyneuro-pathy, organomegaly, endocrinopathy, myeloma, skin changes, GM1 ganglioside autoantibodies)
9 Paraneoplastic (Hodgkin disease, lymphomas)
10 Hereditary motor and sensory neuropathies (HMSNs): motor signs tend to predominate, although there is a sensory component to both.
   10.1 HMSN I (Charcot-Marie-Tooth): hypertrophic demyelinating
   10.2 HMSN II: axonal
11 Diabetes: purely motor involvement occurs but is very rare.

Mixed sensorimotor neuropathy (subacute/chronic)

- Very large differential diagnosis.
- Most sensorimotor neuropathies occur over a subacute to chronic (weeks/months) time course.
- May divide differential by etiology, associated with:
  1 systemic disease,
  2 medications/drugs,
  3 toxins, or
  4 genetics.
- Approach to diagnosis should include narrowing down the differential based on history (temporal course, associated symptoms, other medical diagnoses [diabetes, renal failure, cancer], medication, or toxin exposures, etc.).
- If no specific diagnosis is suspected from history and exam, then work-up for the most common etiologies is reasonable (labs for glucose, renal function, liver function, vitamin B_{12} level, ESR, HIV).
- If symptoms persist or progress, and initial diagnostic work-up is negative, then pursue less common causes (screen for neoplasms, serum protein electrophoresis, urine protein electrophoresis, angiotensin converting enzyme, autoantibodies, screen for toxins, etc.).
- Electrodiagnostic testing (NCV, EMG) can sometimes be helpful to determine whether the neuropathy is primarily demyelinating or axonal, to evaluate the extent of affected nerves/muscles, and, occasionally, to objectively follow the course of the illness.

Sensorimotor neuropathies associated with systemic disease

1 **Diabetes**: distal symmetric sensorimotor neuropathy, mononeuropathy
2 **Uremia**: distal symmetric sensorimotor neuropathy, mononeuropathy
3 **Alcohol-related** (toxin, also associated vitamin deficiency and liver disease)
4 **Vitamin deficiencies**
   4.1 Vitamin B$_1$ (thiamine) deficiency: burning dysesthesias feet > hands, wasting of distal > proximal muscles; axonal neuropathy.
   4.2 Vitamin B$_{12}$ deficiency: subacute combined degeneration, impaired proprioception/vibration, painful paresthesias.
5 **Chronic liver disease**
6 Paraneoplastic
   6.1 Lung
   6.2 Lymphoma
7 Paraproteinemia
   7.1 Multiple myeloma, osteosclerotic myeloma
   7.2 MGUS: monoclonal gammopathy of uncertain significance
   7.3 POEMS syndrome (polyneuropathy, organomegaly, endocrinopathy, myeloma, skin changes)
   7.4 Macroglobulinemia
   7.5 Cryoglobulinemia
8 Infection
   8.1 AIDS-related
   8.2 Leprosy (tuberculoid)
   8.3 Cytomegalovirus
   8.4 Diphtheria
9 Collagen vascular disease
   9.1 Polyarteritis nodosa: mononeuritis multiplex; vasculitis.
   9.2 Sjögren syndrome: anti-Ro and anti-La antibodies, associated xerophthalmia, xerostomia.
   9.3 Wegener granulomatosis: necrotizing lesions of upper/lower respiratory tracts, glomerulonephritis, and antineutrophilic cytoplasmic antigen (ANCA) antibodies.
   9.4 Rheumatoid arthritis, systemic lupus erythematosis, systemic sclerosis: vasculitic neuropathy; rare.
10 Critical illness polyneuropathy: severe sensorimotor polyneuropathy; associated with sepsis, multisystem organ failure, prolonged neuromuscular blocking agents. Rarely, septic emboli from bacterial endocarditis infarct peripheral nerves.
11 Sarcoidosis: chronic sensorimotor neuropathy; other neuropathic manifestations include multiple cranial neuropathies.

Sensorimotor neuropathies associated with medications/drugs

1 Anti-infectives

    1.1 Isoniazid: may induce vitamin B_6 deficiency; usually sensory.

    1.2 Nitrofurantoin: dose-dependent; exacerbated by renal failure.

    1.3 Thalidomide

2 Chemotherapeutic agents

    2.1 Vincristine

3 Antiarrhythmics

    3.1 Amiodarone: dose-dependent

    3.2 Perhexilene dose-dependent

4 Miscellaneous

    4.1 Aurothioglucose: idiosyncratic.

    4.2 Disulfiram: after chronic therapy.

    4.3 Hydralazine: vitamin B_6 antagonist, rarely toxic.

    4.4 Phenytoin: after chronic therapy (decades).

Sensorimotor neuropathies associated with toxins

1 Acrylamide

2 Metals

    2.1 Arsenic: chronic poisoning develops pain and paresthesias, long before weakness and eventually paralysis occurs. Reflexes lost, Mees lines on fingernails. Acute poisoning is overshadowed by systemic symptoms of vomiting, diarrhea.

    2.2 Thallium

3 Carbon disulfide

4 Organophosphates

5 n-Hexanes

Sensorimotor neuropathies associated with genetics (see Chapter 12: Neurogenetics)

1 Hereditary motor and sensory neuropathies (HMSNs).

2 Hereditary liability to pressure palsy: multiple pressure neuropathies.

3 Ataxia-telangiectasia: also recurrent sinopulmonary infections.

4 Refsum disease: retinitis pigmentosum, ichthyosis, sensorineural deafness.

5 Metachromatic leukodystrophy: mixed central and peripheral demyelination.

6 Krabbe disease: usually infantile onset with developmental regression; however, juvenile and adult slower onset dementia, optic atrophy, leukodystrophy.

Primarily sensory neuropathy

- Most of these diagnoses are sensorimotor neuropathies with predominantly sensory symptoms, as opposed to purely sensory neuropathies.

- Sensory neuropathies may also be divided into those associated with:
  1 Systemic disease
  2 Drugs/medications
  3 Toxins
  4 Genetics
- Approach the diagnosis of these neuropathies similarly to chronic sensorimotor neuropathies: first evaluate careful history and examination, then screen for most likely diagnoses. If symptoms persist or progress and no diagnosis is forthcoming, then evaluate for less common etiologies.

Primarily sensory neuropathies associated with systemic disease

1 **Diabetes**: usually sensorimotor, but acute painful polyneuropathy also occurs.
2 **Infection**
    2.1 **Herpes zoster**: painful acute/subacute neuropathy occurring in the cutaneous distribution of CN V, CN VII, or a peripheral nerve root. Motor involvement in <5%. .
    2.2 Lyme disease: painful sensory radiculitis, appears 3 weeks after the erythema migrans. Pain may be patchy and migrate from area to area. Also associated with cranial neuropathy, particularly bilateral facial.
    2.3 Leprosy (lepromatous)
3 **Vitamin deficiency**
    3.1 Vitamin B_{12}: may be predominantly proprioceptive impairment and painful dysesthesias.
    3.2 Vitamin E: severe proprioceptive and vibratory deficits, sensory ataxia.
4 **Hypothyroidism**: painful paresthesias in hands and feet; weakness is uncommon. Entrapment neuropathies are relatively common.
5 **Uremia**: usually sensorimotor neuropathy, sometimes mostly sensory.
6 Acromegaly: entrapment neuropathies common, usually sensorimotor symptoms.
7 Systemic amyloidosis: painful neuropathy with eventual loss of pain and temperature fibers; spared proprioception, and vibratory sense. Autonomic neuropathy is also prominent.
8 Neuralgic amyotrophy (Parsonage-Turner syndrome): painful brachial plexopathy. Occasionally occurs following viral syndrome or post-vaccination.
9 Paraneoplastic
    9.1 Breast carcinoma
    9.2 Small cell lung carcinoma: anti-Hu antibodies
    9.3 Polycythemia vera
10 Paraproteinemia (multiple myeloma)
11 Primary biliary cirrhosis

Primarily sensory neuropathies associated with drugs/medications
1 Chemotherapeutic agents
    1.1 Cisplatin: purely sensory.
    1.2 Vincristine: sensory > motor; usually hands > feet.
2 Anti-infectives
    2.1 Metronidazole: dose-related.
    2.2 Thalidomide
3 Hydralazine
4 Pyridoxine: occurs with megadose intake.
5 Phenytoin: mild, after decades of use.

Primarily sensory neuropathies associated with toxins
1 **Radiation neuropathy/plexopathy**
    ♦ Initial symptoms are predominantly severe pain, followed by paresthesias and sensory loss. Motor involvement is generally late.
    ♦ Onset may be 12 months to many years after radiation therapy.
2 Arsenic: mostly sensorimotor; with acute toxicity, many systemic symptoms.
3 Acrylamide monomer: large fiber sensory neuropathy; sensory ataxia.

Primarily sensory neuropathies associated with genetics (see Chapter 12: Neurogenetics)
1 Hereditary sensory neuropathy: dorsal root ganglion neurons involved.
2 Hereditary amyloid neuropathies: also autonomic neuropathy.
3 Fabry disease: X-linked, painful neuropathy.

DDx by etiology

Cardiovascular manifestations in neuromuscular disorders

- Cardiac manifestations in neuromuscular disorders are common.
- Cardiac involvement can be related to rhythm, conduction disturbances, myocardial dysfunction, or coronary artery disease.
- Early recognition of cardiac symptoms is critically important as some can be fatal if not treated promptly.

Disorders	Cardiac manifestations
Guillain-Barré syndrome	• Arrthythmias • Autonomic dysfunction, including orthostatic hypotension and diaphoresis

Continued

Disorders	Cardiac manifestations
Periodic paralysis	• Arrhythmias (related to K^+ level)
Mitochondrial myopathies	• Cardiomyopathy
Alcoholic myopathy	• Dilated cardiomyopathy
Muscular dystrophies • Duchenne muscular dystrophy • Becker muscular dystrophy • Emery-Dreifuss muscular dystrophy • Limb-girdle type 1B, 1D, 2C, 2E, 2F muscular dystrophy	• Dilated cardiomyopathy • Atrial flutter • Atrial fibrillation • Mitral valve regurgitation
Myotonic dystrophy	• Intraventricular conduction defect, mainly right or left bundle branch block (due to fatty infiltration of the Purkinje-His system) • Stoke-Adams syndrome • Heart failure in 10% of cases
Friedreich ataxia	• Hypertrophic > dilated cardiomyopathies
Charcot-Marie-Tooth disease	• Dilated cardiomyopathy • Heart failure • Cardiac arrhythmias • Conduction abnormalities
Centronuclear myopathy	• Myocardial fibrosis • Dilated cardiomyopathy

Cardiac manifestations are not clearly associated with myasthenia gravis. However, anti-arrhythmic drugs, like procainamide and quinidine, may unmask or worsen the condition.

Hereditary neuropathies (see Chapter 12: Neurogenetics)

Neuropathies with autonomic nervous system involvement

- Some peripheral neuropathies also have involvement of the autonomic nervous system.
- This is clinically relevant because symptoms of autonomic dysfunction may be prominent, including arrhythmias, orthostatic hypotension, hypertension, anhidrosis, etc.

1 Acute

  1.1 **Guillain-Barré syndrome**

  1.2 Acute panautonomic neuropathy (idiopathic or paraneoplastic)

  1.3 Porphyria

  1.4 Toxins (vincristine, vacor)

2 Chronic
   2.1 **Diabetes mellitus**
   2.2 Paraneoplastic sensory neuropathy
   2.3 Human immunodeficiency virus-associated autonomic neuropathy
   2.4 Amyloid neuropathy (familial or primary)
   2.5 Hereditary sensory and autonomic neuropathy (HSAN)

- Critical illness polyneuropathy is the most common neuromuscular complication in the intensive care unit setting.
- Critical illness myopathy may be more common in units that frequently use neuromuscular blocking agents and steroids.
- The first and often the only clinical sign of critical illness polyneuropathy is respiratory muscle weakness, manifested as a difficulty in weaning from the mechanical ventilator.

Neuromuscular disorders in the critically ill

1 **Critical illness polyneuropathy**
- Usually occurs after sepsis.
- Clinical features include severe weakness or absent movement of the limbs or absent tendon reflexes (previously present). Head, face, and jaw movements are relatively preserved.
- **Most patients have no clear-cut signs of neuromuscular disease. This diagnosis should always be considered despite lack of supportive physical signs.**
- Electrophysiological study demonstrates findings consistent with primary axonal degeneration of mainly motor fibers.
- Exact mechanism of polyneuropathy is not known.

2 Critical illness myopathy
- Usually occurs after sepsis or prolonged use of neuromuscular blocking agents and corticosteroids.
- Acute quadriplegia is a frequent finding.
- Electrophysiological study demonstrates neuromuscular transmission defect and/or myopathy.
- No specific treatment available.

3 Axonal motor neuropathy
- Clinical presentation is very similar to critical illness myopathy.
- Diagnosis is made by muscle biopsy showing normal or denervation atrophy of muscle, while thick myosin filament loss is evident in critical illness myopathy.

4 Acute necrotizing myopathy of intensive care
- Usually preceded by transient infection or trauma.

- Severe muscle weakness associated with increased serum creatine kinase and myoglobinuria.
- Positive sharp waves and fibrillation potentials are observed on needle EMG.

5 Cachetic myopathy
  - Usually preceded by severe systemic illness with prolonged recumbency.
  - Diffuse muscle wasting is demonstrated.
  - Electrophysiological study reveals normal finding, while type II fiber atrophy is seen on muscle biopsy.

- Diabetes is one of the most common causes of neuropathy.
- Diabetes can cause multiple types of neuropathy.

Neuropathies associated with diabetes

1 Acute/subacute diabetic neuropathies – usually occur and then recover to some degree over time.
  a Acute painful neuropathy
    - Abrupt onset of burning pain, usually in feet/legs.
    - May last months and then somewhat recover.
    - Not necessarily a prelude to chronic sensorimotor neuropathy.
  b Diabetic amyotrophy
    - Pain.
    - Asymmetric, usually proximal lower extremity weakness.
    - Wasting and atrophy of quadriceps, iliopsoas, and/or adductors.
    - May last years, but can resolve spontaneously.
  c Mononeuropathy
    - Diabetics may have a predisposition to pressure palsies.
    - Conversely, may represent vascular insults.
  d Cranial neuropathy
    - Usually CN III or CN VI.
    - CN III palsy generally spares pupil.
2 Chronic diabetic neuropathies: slowly progressive
  a **Mixed sensorimotor neuropathy**
    - Most common.
    - Distal, symmetric and primarily sensory.
    - Usually small fiber involvement with burning pain.
  b *Autonomic neuropathy*
    - Fairly common but with nonspecific symptoms or may be asymptomatic.
    - Test parasympathetic function by measuring heart rate at rest, with deep breathing, and when standing.
    - Test sympathetic function by checking mean arterial blood pressure in supine to standing positions.

Neuropathies associated with HIV/AIDS

- HIV-positive persons may suffer from a number of different neuropathies.
- The exact type and etiology is generally dependent upon the stage of the HIV infection/AIDS.

1 *Acute demyelinating neuropathy*
   - Occurs early in the course of infection, before the person becomes immuno-compromised.
   - May occur at the time of seroconversion.
   - Similar to AIDP/Guillain-Barré syndrome, but more often associated with:
      - Generalized lymphadenopathy
      - Frequent cranial nerve involvement
      - Higher frequency of other STDs
2 Subacute demyelinating neuropathy
   - Also occurs before evidence of immunocompromise.
   - Clinically indistinguishable from idiopathic CIDP.
   - CSF shows elevated protein, but may also show pleocytosis.
3 **Axonal sensorimotor neuropathy**
   - Occurs once patient develops criteria for AIDS.
   - Painful paresthesia, particularly in the feet.
4 Mononeuritis multiplex
   - Associated with HIV infection itself.
      - May occur at any stage of the disease.
   - Associated with concomitant hepatitis.
   - Associated with CMV
      - Occurs once CD4 count is low (particularly <50).
5 Polyradiculopathy
   - May also occur in association with CMV infection.

Myopathies associated with normal creatine kinase

- In the following myopathies, there is no associated muscle destruction. Therefore, creatine kinase level remains normal.
- Thus, a normal CK level alone does not necessarily exclude a myopathy.

1 Steroid myopathy
   - The long-term use of steroids may cause worsening of muscle strength associated with a normal or unchanged CK level.

- In fact, steroids do not cause histologic signs of myopathy, but rather, selective atrophy of type II muscle fibers.
2 Mitochondrial myopathies
  - Clinical definitions of mitochondrial encephalomyopathy include:
    - Kearns-Sayre syndrome
    - Mitochondrial encephalopathy, lactic acidosis, and stroke-like episodes (MELAS)
    - Myoclonic epilepsy ragged-red fibers (MERRF)
    - Neuropathy ataxia retinitis pigmentosa syndrome
    - Mitochondrial neurogastrointestinal encephalomyopathy syndrome
3 Channelopathies
  - These disorders are caused by mutations in genes that code for chloride, sodium, or calcium channels in muscle fiber membranes.

Myopathies associated with markedly elevated serum creatine kinase

- Sustained serum creatine kinase (CK) elevation is often due to myopathies, less commonly with neurogenic disorders.
- CK-MM is the predominant isoenzyme in myopathies. Many factors are involved in the elevation of CK enzyme including:
  - Severity of disease
  - Course of disease
  - Available muscle mass
  - Myofiber necrosis: the major factor in CK elevation
- Idiopathic hyperCKemia is defined as persistent elevation of serum CK levels of skeletal muscle origin without clinical manifestations of weakness, abnormal neurological examination, EMG, or muscle biopsy. With the advances of genetic tests, it is likely that more patients with this condition will have a defined neuromuscular disease.

1 **Dystrophinopathies**
  - Associated with the highest recorded CK serum concentration.
  - Examples include Duchenne and Becker muscular dystrophy.
2 Rhabdomyolysis and myoglobinuria
3 Malignant hyperthermia (only during attack)
4 Neuroleptic malignant syndrome
5 Polymyositis, dermatomyositis
6 Myoshi distal myopathy (dysferin mutation, AR transmission)
7 Hypothyroid myopathy: may be associated with elevated CK

Specific mononeuropathies and look-alikes

Median nerve disorders

- The median nerve fibers (C6, C7, C8, and T1) pass through the upper, middle, and lower trunks and the lateral and medial cords of the brachial plexus.
- The median nerve innervates pronator teres before entering the forearm between the two heads of this muscle.
- It gives branches to flexor carpi radialis, palmaris longus, and flexor digitorum sublimis and a purely motor branch, **anterior interosseous nerve**, which supplies the flexor pollicis longus, pronator quadratus, and the lateral half of the flexor digitorum profundus.
- The median nerve finally traverses the carpal tunnel under the flexor retinaculum, from which it emerges to innervate the **LOAF** muscles of the hand (first and second **L**umbricals, **O**pponens pollicis, **A**bductor pollicis brevis, and **F**lexor pollicis brevis) as well as giving sensory branches to the volar surface of the lateral three and a half digits and the dorsal portion of the terminal phalanges.

Location of median nerve lesions:

1 **Carpal tunnel syndrome (CTS)**
   - **The most common focal neuropathy**
     - Clinically, it is often bilateral, although the dominant hand is often involved.
     - Sensory complaints are more often diffuse, even extending proximally rather than in the median distribution. Nocturnal exacerbation is a common feature.
     - Symptoms are often elicited by wrist flexion (Phalen sign), by tapping the nerve at the wrist (Tinel sign), and patients often obtain relieve by shaking their wrist (Flick sign).
     - CTS is usually sporadic or related to recurrent activity (repetitive stress syndrome). There are predisposing conditions including previous Colles fracture, rheumatoid arthritis, diabetes mellitus, acromegaly, myxedema, pregnancy, etc.
     - 'Double crush' syndrome describes a concomitant association between CTS and cervical radiculopathy, ranging from 6–48% in various series.
2 Anterior interosseous syndrome
   - The anterior interosseous nerve may be damaged by direct trauma, forearm or humeral fracture, injections, or blood drawing.
   - In fully established syndrome, three muscles are weak; flexor digitorum profundus (second and third digits), flexor pollicis longus, and pronator quadratus.

- The pinch maneuver or 'ring sign' may demonstrate flexion weakness of the distal phalanges of the thumb and index fingers.

3 Pronator teres syndrome
  - The median nerve in the region of the elbow may be injured by occupational pressure, such as carrying a grocery bag.
  - The clinical picture may mimic CTS when the entire median nerve is involved.
  - Distinguishing features are aggravation of symptoms by pronation of forearm, elbow flexion, and weakness of muscles proximal to the wrist. Nocturnal exacerbation is not a typical feature as in CTS.

4 Ligament of Struthers
  - A rare entrapment point can occur under a ligament connecting the medial humeral epicondyle to an anomalous bony spur.

Radial nerve disorders

- The radial nerve receives contribution mainly from C5, C6, C7, C8 which pass through the upper, middle, and lower trunks and posterior cord of the brachial plexus.
- The radial nerve is the largest terminal branch of the brachial plexus and supplies the extensor muscles of the arm and forearm as well as the overlying skin.
- It gives branches to the triceps and anconeus muscles before winding around the spiral groove. Branches to brachioradialis, extensor carpi radialis longus and brevis, and supinator muscles arise prior to the radial nerve's entrance into the posterior compartment of the forearm.
- The radial nerve then continues as a posterior interosseous nerve, which innervates the remaining wrist and finger extensors.
- The superficial radial nerve separates from the main trunk above the elbow and descends to the distal forearm where it supplies the radial aspect of the hand and the proximal dorsum of the first three and a half digits.

Location of radial nerve lesions:

1 **Saturday night palsy**
  - **The most common radial neuropathy.**
  - **The site of entrapment is at the spiral groove of the humerus.**
  - Injured by pressure during obtunded states or sleep and can occur in utero by the umbilical cord or by decreased fetal activity.
  - Predisposing factors include severe muscular exertion, alcoholism, diabetes mellitus and advanced Parkinson disease.

- Clinically, weakness of wrist and finger extension plus brachioradialis weakness sparing the triceps (nerve to triceps exits before the spiral groove). Sensory loss is limited to the dorsum between the lateral two digits.

2 Posterior interosseous nerve syndrome
- The posterior interosseous nerve is the motor branch of the radial nerve distal to the supinator muscle. Its entrapment occurs at the fibrous arch of origin of the supinator muscle.
- The lesions occur in trauma and fracture of the radial head. Tennis elbow has been attributed to a lesion in this area.
- Clinically, there is wrist extension but with radial deviation. This is because the extensor carpi radialis is spared as well as brachioradialis and triceps muscles.
- Theoretically, there should be no sensory changes.

3 Others
- Cheiralgia paresthetica or Wartenberg disease is a term describing an isolated numbness and pain in the distal forearm resulting from direct injury or pressure to the superficial radial nerve, such as wearing a wristwatch. 'Handcuff neuropathy' is a modern term for this condition.
- A proximal lesion in the axilla can occur from crutch misuse, resulting in triceps weakness and forearm sensory changes.

Ulnar nerve disorders

- The ulnar nerve is derived from the C8, T1 roots, lower trunk, and medial cord of the brachial plexus.
- It is palpable behind the medial epicondyle in the ulnar sulcus and then passes between the aponeuritic origin of the two heads of the flexor carpi ulnaris (cubital tunnel) to course deep in the forearm.
- The dorsal sensory branch provides sensory innervation to the ulnar part of the back of the hand and parts of the dorsum of the little and ring fingers.
- The ulnar nerve enters the hand by passing through the canal of Guyon and immediately divides into a superficial sensory and deep motor branch.
- Ulnar neuropathy results in weakness of the ulnar innervated muscles. The medial digits can appear separated with clawing. Testing thumb adduction can cause substituted flexion of the distal thumb for the weak adductor pollicis ('Froment sign').
- The ulnar nerve provides motor innervation to the following muscles:
  - Flexor carpi ulnaris
  - Flexor digitorum profundus (ulnar half)
  - Hypothenar eminence muscles
  - Adductor pollicis
  - Dorsal interossei
  - Ulnar lumbricals

Locations of ulnar nerve lesions:

1 **Medial epicondyle (elbow)**
   * **The most common site for ulnar entrapment and the second most common upper extremity compression neuropathy.**
   * The mechanism of injury is usually recurrent microtrauma, including repeated leaning on an elbow, prolonged bed rest, or a fracture.
   * Transsulcal nerve conduction velocity slowing of greater than 10 m/sec is useful for localization of the lesion in the elbow region.
   * Also called tardy ulnar palsy and Vegas neuropathy (due to prolonged gambling!).

2 Cubital tunnel
   * It is located 1.5 to 4.0 cm below the ulnar sulcus and the two sides of the tunnel are formed by the two heads of flexor carpi ulnaris.
   * Entrapment can occur at the entrance (humeroaponeurotic arcade) or exit (deep flexor aponeurosis) of the cubital tunnel.

3 Guyon canal
   * Less frequent location for ulnar entrapment.

Ulnar neuropathy vs. cervical radiculopathy

* Ulnar neuropathy and lower cervical radiculopathy can present similarly.
* There is considerable overlap in the clinical syndromes involving the C7-T1 nerve roots, often making precise localization difficult if based solely on neurological exam.

	Ulnar neuropathy	Brachial plexus, medial cord	Brachial plexus, lower trunk	C8 radiculopathy
Causes	Compression, usually at ulnar groove, elbow fracture	Traumatic injuries, tumors, neuritis/ plexitis	Traumatic injuries, particularly at birth (Klumpke palsy)	Compression by cervical disc or foraminal stenosis; tumor of nerve root
Wrist flexion	Weak	Weak	Weak	Weak
Finger flexion	Normal	Weak	Weak	Normal
Thumb flexion / opposition	Normal	Weak	Weak	Normal
Interossei weakness / atrophy	Yes (esp. atrophy of 1st dorsal interosseous)	Yes, same	Yes, same	Yes

	Ulnar neuropathy	Brachial plexus, medial cord	Brachial plexus, lower trunk	C8 radiculopathy
Sensory loss	Ulnar aspect of hand, 5th digit and half of 4th	Same as ulnar + palmar aspect of hand and digits 1–4	Similar to medial cord	Same as ulnar + ulnar aspect of forearm
Triceps reflex	No	Partial	No	Partial
Hand shape	Claw hand	Simian hand	Simian hand	Either
Horner syndrome	Never	Never	Can occur	Can occur

Meralgia paresthetica

- Caused by damage to the lateral cutaneous nerve of the thigh.
- Classic symptoms include pain in the lower back, buttock, anterolateral thigh, and lateral knee regions, while paresthesia and hypesthesia usually involve a much more limited area in the anterolateral thigh.
- Aggravated by standing and relieved by sitting.

Associated with:

1 Obesity: symptoms disappear with weight loss.
2 Pregnancy: symptoms disappear with delivery of the baby.
3 Tight workbelts, harnesses.
4 Backpacking, carrying heavy loads using back with waist strap.
5 Diabetes.

Peroneal nerve disorders

- The common peroneal nerve (L4, L5, S1, S2) runs laterally in the popliteal fossa after its origin from the sciatic nerve. It curves around the neck of the fibula and divides into the superficial and common peroneal nerves.
- The deep peroneal nerve divides into terminal, medial, and lateral branches. The lateral (motor) branch innervates extensor digitorum brevis (EDB) and the medial branch (sensory) innervates the first dorsal web space.
- The superficial peroneal nerve provides motor innervation to the peroneus longus and brevis muscles, and sensory supply to the lower lateral leg and dorsum of the foot.
- Peroneal nerve lesion causes foot drop. However, associated physical signs are different depending on the location of the lesion.

Locations of peroneal nerve lesions:
1 **At the neck of the fibula**
   * The common peroneal nerve is vulnerable to compression where it becomes superficial over the lateral aspect of the neck of the fibula.
   * Commonly, pressure is exerted while crossing the legs. It can also occur in patients who have lost a great deal of weight.
   * Other causes include Baker cyst, fracture of the distal femur or midshaft of the fibula.
   * Examination reveals a foot drop with impaired dorsiflexion and foot eversion. **A key feature to differentiate peroneal nerve lesion from L5 radiculopathy is the additional involvement of foot inversion in L5 radiculopathy** (for details see under Foot drop).
2 Anterior tarsal tunnel syndrome
   * The anterior tarsal tunnel is formed by the external retinaculum, bridging the malleoli. Passing through this is the distal portion of the deep peroneal nerve, with motor innervation limited to the EDB and sensory territory limited to the first dorsal web space.
   * This syndrome consists of pain and numbness of the dorsum of the foot, worse at night, with atrophy of the EDB only. It is related to edema, fractures, ankle sprains, or tight boots.
   * **Although sensory complaints in the foot are not rare, it is rare for the cause to be ankle lesions. More commonly, it is caused by a L5, S1 or common peroneal nerve lesions.**
3 Less commonly, a sciatic nerve lesion can selectively involve the peroneal fibers. Involvement of the short head of biceps femoris in addition to the peroneal nerve innervated muscles is the clue to this localization.

Foot drop

* Foot drop is defined as severe weakness of ankle dorsiflexion with intact plantar flexion. Foot drop is different from flail foot, in which there is no or minimal ankle or foot movements in all directions, including severe weakness of ankle dorsiflexion, plantar flexion, and intrinsic foot muscles.
* Foot drop is a direct effect of tibialis anterior muscle weakness, often associated with weakness of toe extension due to weakness of extensor hallucis and extensor digitorum longus and brevis.
* Unilateral foot drop is caused by disorders distinct from those leading to bilateral foot drop. Most cases of bilateral foot drop are caused by generalized disorders, such as myopathy or motor neuron disease, whereas unilateral foot drop is often due to a focal disorder, such as mononeuropathy or radiculopathy.

	Peroneal neuropathy	L5 radiculopathy	Sciatic neuropathy	Lumbar plexopathy
Causes	Compression	Disc herniation, lumbar stenosis	Hip surgery	Prolonged labor, pelvic fracture
Ankle inversion	Normal	Weak	Normal or mildly weak	Weak
Toe flexion	Normal	Weak	Normal or mildly weak	Weak
Plantar flexion	Normal	Normal	Normal or mildly weak	Normal
Ankle jerk	Normal	Normal	Normal or depressed	Normal or depressed
Sensory loss	Distal 2/3 of lateral leg, dorsum of foot	Big toe	Entire lateral leg and dorsum of foot	L5 dermatome
Pain	Rare, deep pain	Radicular pain	Can be severe	Radicular pain

Unilateral foot drop
- Peroneal neuropathy and L5 radiculopathy are by far the two most common causes.
1 **Peroneal neuropathy**
2 **L5 radiculopathy**
3 Motor neuron disease
4 Multifocal motor neuropathy
5 Poliomyelitis
6 Parasagittal lesions

Bilateral foot drop
- Less common than unilateral foot drop.
- Cauda equina or conus medullaris lesions are the most common causes of bilateral foot drop.
1 **Cauda equina lesions**
2 **Conus medullaris lesions**
3 Myopathies
   - Distal myopathies, e.g. Welander myopathy, etc.
   - Facioscapulohumeral dystrophy
   - Scapuloperoneal muscular dystrophy
4 Neuropathies
   - Bilateral peroneal neuropathies
   - Bilateral sciatic neuropathy
   - Multifocal motor neuropathy with conduction block
   - Hereditary neuropathy with liability to pressure palsy
5 Motor neuron disease
6 Bilateral parasagittal lesions

Chapter 9

Neuro-ophthalmology and Neuro-otology

Cardinal positions of gaze

- There are seven extraocular muscles: four rectus muscles, two oblique muscles, and the levator palpebrae superioris muscle.
- The recti and obliques move the globe, whereas the levator primarily moves the eyelid and only indirectly affects ocular motility.
- The medial rectus (MR) and the lateral rectus (LR) muscles have only horizontal actions, MR-adduction and IR-abduction.
- The superior rectus (SR) and the inferior rectus (IR) muscles insert on the globe from a more lateral position and hence provide more complex motility. The primary action of the SR is elevation and its secondary actions are adduction and intorsion. The primary action of the IR is depression and its secondary actions are adduction and extorsion.
- The primary action of the superior oblique (SO) muscle is intorsion; secondarily, depression and abduction. The primary action of the inferior oblique (IO) muscle is extorsion; secondarily, elevation and abduction.

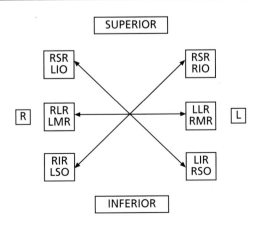

The muscles listed in each box represent the muscles of each eye that must contract to move both eyes conjugately in the direction of gaze indicated. **295**

Ocular problems

Pupillary abnormalities

Fixed dilated pupil

- Fixed dilated pupil is one of the most common neuro-ophthalmologic consultations from the emergency room.
- Pharmacologic blockade is the most common cause of a fixed dilated pupil in an otherwise normal healthy patient.
- A fixed dilated pupil in an awake patient is NOT due to herniation.

1 **Pharmacologic blockade**
   - Results from purposeful or inadvertent instillation of atropine-like drugs into the eyes, for example, scopolamine.
   - It can be differentiated from a dilated pupil accompanying an oculomotor nerve palsy or Adie syndrome by the absence of ptosis or eye movement abnormalities, and also by the failure of the pupil to constrict after pilocarpine 0.5–1% instillation. These drops would cause constriction of a mydriatic pupil accompanying an oculomotor nerve palsy.
2 **Oculomotor nerve palsy**
   - Because parasympathetic fibers are located in the peripheral (superficial) portion of the oculomotor nerve as it exits the brainstem, they are typically affected by a compressive lesion and spared by a vasculopathic lesion (e.g. diabetes mellitus).
   - When an acute third nerve palsy is accompanied by pupillary mydriasis, an aneurysm at the junction of the internal carotid and posterior communicating arteries must be vigorously and urgently investigated with appropriate neuroimaging.
3 Tonic pupil (Holmes-Adie pupil)
   - Adie tonic pupil is typically seen as unilateral mydriasis in an otherwise healthy young woman.
   - Acutely the pupil is large, but it diminishes in size over months to years. The pupil shows sluggish or no reaction to light and a slow (tonic) near response. At the slit-lamp, slow vermiform contractions of the iris help in making the diagnosis.
   - The precise cause is unknown but postganglionic parasympathetic denervation is present.
   - The condition can be diagnosed by its hypersensitivity to weak miotic eye drops; Adie pupil constricts to 0.05–0.1% with pilocarpine eye drops, which affect a normal pupil only minimally.

4 Others
    4.1 Traumatic sphincter iris rupture
    4.2 Acute angle-closure glaucoma

Argyll-Robertson pupil

- Pupils are small, irregular, and unequal.
- Normal afferent visual system.
- Light-near dissociation: light reflex is absent, but accommodation and convergence are intact.
- Little response to atropine or physostigmine.

Causes:
1 **Neurosyphilis: almost pathognomonic**
2 **Diabetes mellitus**
3 Multiple sclerosis
4 Other infectious/inflammatory causes
    4.1 Brainstem encephalitis
    4.2 Lyme disease
5 Others
    5.1 Pinealoma
    5.2 Syringobulbia
    5.3 Chronic alcoholism
Any chronic lesions involving the rostral midbrain can cause Argyll-Robertson pupil.

Horner syndrome (see Chapter 2: Clinical syndromes)

Light-near dissociation

- Light-near dissociation refers to an absent or impaired light reflex with preserved accommodation and convergence.
- The near-reflex pathway subserves pupillary constriction when fixating at a close target. The final common pathway is mediated through the oculomotor nerve with a synapse in the ciliary ganglion. Its central fibers are located more ventrally in the midbrain than those of the light-reflex pathway; ventral to the Edinger-Westphal nuclei. Unlike the light-reflex pathway which is entirely subcortical, the near-reflex pathway sends fibers to the cortex bilaterally.

1 **Diabetes mellitus**
  * Probably the most common cause of light-near dissociation due to presumed small vessel disease.
2 **Dorsal midbrain syndrome** (Parinaud syndrome)
  * Physical signs include:
    ▪ Mid-dilated pupils with light-near dissociation
    ▪ Upgaze palsy
    ▪ Eyelid retraction
    ▪ Convergence-retraction nystagmus
  * Most common causes:
    2.1 **Pineal-region tumor** compressing the dorsal midbrain
    2.2 **Hydrocephalus**
    2.3 Syringobulbia
    2.4 Multiple sclerosis
    2.5 Stroke
3 **Argyll-Robertson pupil**
  * Physical signs: both pupils are miotic, asymmetric in size, and irregular in shape.
  * Although rare, a classic syndrome of neurosyphilis.
4 Adie pupil
  * Large, regular, circular pupil, poorly reactive to light.
  * Strong, persistent stimulus will cause slow tonic constriction. Slow redilation.
5 Afferent visual pathway lesion
  * Pupil usually dilated, poorly reactive, loss of consensual response.
  * Due to lesions in optic nerve, chiasm: multiple sclerosis, optic neuritis.
6 Others
    6.1 Amyloidosis; due to associated autonomic neuropathies
    6.2 Bilateral optic atrophy
    6.3 Brainstem encephalitis, Miller-Fisher variant of Guillain-Barré syndrome
    6.4 Lyme disease
    6.5 Wernicke encephalopathy, chronic alcoholism

Relative afferent pupillary defect

* The swinging flashlight test is used to detect the presence of a relative afferent pupillary defect (RAPD or Marcus Gunn pupil). During the swinging flashlight test, the examiner alternately and briskly illuminates each eye several times, noting pupillary response. A normal consensual response is for the pupils to become initially constricted and to remain so as the light is swung from eye to eye.

- Swinging the light to the eye with optic nerve disease may show no pupillary change in that eye if the pupil is immobile. In such a situation, the degree of consensual response in the normal eye reflects optic nerve activity in the affected eye, and swinging the light to the intact eye should result in further pupillary constriction.
- RAPD is not seen with symmetric damage to the anterior visual pathways, and it is not present in patients with cataract or other media opacities, refractive errors, functional visual loss, or cortical lesions.
- The RAPD is proportional to the amount of visual loss, graded +1 to +4, with +4 indicating an amaurotic pupil.

1 **Asymmetric optic nerve disease**
   1.1 Optic neuritis, multiple sclerosis
   1.2 Optic atrophy
   1.3 Optic nerve compression
   1.4 Optic nerve tumor: glioma
2 Extensive retinal damage
   2.1 Ischemia: retinal infarction
   2.2 Infectious: chorioretinitis

Retinal problems

Optic disc swelling

- When optic disc swelling is associated with increased intracranial pressure, it is termed papilledema. The majority of papilledema is bilateral.
- Papilledema takes days to develop, so at an early stage a patient might have normal fundoscopic examination (except for loss of venous pulsations), despite other clinical signs of increased intracranial pressure.

1 Exclude **pseudopapilledema,** which can occur in:
   ◆ Optic nerve drüsen (hyaline bodies of the optic nerve head, does not occur in children younger than 12 years old).
   ◆ Normal variations; normal individuals can have blurring of the nasal disc margins (but not the temporal margins).
2 *Papilledema*
   ◆ Because it is usually caused by diffuse increased intracranial pressure, true papilledema is generally bilateral. This should be distinguished from a focal process in the optic nerve that causes papillitis, which is usually unilateral.

- *Increased intracranial pressure* may be due to many causes:
  2.1 *Focal cerebral process: tumor, abscess, hematoma*
  2.2 *Diffuse cerebral process: trauma, anoxia, infections, e.g. encephalitis*
  2.3 *Obstruction of CSF flow* causing increased pressure
    - *Obstructive hydrocephalus* can result in papilledema.
    - (Patients with normal pressure hydrocephalus do not have optic disc swelling.)
  2.4 Pseudotumor cerebri (benign intracranial hypertension)
3 Unilateral optic disc swelling
  - Usually results from local lesions rather than diffuse process, as above.
    3.1 Papillitis or optic neuritis
      3.1.1 Demyelination
        3.1.1.1 **Optic neuritis**
        3.1.1.2 Devic disease (bilateral optic neuritis and myelopathy)
      3.1.2 Inflammation (could be either unilateral or bilateral)
        3.1.2.1 Sarcoidosis
        3.1.2.2 Behçet disease
        3.1.2.3 *Temporal arteritis*
      3.1.3 *Infections* (could be either unilateral or bilateral) causing neuroretinitis – varicella zoster virus, Epstein-Barr virus, Lyme disease, syphilis, toxoplasmosis, and cytomegalovirus
    3.2 *Anterior ischemic optic neuropathy* (posterior ischemic optic neuropathy does not cause optic disc swelling)
    3.3 Focal mass lesions
      3.3.1 Optic nerve compression from local structures (lymphoma, meningioma, metastasis)
      3.3.2 Foster-Kennedy syndrome (associated with anosmia)
        - Optic atrophy on one side and papilledema on the other.

Disc swelling: optic neuropathy vs. papilledema

- Disc swelling due to raised intracranial pressure (papilledema) is usually bilateral and approximately equal in both eyes.
- Unilateral disc swelling is most commonly caused by local pathology within the optic nerve or orbit.

Papilledema	Optic neuropathy
Usually bilateral	Can be bilateral or unilateral
Optic nerve function is usually preserved at the initial presentation	Patients usually have impaired visual acuity, color vision, or visual field (VF) defects

Papilledema	Optic neuropathy
Early findings include optic disc swelling with later optic atrophy	Associated clinical signs: • Impaired visual acuity • VF defect • Relative afferent papillary defect (RAPD)
Common causes: • Space occupying lesions • Pseudotumor cerebri • Toxic-metabolic causes • Malignant hypertension • Cerebral venous thrombosis	Common causes: • Inflammatory diseases • Autoimmune diseases • Infections • Toxic/nutritional
Neuroimaging usually reveals abnormalities	Neuroimaging may be normal. The abnormalities may be restricted to the optic nerves only. MRI of orbits with T1-fat suppression is the investigation of choice
	VEP: significant delayed P100 waveform

Papilledema vs. pseudopapilledema

- In assessing an elevated optic disc, physicians must first determine whether there is acquired disc edema, or whether the disc appearance is of pseudopapilledema.
- Whether the fiber layer is hazy, obscuring retinal vessels as with edema, or seems normal, as is usual in pseudopapilledema, is an important distinguishing feature.
- The evaluation for the presence of spontaneous venous pulsation is of limited value because pseudopapilledema also does not show spontaneous venous pulsation.
- Hemorrhages can also occur in both settings.

Features	Papilledema	Pseudopapilledema
Disc color	Hyperemic	Pink, yellowish
Disc margins	Indistinct early at superior and inferior poles	Irregularly blurred
Disc elevation	Minimal	Minimal to marked with center of the disc most elevated
Vessels	Normal distribution, absent spontaneous venous pulsation	Emanate from the center with frequent anomalous patterns, spontaneous may be absent
Nerve fiber layer	Dull as a result of edema	No edema, glistening fiber layer
Hemorrhages	Splinter	Subretinal, retinal, and vitreous

Modified from: Beck R.W., Smith C.H. *Neuro-Ophthalmology: A Problem-Oriented Approach*. Boston, Little Brown, 1988.

Retinitis pigmentosa

- Affects all the retinal layers, both the neuroepithelium and pigmented epithelium.
- Individually, the causes are rare; however, storage disorders and mitochondrial disorders cause many cases of retinitis pigmentosa in children. Specific diagnosis can be made by considering associated features.
- Clinical features:
  - Nyctalopia (impairment of night vision)
  - Visual field constriction
  - Late color vision impairment
  - Metamorphopsia (distorted vision)
- Exam findings:
  - Pigmentary deposits ('bone corpuscles')
  - Disc pallor and attenuated vessels
  - Pigment spares the fovea

1 **Storage diseases**
    1.1 Neuronal ceroid lipofuscinosis: myoclonic seizures, dementia
    1.2 Refsum disease: polyneuropathy, ichthyosis
    1.3 Abetalipoproteinemia (Bassen-Kornzweig disease): acanthocytosis
    1.4 Mucopolysaccharidoses: coarsened facies, organomegaly, Hurler disease, Hunter disease, Scheie disease
2 **Mitochondrial disorders**
    2.1 Kearne-Sayre syndrome: progressive external ophthalmoplegia, heart block
    2.2 Progressive external ophthalmoplegia
    2.3 Neuropathy, ataxia, retinitis pigmentosa syndrome
3 Neurodegenerative disease – Friedreich ataxia, spinocerebellar degeneration, Hallervorden-Spatz disease, familial spastic paraplegia, Chediak-Higashi syndrome
4 Peroxisomal disorders – Zellweger disease, neonatal adrenoleukodystrophy, infantile Refsum disease
5 Toxic retinopathy: may be caused by thioridazine or chloroquine
6 Post-infectious retinopathy: congenital rubella, syphilitic retinitis
7 Cancer-associated retinopathy: pigmentary changes may be sparse initially
    7.1 Small cell lung carcinoma: most common
    7.2 Others: endometrial/uterine, breast, prostate
    7.3 Cutaneous melanoma-associated retinopathy
8 Others
    8.1 Usher syndrome
    8.2 Cockayne syndrome
    8.3 Lawrence-Moon-Biedl syndrome
    8.4 Bardet-Biedl syndrome

Visual disturbances

Amaurosis fugax

- Amaurosis fugax or transient monocular blindness are terms used interchangeably to describe the abrupt onset, over seconds, of loss of vision (greyish haze or black) in one eye.
- Typically, the symptoms arise spontaneously, without provocation, but they may be precipitated by white or bright light, change in posture, exercise, or hot bath, particularly in patients with severe carotid occlusive disease. The visual loss is usually painless and complete immediately. Patients tend to describe it as if a blind or shutter had come down from above.
- The two most common causes are ipsilateral carotid embolism (less likely from the heart) and thrombosis of the posterior ciliary artery. However, there are other causes of amaurosis fugax, which are important to differentiate as the prognosis and treatment of the specific diagnoses are distinct.

1 **Retinal causes: most common**
    1.1 **Retinal ischemia/infarction**: usually due to low retinal perfusion from internal carotid artery embolism or thrombosis of posterior ciliary artery.
    1.2 Conditions resulting in high resistance to retinal perfusion can also cause similar symptoms including:
        1.2.1 Glaucoma
        1.2.2 Retinal vein occlusion
        1.2.3 Increased blood viscosity
    1.3 Paraneoplastic retinopathy and chorioretinitis can produce similar symptoms on occasion.
    1.4 Retinal migraine is an infrequent cause and probably a diagnosis of exclusion.
2 Optic nerve lesions
    2.1 *Anterior ischemic optic neuropathy (AION)*
    2.2 *Giant cell arteritis*
    2.3 Optic neuritis with Uthoff phenomenon (neurological worsening after exercise or increase in temperature)
3 Ocular diseases
    3.1 *Vitreous hemorrhage*
    3.2 Lens subluxation
    3.3 Cataract

Tunnel vision

- Tunnel vision describes a concentric diminution of the visual field.
- Although tunnel vision may imply a hysterical cause, there are many organic etiologies associated with tunnel vision and these should be excluded before the diagnosis of hysteria is made.
- A useful clue to distinguishing hysterical from organic tunnel vision is that the area of the visual field will increase with distance from the object in organic visual field defect.

1 Ocular disease
   1.1 Glaucoma
2 Retinal lesions
   2.1 Chorioretinitis
   2.2 Retinitis pigmentosa
3 Optic nerve lesions
   3.1 Optic neuritis
4 Cerebral process/lesions
   4.1 Bilateral lesions of the anterior calcarine cortex
   4.2 Migraine
5 Hysteria
   • Should be a diagnosis of exclusion.

Nonorganic visual disturbances

- Functional visual problems may represent up to 5% of an average ophthalmologist's practice. A careful history and physical examination is needed.
- Different tests are necessary for different functional visual disturbances. For example, if a patient complains of tunnel vision, confrontational visual field testing can be useful. Normally (in an organic disturbance), the area of visual field defect increases with increasing distance from the object.
- The use of visual-evoked potentials (VEPs) to diagnose functional visual loss can be frustrating. Factitious abnormalities in VEPs are easily induced by subjects who fix eccentrically on the target, or who converge and accommodate to blur vision. **An abnormal VEP is therefore not diagnostic of an organic visual disturbance**.
- Approximately 50% of patients with functional visual disturbances will improve with time and reassurance.
- Functional visual disorder should always be a diagnosis of exclusion, arrived at only after organic causes have been carefully ruled out.

Some forms of nonorganic visual disturbances have been described.
1 **Visual field loss**: usually of four common types
  * Tunnel vision
  * Spiral vision
  * Star-shaped vision
  * Isopter inversion (visual field plotted with a larger test object is smaller than the visual field plotted with a smaller test object)
2 **Visual acuity loss**: can be either unilateral or bilateral
  * Examination of pupils, optokinetic nystagmus, and the use of a mirror to induce eye movement via the pursuit reflex may be useful.
3 **Diplopia**: particularly monocular diplopia
4 Convergence insufficiency
5 Convergence spasm
6 Color perception abnormalities
7 Voluntary nystagmus
8 Pharmacologic pupils
9 Loss of depth perception

Eye movement abnormalities

Diplopia/external ophthalmoplegia

Horizontal gaze palsies

* Supranuclear structures coordinate the action of muscle groups and control conjugate eye movements. The final common pathway for horizontal conjugate gaze starts in the abducens nucleus that contains motor neurons and internuclear neurons. The axons of the internuclear neurons cross to the contralateral side in the lower pons and, after ascending in the medial longitudinal fasciculus (MLF), synapse in the portion of the oculomotor nucleus that innervates the medial rectus muscle.
* This final pathway is controlled by the vestibular system, the optokinetic system, the smooth pursuit system, and lastly the saccadic system. Therefore, an excitatory horizontal vestibulo-ocular impulse originating in the horizontal canal is relayed from the ipsilateral medial vestibular nucleus to the contralateral abducens nucleus, resulting in conjugate horizontal deviation of the eyes to the contralateral side. A lesion anywhere along the above pathway can cause horizontal gaze palsy.

- In general, unilateral restriction of voluntary horizontal conjugate gaze to one side is usually due to contralateral frontal or ipsilateral pontine damage. Clinically, pontine lesions can be differentiated from supranuclear lesions by oculocephalic or doll's eyes maneuver or caloric stimulation. This procedure will overcome gaze deviations induced by supranuclear lesions, but not pontine lesions.
- MR imaging is the procedure of choice in evaluating horizontal gaze palsies.
- EEG is recommended in patients with intermittent conjugate gaze deviation with horizontal gaze palsies and evidence of contralateral cortical lesions.

1 **Frontal lobe destructive lesion (infarct, tumor, abscess, hemorrhage, etc.)**
   - Eye deviation TOWARD the side of the lesion or paresis of gaze AWAY from the lesion.
   - Impaired voluntary pursuit; slow reflex pursuit intact.
   - Can be overcome by reflex maneuvers (oculocephalic, oculovestibular).
   - May have associated hemiparesis contralateral to lesion.
2 **Pontine lesion (infarct, tumor, demyelinating, etc.)**
   - Eye deviation AWAY from the side of the lesion.
   - Eye deviation unable to be overcome by reflex maneuvers.
   - May have associated facial palsy ipsilateral to the lesion and/or hemiparesis contralateral to the lesion.
3 Frontal lobe irritative lesion (triggering seizures, for example)
   - Transient eye deviation AWAY from the epileptic focus DURING A SEIZURE.
   - Post-ictally or interictally, eye deviation may be TOWARD the lesion (like 1, above).
4 Parietal lobe lesion
   - Saccadic latencies may be increased bilaterally.
5 Occipito-temporal lobe lesion
   - Reflex pursuit deficits toward the side of the lesion.
6 Thalamic lesion
   - Eye deviation AWAY from the side of the lesion.
   - May have pursuit deficit toward the side of the lesion.
7 Cerebellar lesions
   - Can be associated with impairments of both pursuit and saccades.
8 Other (nonlateralized) conditions
   - 8.1 *Neuromuscular disorders*: fatigable gaze palsy
      - 8.1.1 Myasthenia gravis: ptosis, proximal/bulbar weakness
      - 8.1.2 Botulism: constipation
   - 8.2 *Guillain-Barré syndrome*: Miller-Fisher variant: ophthalmoplegia, ataxia, areflexia

8.3 Drugs, medications: phenothiazines

8.4 Neurodegenerative disorders: often with vertical gaze palsy

    8.4.1 Progressive supranuclear palsy: impaired upgaze, axial rigidity

    8.4.2 Huntington disease: chorea, psychiatric disorders

    8.4.3 Wernicke syndrome

    8.4.4 Wilson disease

8.5 Cranial neuropathy/ies (may be isolated or in combination, ipsilateral or bilateral)

    8.5.1 *Infection*: tuberculous or fungal meningitis

    8.5.2 Neoplasm: carcinomatous meningitis

8.6 Ocular myopathy: progressive external ophthalmoplegia

8.7 Ophthalmoplegic migraine: episodic gaze palsy associated with headache

9 Pseudoparalysis of ocular muscles: thyroid ophthalmopathy

Transient diplopia

- Diplopia may only occur in certain directions of gaze and fluctuate during the day.
- Intermittent, transient, and paroxysmal diplopia is one of the common presenting symptoms in eye movement disorders encountered by clinical neurologists and ophthalmologists. The diagnosis depends upon an awareness of the potential causes, on careful history-taking, and astute physical examination. In some cases, important physical signs may be easily overlooked or absent on examination between attacks.
- One of the most common causes of intermittent diplopia is myasthenia gravis (MG). MG should be considered and excluded in every case presenting with ptosis and/or ocular motor weakness without pupillary involvement.
- It is useful to classify the causes of intermittent diplopia based on symptom duration.

Duration	Differential diagnosis

Seconds to minutes	1 Myasthenia gravis: usually longer duration
	2 Superior oblique myokymia: aberrant trochlear nerve/superior oblique muscle function resulting in episodes of oscillopsia and diplopia
	  • Usually idiopathic
	  • Rarely due to vascular compression, pontine tumor, or MS
	3 Ocular neuromyotonia: intermittent extraocular muscle spasm
	  • Usually following radiation for skull base tumor
	4 Near-reflex accommodation spasm
	  • Usually functional
	  • Rarely due to brain trauma, seizure, binocular disruption

Continued

Duration	Differential diagnosis
Seconds to minutes (*continued*)	5 Retinal hemifield slip phenomena: associated with initiation of visual pursuit of a moving object
	6 Drugs/medications
	7 Oculomotor palsy cyclic spasm
	• Etiology may be congenital or like ocular neuromyotonia, above
	8 Multiple sclerosis – usually longer duration
Minutes to hours	1 **Myasthenia gravis**
	2 *Vertebro-basilar insufficiency*
	3 Ophthalmoplegic migraine: individual attack
	4 Restrictive orbitopathies
	5 Brown syndrome: congenital or acquired restriction of superior oblique muscle or pulley
	6 Drugs/medications
Days to weeks	1 **Myasthenia gravis**
	2 Ophthalmoplegic migraine: recurrent attacks
	3 Multiple sclerosis: relapsing/remitting episodes
	4 Restrictive orbitopathies
	5 Brown syndrome

Vertical diplopia

- Patients with vertical diplopia complain of seeing two images, one atop or diagonally displaced from the other.
- If the patient complains of vertical diplopia at primary gaze, at least one of the vertically acting extraocular muscles is hypoactive: the right/left inferior/superior rectus, inferior/superior oblique muscles, for example.
  - If vertical separation is worse on looking to the right, possibilities are hypoactive right SR/IR or left SO/IO.
  - If separation is worse on looking to the right and down, then possibilities are hypoactive right IR/left SO.
- Patients with binocular vertical diplopia usually adopt a compensatory head, face, or chin position to move their eyes into a gaze angle that achieves binocular single vision. Hypoactive superior/inferior rectus is compensated by chin flexion/extension, while hypoactive superior/inferior oblique causes angular head tilt.
- A three-step test for evaluation of vertical diplopia:
  1 Determine if there is hypertropia in the primary position. If there is right hypertropia, possibilities are right IR/SO or left SR/IO.
  2 Compare the amount of vertical deviation in the right/left gaze. If the right hypertropia increases on left gaze, possibilities are right SO or left SR.
  3 Compare the vertical deviation in right head tilt and left head tilt. If vertical deviation is increased with right head tilt, the possibility is right SO (Bielschowsky maneuver).

1 Supranuclear causes:
  1.1 Skew deviation: **brainstem or cerebellar lesion** not directly affecting the oculomotor nuclei (ischemia, tumor, elevated intracranial pressure, etc.)
  1.2 Supranuclear monocular elevation paresis
  1.3 Wernicke syndrome
  1.4 Dissociated vertical deviation
    ▪ Covering one eye results in upward deviation of the same eye; usually bilateral.
    ▪ May occur during periods of inattention.
    ▪ Attributed to early disruption of visual fusion (strabismus, congenital cataract).
2 Ocular motor nerve dysfunction
  2.1 **Cranial nerve (CN) palsies:** see Chapter 2: Clinical syndromes)
  2.2 Superior oblique myokymia
  2.3 Decompensation of a long-standing phoria
3 Neuromuscular junction disorders
  3.1 *Myasthenia gravis*
  3.2 *Botulism*
4 Orbital (mechanical processes causing vertical misalignment) or ocular (pathology in the globe) disease
  4.1 Orbital floor blowout fracture
  4.2 Orbital tumors
  4.3 Brown syndrome
  4.4 Graves disease
  4.5 Direct trauma to the eyes
  4.6 Retinal diseases
  4.7 Corneal or lens disease
    ▪ Usually overlapping images rather than two discrete images
    ▪ Monocular diplopia

Signs associated with diplopia

- There are many causes of diplopia. The useful signs below may help localize the lesion as well as determine the possible etiology.

Features	Possible diagnosis
Extraocular muscle fatigue Lid fatigue Weakness of neck flexors, bulbar muscles	Myasthenia gravis
Narrowing of palpebral fissure on adduction as well as abduction deficits	Duane retraction syndrome

Continued

Features	Possible diagnosis
Paradoxical elevation of the upper lid on attempted adduction or downward gaze (aberrant reinnervation)	Old third nerve palsy as a result of trauma or compressive lesion
Horner syndrome Ophthalmoplegia Impaired sensation of V1	Superior orbital fissure syndrome Anterior cavernous sinus lesion
Horner syndrome Ophthalmoplegia Impaired sensation of V1, V2 and/or V3	Posterior cavernous sinus lesion
Proptosis	Orbital lesions, e.g. thyroid disease, inflammation, infiltrative lesions, or carotico-cavernous fistula
Ophthalmoplegia, nystagmus, ataxia and confusion	Wernicke encephalopathy
Crossed hemiparesis, spinothalamic signs	Brainstem syndromes
Facial pain, hearing loss, ipsilateral lateral rectus weakness	Gradenigo syndrome

Internuclear ophthalmoplegia

- Syndrome caused by a lesion in the medial longitudinal fasciculus (MLF). With the gaze directed away from the side of the lesion, the ipsilateral (adducting) eye will not adduct and the contralateral (abducting) eye demonstrates horizontal nystagmus.
- Due to disconnection between the third nerve (and, therefore, the medial rectus) from the sixth nerve nucleus (abducens) of the opposite (contralateral to lesion) side.
- Abduction in either eye is normal, whereas adduction is impaired: dissociation of eye movements. Saccades may be slow before adduction is impaired.
- Diplopia is not a presenting complaint.
- May be bilateral.

1 **Multiple sclerosis**
   - More likely etiology of INO in adulthood/middle age.
   - Often bilateral.
2 *Vascular brainstem lesion*
   - More likely etiology of INO in elderly or person with vascular risk factors.
   - Often unilateral.
3 Pontine glioma

- More likely etiology of INO in a child.
4 Inflammatory lesions of the brainstem
5 *Myasthenia gravis*: unusual

One-and-a-half syndrome

- In the 'one-and-a-half' syndrome, there is a conjugate gaze palsy to one side ('one') and impaired adduction on looking to the other side ('a half'). As a result, the only horizontal movement remaining is abduction of one eye, which may exhibit nystagmus in abduction.
- The responsible lesion involves the PPRF or abducens nucleus and the adjacent MLF on the side of the complete gaze palsy.
- Patients with one-and-a-half syndrome often have exotropia of the eye opposite the side of the lesion, called paralytic pontine exotropia.
- Most patients with a one-and-a-half syndrome have other signs and symptoms of brainstem involvement. A patient with isolated one-and-a-half syndrome, especially with variable ocular motor paresis or ptosis, should have a tensilon test to investigate the possibility of myasthenia gravis. MG can cause pseudo one-and-a-half syndrome!

1 **Brainstem infarction**
- The most common cause in the elderly.
2 **Multiple sclerosis**
- The most common cause in young adults.
3 Trauma
4 Postoperatively after posterior fossa procedure
5 *Basilar artery aneurysm or brainstem arteriovenous malformations*
6 *Myasthenia gravis* – pseudo one-and-a-half syndrome

Nystagmus

Downbeat nystagmus

- Downbeat nystagmus is always of central origin and localizes the lesion to the cervicomedullary junction. Characteristically, the nystagmus increases in amplitude with lateral gaze.
- Most cases of downbeat nystagmus are associated with Chiari malformation and various forms of cerebellar degeneration.
- Its pathophysiology is not well understood and many cases have no identifiable cause.

1 **Cervicomedullary lesions**
   1.1 **Arnold-Chiari malformation**
   1.2 **Spinocerebellar degeneration**
   1.3 Syringobulbia
   1.4 Basilar invagination
   1.5 Floccular lesions
2 **Undetermined cause/idiopathic**
   • Represents a significant number of patients
   • Diagnosis of exclusion
3 Non-structural causes
   3.1 Wernicke-Korsakoff syndrome
   3.2 Lithium intoxication
   3.3 Paraneoplastic syndrome

Upbeat nystagmus

> • Upbeat nystagmus is usually worse on upgaze (Alexander law) and, unlike downbeat nystagmus, it does not increase on lateral gaze.
> • Damage to the central projections to the anterior semicircular canals, which tend to deviate the eyes superiorly, has been suggested to explain upbeat nystagmus.
> • MR imaging is warranted in most cases of upbeat nystagmus to rule out structural lesions, not only posterior fossa lesions but also in the anterior visual pathway (especially in children).
> • The treatment of upbeat nystagmus is directed at the etiology. However, clonazepam, a GABA-A agonist and baclofen, a GABA-B agonist, have been shown to reduce nystagmus velocity and oscillopsia. Anticholinergics may be considered in some cases.

1 **Primary cerebellar degeneration and atrophy**
2 Posterior fossa masses
3 *Medullary lesions or diffuse brainstem lesions*
4 Others
   4.1 Congenital, e.g. cases associated with congenital anterior visual pathway disorders
   4.2 Transient finding in otherwise normal healthy neonates
   4.3 Middle ear disease
   4.4 *Organophosphate poisoning*
   4.5 Anticonvulsant intoxication
   4.6 Tobacco-induced

Periodic alternating nystagmus

- With periodic alternating nystagmus (PAN), the eyes exhibit primary position nystagmus, which after 60 to 120 seconds stops for a few seconds and then starts beating in the opposite direction. Horizontal jerk nystagmus in the primary position that is not associated with vertigo is usually PAN.
- PAN may be associated with periodic alternating oscillopsia, periodic alternating gaze, or periodic alternating skew deviation.
- PAN is thought to be caused by dysfunction of the GABA-ergic velocity storage mechanism and may be controlled by the GABA-B agonist baclofen.
- In acquired cases, if MR imaging is normal and the patient has a history of subacute onset of progressive cerebellar signs and symptoms, Creutzfeldt-Jakob disease should be considered and an EEG should be performed.

1 **Acquired causes: most common**
   1.1 **Lesions at the craniocervical junction**, e.g. Arnold-Chiari malformation
   1.2 Multiple sclerosis
   1.3 Cerebellar degeneration
   1.4 Cerebellar masses
   1.5 Ataxic-telangiectasia
   1.6 *Brainstem infarction*
   1.7 Anticonvulsants
2 Congenital
   - Less common than acquired causes
   - Patients may also respond to baclofen
   - Associated with albinism

Ptosis

- Ptosis is present when the upper eyelid is less than 2 mm from the center of the pupil.
- A number of conditions may cause downward displacement of the eyelid without true ptosis.
- Ptosis may be classified into mechanical, neurogenic, myogenic, and neuromuscular junction causes. However, the list below includes only common causes of unilateral and bilateral ptosis.

Unilateral ptosis:
1 **Third nerve palsy**: see Chapter 2 for specific differential.
2 Horner syndrome: see Chapter 2 for specific differential.

3 *Myasthenia gravis*
4 Congenital or idiopathic

Bilateral ptosis:
1 *Myasthenia gravis*
2 Myotonic dystrophy
3 Oculopharyngeal muscular dystrophy
4 Mitochondrial dystrophy (e.g. Kearns-Sayre Syndrome)
5 Tabes dorsalis
6 Congenital
7 Bilateral Horner syndrome (e.g. in syringomyelia)

Strabismus or squint

- Strabismus refers to a muscle imbalance that results in a misalignment of the visual axes of the two eyes.
- It may be caused by weakness of an individual eye muscle (paralytic strabismus) or by an imbalance of muscular tone, presumably due to a faulty 'central' mechanism that normally maintains a proper angle between the two visual axes (nonparalytic strabismus).
- Almost everyone has a slight tendency to strabismus, i.e. to misalign the visual axes when a target is viewed with one eye. This tendency is termed *phoria* and is normally overcome by the fusion mechanisms.
- A misalignment that is manifest during binocular viewing of a target and cannot be overcome, even when the patient is forced to fixate with the deviant eye, is called a *tropia*.
- Paralytic strabismus is primarily a neurological problem, whereas nonparalytic strabismus or comitant strabismus is more an ophthalmological problem.

Nonparalytic strabismus	Paralytic strabismus
Degree of deviation remains the same throughout all directions of movement	Degree of deviation of the eyes increases as the eyes move in the direction of the pull of paretic muscle
Usually ophthalmological problem	Usually neurological problem
Each eye shows a full range of movement when the other is covered	Affected eye shows the same restriction of movement when used alone or when both eyes are used together
One eye frequently shows opacity of the media or severe refractive error	Not usually present
The patient does not complain of diplopia	The patient usually complains of diplopia (if nerve lesions occur after infancy)

Hearing loss

Deafness

- Deafness is defined as a reduction in auditory acuity. This is a problem of immense proportion; at least 28 million Americans of all ages have a significant degree of deafness.
- In approximately 50% of affected children and 33% of affected adults, the deafness is hereditary.
- In clinical practice, Rinne and Weber tests are of value in differentiating conductive from sensorineural deafness. In the Weber test, sound is localized to the normal ear if sensorineural deafness is present, while it is reversed in conductive deafness. In the Rinne test, if sound cannot be heard by air conduction after bone conduction has ceased, then conductive hearing loss is present.
- In general, early sensorineural deafness is characterized by a partial loss of perception of high-pitched sounds and conductive deafness by a partial loss of low-pitched sounds.

1 Conductive deafness
   - Due to a defect in the mechanism by which sound is transformed and conducted to the cochlea.
     1.1 **Chronic otitis media**: common in children
     1.2 **Impacted cerumen**
     1.3 **Otosclerosis**: main cause of deafness in early adult life
     1.4 Trauma
        1.4.1 Temporal bone fracture
        1.4.2 Ruptured tympanic membrane
2 Sensorineural deafness or nerve deafness
   - Due to disease of the cochlea or of the cochlear division of the eighth cranial nerve.
   - Cochlear hearing loss can be recognized by eliciting the symptoms of recruitment and diplacusis. There is a heightened perception of loudness, or recruitment.
     2.1 **Hereditary or genetic sensorineural hearing loss**
        - Most common in children and young adults.
        - Many individual syndromes described; all types of inheritance patterns.
     2.2 **Presbyacusis**: usually high-frequency; most common in the elderly
     2.3 **Loud noises**, especially chronically: usually high-frequency
     2.4 Infection

2.4.1 Cochlear infection: congenital rubella, post-bacterial meningitis, mumps, chronic infection spreading from middle ear to inner ear; rarely measles vaccination, mycoplasma, scarlet fever

2.4.2 Auditory nerve damage: syphilitic or other chronic meningitides

2.5 Drugs/medications

2.5.1 Permanent impairment: streptomycin, kanamycin, neomycin, gentamycin

2.5.2 Transient dysfunction: quinine, aspirin

2.6 Ménière disease: usually with tinnitus and vertigo

2.7 Cerebellopontine angle tumor

3 Central deafness

- Due to lesions of the cochlear nuclei and their connections with the primary auditory receptive areas in the temporal lobes.
- Complete tone deafness, probably inherited as an autosomal dominant trait, is also a cause of central deafness.
- Since the cochlear nucleus is connected with the cortex of both temporal lobes, hearing is unaffected by unilateral cerebral lesions.
- Deafness due to brainstem lesions is very rare.

Sensory vs. neural lesions in sensorineural hearing loss

- Major emphasis has been placed on the problem of differentiating cochlear dysfunction from lesions of the eighth cranial nerve.
- Although many referrals for audiometric evaluation are made for this reason, even the more sophisticated special auditory tests may not be able to determine the specific pathology underlying the disorder.
- MRI may be necessary to locate the presence of a structural abnormality.

Cochlear disorders	Neural disorders
Unilateral hearing loss with mainly **low**-frequency impairment	Unilateral hearing loss with mainly **high**-frequency impairment
No brainstem signs	Other brainstem signs may be present, e.g. ipsilateral ataxia
Normal speech	Poor speech discrimination
Absence of otoacoustic emissions (OAEs)	OAEs are present. Usually presence of transient-evoked OAEs (TEOAEs) with hearing loss greater than 30–50 dB
Normal acoustic reflexes	Elevated or absent acoustic reflexes
Reflex decay absent	Reflex decay present
All waves delayed on BAERs	Slow wave I–III, I–IV on BAERs

Tinnitus

- Tinnitus refers to sounds originating in the ear, i.e. for which there is no external source. Although usually 'ringing' in character, this is not necessarily so.
- Tinnitus is a remarkably common symptom, affecting more than 37 million Americans.
- Most often, tinnitus signifies a disorder of the tympanic membrane, ossicles of the middle ear, inner ear, or the eighth cranial nerve. A majority of patients who complain of tinnitus have some degree of deafness as well.
- Tinnitus that is localized to one ear and is described as tonal is usually associated with an impairment of cochlear or neural function. Tinnitus due to middle ear disease tends to be more constant than the tinnitus of sensorineural deafness.
- Tinnitus that is unilateral, pulsatile, or fluctuating and associated with vertigo must be investigated by appropriate neurological and audiologic studies.

Two basic types of tinnitus are recognized:

Tonal tinnitus	Nontonal tinnitus
Subjective tinnitus: heard only by patient	Objective tinnitus: under certain conditions, able to be heard by examiner
	Pulsatile tinnitus
More common	Less common
Diseases of the middle or inner ear; possibly related to overactivity or disinhibition of hair cells adjacent to the part of the cochlear that has been injured.	Not due to a primary dysfunction of the auditory neural mechanism. The origin is in the contraction of muscles of the eustachian tube, middle ear, palate, or pharynx
	Caused by:
	1 **Carotid disease**
	2 **Pseudotumor cerebri**
	3 **Glomus tumor**
	4 Palatal myoclonus – rare

Hyperacusis

- Hyperacusis refers to abnormal perception of sounds as being loud or painful sensitivity to loud sounds.
- This is a common symptom and is not associated with increased keenness of hearing to quiet sound stimuli.

1 **Migraine**: probably the most common cause of hyperacusis
2 Any process resulting in meningeal or cerebral irritation
   2.1 Meningoencephalitis
   2.2 Aseptic meningitis
3 Involvement of the nerve to the stapedius muscle
   ♦ The nerve to the stapedius muscle is a small branch of the facial nerve, exiting at a level below the geniculate ganglion but above the junction with the chorda tympani.
   ♦ Usually accompanied by lower motor neuron facial palsy.
   ♦ Can be tested by applying a stethoscope in the patient's ear. A tuning fork at the bell is louder on the side of the paralyzed stapedius muscle.

Dizziness and balance problems

Dizziness: episodic

* The majority of causes of dizziness are due to non-neurological conditions, for example cardiac diseases or systemic conditions.
* Patients who have predominantly presyncope or actual syncope should have cardiac evaluation as well as orthostatic blood pressure assessment.
* Attention should also focus on systemic conditions that could give rise to a general feeling of malaise and weakness, which the patient may interpret as a disorder of balance.

Single episode	Recurrent episodes	Chronic disequilibrium
• **Acute peripheral vestibulopathy: infectious, inflammatory**	• **Migraine: in young adults**	• **Drugs, ototoxicity**
• Air travel	• **Benign positional paroxysmal vertigo (BPPV): in elderly**	• **Multiple sensory deficits**
• Trauma	• Ménière disease	• Uncompensated peripheral vestibulopathy
• Perilymph fistula	• Peripheral vestibulopathy	• Multiple sclerosis
• Ramsay Hunt syndrome	• *Vertebrobasilar insufficiency*	• *Brainstem infarcts*
• *Syncope and presyncope*	• *Syncope and presyncope*	• Chronic mastoiditis
	• Complex partial seizure	• Autonomic neuropathy
		• Cerebellar degeneration

Ref: Modified from Troost B.T. 'Dizziness and vertigo' in *Neurology in Clinical Practice.*

Vertigo

- Vertigo refers to a hallucination of movement. A careful history and physical examination is usually enough to separate true vertigo from dizziness or other types of pseudovertigo.
- Patients with true vertigo usually complain that objects in the environment spin around or move rhythmically in one direction, or that they experience a sensation of whirling of the head and body.
- More commonly, vertigo suggests the disease originates in the vestibular end organs, the vestibular division of the eighth nerve, or the vestibular nuclei of the brainstem and their connections. The differentiation can usually be made based on the form of vertiginous attack, the nature of associated symptoms, and signs and tests of labyrinthine function.
- Lesions in the cerebral cortex, eyes, cerebellum, and perhaps cervical muscles may give rise to vertigo. However, these are not common causes of vertigo, and vertigo is rarely the dominant manifestation of disease in these parts.
- The three most common causes of peripheral vertigo are Ménière disease, benign paroxysmal positional vertigo, and vestibular neuritis.

1 **Peripheral vertigo**: the most common cause of true vertigo

  1.1 **Ménière disease**
- Ménière disease is characterized by attacks of vertigo associated with fluctuating tinnitus and deafness.
- Vertigo in Ménière disease is characteristically abrupt and lasts for several minutes to an hour or longer. It is whirling or rotational in type and usually so severe that the patient cannot stand or walk.
- Associated symptoms include nausea, vomiting, low-pitched tinnitus, a feeling of fullness in the ear and a diminution of hearing. Nystagmus is horizontal with a rotatory component and the slow phase to the side of the affected ear.

  1.2 **Benign paroxysmal positional vertigo (BPPV)**
- This disorder is characterized by paroxysmal vertigo and nystagmus that occur only with the assumption of certain critical positions of the head, usually lying down or rolling over in bed, bending over and straightening up, and tilting the head backwards.
- Vertigo lasts for less than a minute and the examination shows no abnormalities in hearing or any lesions in the ear or elsewhere.
- The diagnosis is can be made by performing a Dix and Hallpike test.

  1.3 **Vestibular neuritis**

- A distinctive disturbance of vestibular function, characterized clinically by a paroxysmal and usually single attack of vertigo, and by a conspicuous absence of tinnitus or deafness. The vertigo usually lasts hours to days, initially associated with vomiting.
- When the hearing loss is present, the entire labyrinth is assumed to be involved, and the term labyrinthitis is used.

1.4 Post-traumatic vertigo

- Post-traumatic vertigo usually immediately follows head trauma. The symptoms can be those of general vestibulopathy or benign positional vertigo.
- The prognosis is generally good, although vertigo sometimes can be delayed after the onset of injury, thought to be due to cupulolithiasis.

1.5 Drug toxicity

- Common vestibulotoxic agents include aminoglycosides.
- Patients usually report progressive unsteadiness, particularly when visual input is diminished. Vestibular testing shows progressive loss of bilateral vestibular function.

1.6 *Labyrinthine ischemia, vertebrobasilar insufficiency*

- Usually associated with other brainstem signs.
- Isolated vertigo is very rarely due to brainstem ischemia.

2 Central causes of vertigo

- Less common, compared to peripheral or systemic causes of vertigo.
- The vertiginous symptoms are usually less prominent and additional neurological signs are usually present on examination.

2.1 *Brainstem ischemia or infarction*

- In general, brainstem TIAs should be accompanied by neurological symptoms or signs, in addition to vertigo or dizziness, for a clear diagnosis of central vertigo to be made. However, isolated vertigo lasting for many minutes may be due to posterior circulation dysfunction.
- Other symptoms are clumsiness, loss of vision, diplopia, perioral numbness, ataxia, and dysarthria.
- Severe vertigo can be an initial symptom of cerebellar infarction. In order to differentiate it from labyrinthine disease, direction of nystagmus and severe ataxia are important findings supportive of cerebellar dysfunction.

2.2 Cerebellopontine angle tumors

- Tumors of the cerebellopontine angle rarely present with isolated vertigo.
- The most common tumor is schwannoma, arising on the vestibular portion of the eighth cranial nerve.
- The most common symptoms associated with the schwannoma is progressive hearing loss and tinnitus. Vertigo is present in 20% of cases.

2.3 Posterior fossa lesions
  - Posterior fossa lesions in different locations are unusual causes of isolated vertigo. The symptoms are usually positional vertigo of central type.
2.4 Temporal lobe epilepsy: a rare cause of vertigo
3 Systemic causes
  3.1 Drugs
  3.2 *Hypotension*
  3.3 Endocrine disorders: diabetes mellitus and hypothyroidism
  3.4 Multiple afferent sensory loss

Peripheral vs. central positional vertigo

- Peripheral causes of vertigo result from dysfunction of vestibular end organs, including semicircular canals, utricle, and saccule, while central vertigo results from dysfunction of the vestibular portion of the eighth cranial nerve (C-P angle lesions), vestibular nuclei, and their connections.
- Differentiation between central and peripheral causes is critically important as the work-up and management is significantly different between the two conditions.
- As the central etiology represents more serious conditions, the assessment for central vertigo should be included in patients who may have only partial features of central vertigo.
- The duration of vertigo and direction of nystagmus are useful clues to differentiate peripheral from central causes.

Features	Peripheral vertigo	Central vertigo
Site of lesions	Semicircular canals Utricle Saccules	Vestibular portion of CN VIII Vestibular nuclei and connections
Intensity of signs and symptoms	Severe Marked vertigo Nausea	Usually mild Less intense vertigo
Associated symptoms	Not often May be none Hearing loss may be present	Ataxia, diplopia, slurred speech, weakness and numbness Rarely for isolated vertigo to be caused by central lesions Hearing loss is rare
Duration	**< 2 minutes**	**Symptoms may persist with long duration**

Continued

Features	Peripheral vertigo	Central vertigo
Latency (time to onset of vertigo and nystagmus)	0–40 seconds (average 7–8 seconds)	No latency Begins immediately
Fatigability (lessening signs and symptoms after repetitive maneuvers)	Yes	No
Nystagmus	**Direction fixed**, torsional, up, upper poles of eyes toward the ground	**Direction changing, variable**
Reproducibility	Less consistent	More consistent

Chapter 10

Neuro-oncology

General information

Epidemiology

Frequency of primary CNS neoplasms by type

- Primary CNS neoplasms are classified histologically based on the presumed normal CNS cell type.
- In some neoplasms, the cell-of-origin remains unknown.
- Frequently, a neoplasm is a mixture of different cell types.
- Primary CNS tumors rarely metastasize outside the CNS.
- Morbidity in intracranial tumors is principally a feature of expansion of intracranial contents within a closed space. In severe cases, this leads to herniation and compression of the respiratory drive center.
- Determination of malignancy is generally based on five histological features:
  - nuclear atypia,
  - cellular pleomorphism,
  - mitoses,
  - vascular proliferation, and
  - necrosis
- Approximately 85% are intracranial, and 15% spinal
- Cumulatively, astrocytomas (combining astrocytomas and glioblastoma multiforme) represent about 30% of intracranial tumors in adults. The majority (70%) of gliomas in adults are supratentorial.
- By contrast, in children, glioblastoma is rare, but astrocytomas are very common (up to 48% of some series). Common pediatric astrocytoma variants include the brainstem astrocytoma and the pilocytic astrocytoma. Medulloblastomas (44%) and ependymomas (8%) are also more frequent in children. The majority of pediatric gliomas (70%) are infratentorial.
- Primary CNS lymphoma has increased in incidence, particularly in persons with impaired immunity (HIV, organ transplant recipients, other immunodeficiency states).

Histological type	Children	Adults
Astrocytoma	25–33%	10–15%
Glioblastoma	3–5%	20–25%
Medulloblastoma	18–19%	–
Meningioma	–	20–30%

Histological type	Children	Adults
Ependymoma	5–7%	2%
Craniopharyngioma	3–6%	–
Pituitary	1–10%	4–8%
Nerve sheath tumor	–	2–7%
Oligodendroglioma	2–4%	**4%**
Germ cell tumor	3–7%	–
Lymphoma	–	2–3%
Others	25–30	10–12%

'–' signifies <2%. Modified from Schoenberg B.S., *et. al.*, *Mayo Clin Proc* 51: 51–56, 1976 and Rowland, Merritt's *Textbook of Neurology*, 9th edition, 1995.

Specific histological types

WHO classification of gliomas

- Gliomas represent the most frequently encountered primary CNS neoplasms.
- They may cause pathology via widespread paranchymal invasion (diffuse gliomas) or compressive mass effect (ependymomas).
- Gliomas demonstrate anaplastic transformation, defined as the tendency to become increasingly malignant over time.
- They histologic classification is frequently complicated by a tendency toward heterogeneous composition.

1 Astrocytic tumors:
    1.1 Astrocytoma
        1.1.1 Fibrillary
        1.1.2 Protoplasmic
        1.1.3 Gemistocytic
    1.2 Anaplastic (malignant) astrocytoma
    1.3 Glioblastoma
        1.3.1 Giant cell
        1.3.2 Gliosarcoma
    1.4 Pilocytic astrocytoma
    1.5 Pleomorphic xanthoastrocytoma
    1.6 Subependymal astrocytoma

2 Oligodendroglial tumors:
   2.1 Oligodendroglioma
   2.2 Anaplastic (malignant) oligodendroglioma
3 Ependymal tumors:
   3.1 Ependymoma
      3.1.1 Cellular
      3.1.2 Capillary
      3.1.3 Clear cell
   3.2 Anaplastic (malignant) ependymoma
   3.3 Myxopapillary ependymoma
   3.4 Subependymoma
4 Mixed gliomas:
   4.1 Oligo-astrocytoma
   4.2 Anaplastic (malignant) oligo-astrocytoma
   4.3 Others

Pilocytic astrocytomas: location

- Peak incidence is 10 years old with ~80% occurrence in 1st two decades.
- Often midline, occurring in the thalamus, hypothalamus, cerebellum, optic chiasm, and brainstem.
- Clinical symptoms related to location. Neurological signs and symptoms progress slowly (in the absence of obstructive hydrocephalus). Symptoms include: headache (50%), seizures (50%), visual changes (20%), and weakness (20%). Signs include: papilledema, hemianopsia, and weakness.
- Most common astrocytic cerebellar neoplasm in children.
- Relatively benign, with excellent prognosis if surgical resection is possible.

Location	Frequency
Cerebral	~32%
Basal ganglia/thalamus	~21%
Cerebellum	~20%
Brainstem	~12%

Modified from Greenberg H.S., Chandler W.F., and Sandler H.M., *Brain Tumors*, 1999.

Malignant astrocytomas: location and presenting symptoms

- Classified by the World Health Organization (WHO) by increasing malignancy as:
  - low-grade astrocytoma (grade II),
  - anaplastic astrocytoma (grade III), and
  - glioblastoma (grade IV)
- The most common adult brain tumor, ~30–45% of primary brain tumors.
- More common in men than in women.
- More common in whites than in blacks.
- Genetic factors in glioblastoma multiforme include loss of chromosome 10 and duplication of epidermal growth factor receptor gene (EGFR) on chromosome 7.
- Prognosis generally poor for grade III and grade IV tumors.

Location of tumor	%
Frontal	~20
Temporal	~17
Parietal	~15
Occipital	~3

Symptom	~% initial symptoms	~% at presentation for medical care
Headache	38	78
Seizure	18	30
Weakness	8	43
Altered mental status	7	42
Dysphagia	5	30
Visual changes	4	39
Altered level of consciousness	2	36
Sensory disturbance	2	14
Gait disturbance	1.5	19
Nausea/emesis		33

Modified from Greenberg H.S., Chandler W.F., and Sandler H.M., *Brain Tumors*, 1999.

Ependymomas: presenting symptoms

- Ependymomas account for approximately 5% of all intracranial tumors, though in children they are the third most common intracranial neoplasm.
- Ependymomas account for 33% of intracranial neoplasms in children younger than 3 years.
- Ependymomas account for 67% of all spinal intramedullary and intradural tumors.
- Can occur in any portion of the ventricular system, including the spinal central canal, although they occur in greatest frequency in the fourth ventricle.
- Hydrocephalus frequently develops and often accounts for initial symptoms.

Symptom	% of patients reporting early	% of patients reporting at diagnosis
Nausea/emesis	29	100
Headache	33	86
Dizziness	9	43
Diplopia	5	48
Gait ataxia	5	48
Hemiparesis	5	9

Modified from Rawlings *et al.*, *Surgical Neurol* 29: 272–281, 1988.

Meningiomas: location and cranial nerve symptoms

- Meningiomas are classified by their site of attachment.
- Due to their tendency to extend, cranial nerve pathology may or may not accurately predict actual primary meningioma location.

Attachment	% of meningiomas
Parasagittal and falx cerebri	25
Convexity	20
Sphenoid ridge	20

Continued

Attachment	% of meningiomas
Olfactory groove	10
Suprasellar	10
Posterior fossa	10
Middle fossa	3
Intraventricular	2

Attachment	Common CN affected	Signs & symptoms
Inner sphenoid ridge	VI, III, IV, V_1	Visual loss, optic atrophy
Olfactory groove	I, II	Anosmia, visual loss, altered mental status, seizures
Cavernous sinus	II, IV, VI, V_1, V_2	Occulomotor pathology, facial sensory disturbances
Cerebellopontine angle	V, VII, VIII, IX, X	Tinnitus, vertigo, facial paralysis, cerebellar pathology, brainstem signs
Middle and rostral clivus	III, V, VI, VII, VIII	Multiple
Posterior clivus	IX, X, XI, XII	Multiple
Cerebellar convexity/tentorium	None	Cerebellar signs, visual loss/ hemianopia
Foramen magnum	VIII, IX, X, XI, XII	Cervical and upper extremity sensory disturbances and weakness

Modified from Hildebrand J., and Brada M., *Differential Diagnosis in Neuro-oncology*, 2001.

Intracranial metastases

- Metastasis may occur to brain parenchyma, to dura, or to leptomeninges. Different types of tumors metastasize preferentially to these locations.
- Up to 25% of patients with systemic cancer develop metastases to one of these locations.
- Parenchymal metastases are usually multifocal and located preferentially near the gray-white junction.
- Dural metastasis is distinct from leptomeningeal metastasis.
- Leptomeningeal metastasis is defined as neoplastic invasion of the pia mater and arachnoid.
- Occurs in approximately 5% of all cancer patients.
- Typically due to hematogenous spread, but may also occur via direct invasion from vertebral metastases, shedding in the CNS, and invasion of nerve sheaths. Iatrogenic metastases may occur after surgical resection.
- Clinical manifestations are extremely variable and frequently multifocal.

- Diagnosis should include CSF studies with cytometry (for meningeal metastasis) and imaging (for all types of metastasis).
- Solitary brain metastasis is a term used to signify cases when no other bodily metastasis (in or out of the brain) is known.

Metastatic tumors to the brain (sites of primary neoplasm)	%
Lung	46%
Breast	13%
GI	9%
Leukemia	7%
GU	7%
Upper respiratory tract	3%
Melanoma	3%
Sarcoma	3%
Others (liver, endocrine, pancreas, etc.)	9%

- Most common parenchymal metastases
  - Lung
  - Melanoma
  - Breast
  - Renal
  - Lymphoma
  - Prostate rarely metastasizes to brain
- Most common dural metastases
  - Prostate
  - Breast
  - Some sarcomas
- Most common leptomeningeal metastases
  - Breast (~41%)
  - Lung (~32%)
  - Skin (includes melanoma) (~10%)
  - GI (~5.5%)
  - GU (~4.5%)
- Most common hemorrhagic metastases
  - Lung
  - Renal
  - Choriocarcinoma
  - Melanoma
- Primary CNS tumors that 'metastasize' within the CNS
  - Glioblastoma
  - Medulloblastoma

- Choroid plexus papilloma
- Ependymoma
- Less common (meningioma, germinoma, pineoblastoma)

Circumscribed, noninfiltrating brain tumors

- Most primary brain tumors, including gliomas and lymphomas, diffusely infiltrate the brain parenchyma.
- A few varieties of neoplasm are well-circumscribed and do not generally invade brain parenchyma.

1 Metastasis
  - Typically show a sharp 'pushing' interface with brain parenchyma.
  - Often multiple, located at gray-white junction.
2 Meningioma
  - Well-circumscribed, firmly attached to dura and may involve adjacent bone.
  - Exert symptoms by compressing adjacent structures, including cranial and peripheral nerve roots.
3 Central neurocytoma and subependymoma
  - Both tumors grow exophytically into the ventricles.
4 Plemorphic xanthoastrocytoma
  - One of the 'circumscribed' astrocytic neoplasms.
5 Infectious lesions: brain abscesses and granulomas may occasionally mimic these types of tumors.

Differentials (in order of frequency)

By age and location

Common brain tumor types by location and age

- Location of primary CNS tumors is predictive of tumor type.
- Predictive tumor type by location is also influenced by patient age.

The top three tumors by location are listed below
Pediatric tumors
1 Cerebral hemisphere
  1.1 **Astrocytoma**
  1.2 Ependymoma

1.3 Oligodendroglioma
2 Temporal lobes
  2.1 **Ganglioma**
  2.2 Oligodendroglioma
  2.3 Pleomorphic xanthoastrocytoma
3 Cerebellum
  3.1 **Medulloblastoma**
  3.2 Astrocytoma (often pilocytic)
  3.3 Dermoid cyst
4 Corpus callosum
  4.1 **Astrocytoma**
  4.2 Oligodendroglioma
  4.3 Lipoma
5 Ventricles
  5.1 **Medulloblastoma**
  5.2 Ependymoma
  5.3a Choroid plexus papilloma
  5.3b Meningioma
6 Cerebellopontine angle
  6.1 **Ependymoma**
  6.2 Choroid plexus papilloma
  6.3 Meningioma

Adult tumors
1 Cerebral hemisphere
  1.1 **Astrocytoma**
  1.2 Glioblastoma multiforme
  1.3 Meningioma
2 Temporal lobes
  2.1 **Ganglioma**
  2.2 Oligodendroglioma
  2.3 Pleomorphic xanthoastrocytoma
3 Cerebellum
  3.1 **Hemangioblastoma**
  3.2 Astrocytoma
  3.3 Medulloblastoma
4 Corpus callosum
  4.1 **Astrocytoma**
  4.2 Glioblastoma multiforme
  4.3 Oligodendroglioma
5 Ventricles
  5.1 **Ependymoma**
  5.2 Choroid plexus papilloma

Supratentorial tumors: adult

- The vast majority (70%) of adult tumors occur supratentorially.
- Supratentorial tumors exert symptoms based on the location. Frontal and non-dominant temporal lobes represent regions relatively silent to tumor growth, and thus, large tumors can present in these regions.
- Symptoms also tend to be more prominent with rapidly growing masses. Indolent tumors such as meningiomas and oligodendrogliomas may have only subtle or slowly progressive symptoms.
- Common symptoms of supratentorial tumors include headache, seizure, focal neurological deficit (weakness, numbness, hemianopia, aphasia).

1 **Metastasis**
- One of the most common masses in the supratentorial space in adults, accounting for up to 40% of all intracranial neoplasms.
- Most frequently multiple, although solitary metastases occur in 30–50% of cases. The common primary tumors are breast, lung, kidney, melanoma, and lymphoma.
- Metastases are often well-defined masses that show enhancement and edema. They are usually located at the gray matter-white matter junction. Most masses follow the flow of carotid arteries (80%) and vertebrobasilar arteries (20%).
- Metastases are typically hypodense on CT imaging. They are also hypodense on T1WI, but may be of variable signal intensity on T2WI.
- Nearly all metastases enhance following contrast administration. The number of lesions may increase with increasing contrast dosage.

2 **Astrocytoma, anaplastic astrocytoma, and glioblastoma multiforme (GBM)**
- 30–40% of all supratentorial tumors in adults. Male > female.
- GBM is the most common and lethal brain tumor (2 year survival <10–15%).
- Pathological criteria for grading gliomas include number of mitoses, presence of necrosis, vascular endothelial proliferation, nuclear pleomorphism, and cellular density.
- Histological grade seems roughly to parallel patients' age in the adults; the older the patient is, the more likely a higher grade glioma. Other features that

are associated with higher grade include ring enhancement, enhancement in general, mass effect, and intratumoral necrosis.

- ◆ GBM is the most common tumor to have intratumoral hemorrhage and seeding. Multicentricity occurs in 4–6% of cases.

3 Oligodendroglioma

- ◆ 4–7% of all intracranial gliomas, with a high rate of calcification (40–70%).
- ◆ The tumor, when pure, is more responsive to therapy, but the histology is usually mixed with the astrocytic form.

4 Meningioma

- ◆ Female > male.
- ◆ Most common supratentorial locations are the falx cerebri and the hemispheric convexities. Meningiomas may also present in the olfactory groove, suprasellarly, and along the sphenoid wing.
- ◆ Rarely invading brain parenchyma, meningiomas exert symptoms primarily by compression of adjacent structures.

5 Pituitary adenoma

- ◆ When extending into the suprasellar region, these tumors may cause compression of the optic chiasm, resulting in bitemporal hemianopia.
- ◆ Macroadenomas (>1 cm) present with headache, visual loss, and endocrinopathy. Microadenomas (<1 cm) usually present with endocrinopathy.

6 Lymphoma

- ◆ The most common type of CNS lymphoma is diffuse histiocytic (large B cell) lymphoma, often associated with immunodeficiency states, including AIDS, transplantations, etc.
- ◆ Primary lymphoma of the CNS usually occurs in the deep gray matter nuclei in the supratentorial space. Coating the ventricles as well as spreading across the corpus callosum is very suggestive of lymphoma. The important DDx in primary CNS lymphoma is cerebral toxoplasmosis.
- ◆ Secondary lymphoma usually involves the leptomeninges and the CSF. Hydrocephalus may be the only sign.

7 Germ cell tumors

- ◆ More common in young men.
- ◆ Account for about 33% of pineal region tumors. Also occur in suprasellar region.
- ◆ Range from benign (teratoma, dermoid, epidermoid, lipoma) to moderate (germinoma) to highly malignant (choriocarcinoma, embryonal cell carcinoma, teratocarcinoma, endodermal sinus tumors).
- ◆ Symptoms are based on location or through endocrine dysfunction.
  - ▪ Increased ICP/hydrocephalus: headache, nausea, vomiting, papilledema.
  - ▪ Brainstem/cerebellar compression: gait disturbance, Parinaud syndrome (upgaze paralysis, light-near dissociation), lid retraction.
  - ▪ Endocrine dysfunction (5%): diabetes insipidus, precocious puberty.

8 Pineal cell tumors
   - Occur predominantly <40 years, no gender preference.
   - Range from pineoblastomas to pineocytomas. Symptoms based on location.
9 Subependymal giant cell astrocytomas
   - Classically, the lesion is seen in 10- to 20-year-old patients with tuberous sclerosis. It may occur in isolation with an atypical variant.
   - They usually occur near the foramen of Monro with marked enhancement.

Infratentorial tumors: pediatric and adult

- Also described as posterior fossa tumors.
- The most common site of CNS tumors in the pediatric population, accounting for two-thirds of childhood brain tumors.
- Account for approximately 15–20% of intra-axial tumors in the adult population.
- Metastatic tumors (not primary CNS) are the most common posterior fossa tumors in adults.
- Signs and symptoms may include headache, papilledema, emesis, disequilibrium, cerebellar and gait ataxia, speech difficulty, and nystagmus.

Pediatric infratentorial tumors
1 Primitive neuroectodermal tumors (PNET)
   1.1 **Medulloblastoma (15–30% of all pediatric brain tumors, 30–40% posterior fossa tumors)**
       - Age of onset 4–8 years. Most common brain tumor in children.
       - Occurs in midline and obstructs 4th ventricle. Symptoms of increased ICP may initially mimic GI distress. Eventually, gait ataxia, squint, positional dizziness, and nystagmus occur.
       - Highly radiosensitive (however, beware CNS radiation in young children). Surgery, radiation, and chemotherapy provide 5 year survival >67%.
       - May 'metastasize' via CSF.
   1.2 Ependymoblastoma: PNET with ependymal differentiation, occur in cerebral hemispheres.
   1.3 Cerebral neuroblastoma: localized solid or cystic cerebral mass.
   1.4 Pinealoblastoma: located in pineal region.
   1.5 Medulloepithelioma
   1.6 Pigmented medulloblastoma
2 **Cerebellar astrocytoma, usually pilocytic (16–24% of all peds)**
   - Age of onset usually after 3 years.
   - Headache is initial symptom in school-age children. Younger children may present with unsteadiness and vomiting.

- Signs: papilledema (83%), ataxia (72%), dysmetria (50%), nystagmus (22%).
- Resection. Good prognosis; 5 year survival 92%, 25 year survival 88%.

3 **Brainstem glioma (4–20% of all peds)**
  - Age at onset 2–13 years.
  - Presentation with cranial neuropathy(ies) and corticospinal tract signs. Dysphagia and hoarseness also occur.
  - Radiation therapy. Poor prognosis.

4 **Ependymoma (6–12% of all peds, 30% in <3 year olds)**
  - Age of onset early childhood.
  - Occurs in 4th ventricle. Presents like medulloblastoma, mostly symptoms of increased ICP (66%). Cerebellar signs lacking early.
  - Surgical resection and shunting. Radiation helps (but again, caution).
  - May 'metastasize' via CSF.

5 Choroid plexus papillomas (1–4% of all pediatric intracranial tumors, 50% in <1 year olds)
  - Presentation is usually hydrocephalus, occasionally aggravated by hemorrhage. May be in 4th or lateral ventricles.
  - Surgical excision and shunting.

6 Hemangioblastoma, cerebellar
  - Onset before age 15 years is unusual. Retinal tumors can present earlier.
  - All children with cerebellar hemangioblastoma have von Hippel-Lindau syndrome (autosomal dominant inheritance). Also retinal hemangioblastoma (up to 50%), renal cell carcinoma (28%), pheochromocytoma (7%).
  - Cerebellar hemisphere location. Headache and ataxia.
  - Surgical resection curative in 80% of cases.

Adult infratentorial tumors

1 **Metastasis**
  - Most common infratentorial tumor in adults. Usually breast, lung, prostate, or head and neck tumors and lymphoma.
  - Symptoms are usually localized pain and cranial neuropathy.
  - Work-up includes MRI with contrast and lumbar puncture for cytology.
  - Therapy with radiation is palliative.

2 **Hemangioblastoma**: see above.

3 **Acoustic neuroma**
  - 5–10% of all intracranial tumors; most common adult tumor at the cerebellopontine angle.
  - Age of onset averages 50 years. No gender preference.
  - Occur bilaterally in less than 5% of cases: these are due to neurofibromatosis.
  - Symptoms of insidious hearing loss (97%), tinnitus (70%), and gait unsteadiness (70%) are common. Other common signs/symptoms include headache (38%), nystagmus (34%), and facial numbness (33%).

4 Ependymoma
  ◆ Supratentorial location more likely in adulthood; 4th ventricular ependymomas rare in adults.
5 Meningioma
  ◆ Several distinct infratentorial locations: see Meningiomas, above.
    • Posterior surface of petrous bone, clivus, foramen magnum, tentorium, or cerebellar convexity.
  ◆ Symptoms based on location: cranial neuropathy, hydrocephalus, craniocervical pain and spastic quadriparesis (foramen magnum), contralateral hemianopia (tentorium), dysmetria/ataxia (cerebellar).
6 Others
  6.1 Craniopharyngioma
  6.2 Chordoma
  6.3 Pontine glioma
  6.4 Pineal region tumors can extend into the infratentorial space.

Tumors in particular brain regions

- The location of the tumor can narrow the differential diagnosis. Tumor location can be discerned from presenting symptoms as well as from neuroimaging.
- Suprasellar/sellar tumors can present with headache, visual disturbance, and endocrinopathy. These tumors can extend posteriorly and cause cranial neuropathies.
- Pineal region tumors can present with headache, nausea, vomiting, impaired upgaze, gait disturbance/ataxia, pupillary abnormalities, and endocrinopathy.
- Intraventricular tumors typically present with signs of hydrocephalus, including headache, nausea, and vomiting.
- Cerebellopontine angle tumors present with hearing loss, disequilibrium, tinnitus, headache, facial numbness, reduced corneal response, and nystagmus.

Sellar/suprasellar tumors
1 **Pituitary adenoma**
2 Craniopharyngioma
3 Meningioma: arise from diaphragma sellae, sphenoid wing, tuberculum sellae
4 Others: chordoma, optic glioma, hypothalamic glioma, germinoma, dermoid, metastasis, nasopharyngeal carcinoma
5 Non-tumor masses: Rathke cleft cyst, sphenoid mucocoele, aneurysm, empty sella

Pineal region tumors

1 **Germ cell tumors**: 57% (most malignant: choriocarcinoma, embryonal cell carcinoma, endodermal sinus tumor, teratocarcinoma > **germinoma** > teratoma, dermoid, epidermoid, lipoma: most benign of GCTs)
2 **Gliomas**: 43% (usually astrocytoma)
3 **Pineal cell tumors**: 35%
4 Meningioma: 9%
5 Metastasis, other: 6%
6 Pineal cyst: 3%

Intraventricular tumors

1 **Medulloblastoma** (most common intraventricular tumor in children): 4th ventricle in kids; cerebellum, etc. in adults.
2 Ependymoma: 4th ventricle location in kids; 3rd/lateral ventricles in all ages.
3 Choroid plexus papilloma: lateral and 4th ventricles.
4 Neurocytoma: 3rd/lateral ventricles. Age of onset 15–40 years.
5 Colloid cyst: classically 3rd ventricle; positional headache or even drop attacks. Also mental symptoms from damage to limbic system and fornix.
6 Meningioma: any ventricle.

Cerebellopontine angle tumors

1 **Acoustic neuroma**
2 Meningioma
3 Cholesteatoma (epidermoid)
4 Others: trigeminal or other cranial neuroma, choroid plexus papilloma (extending through foramen of Luschka), brainstem glioma
5 Other non-tumor masses include arachnoid cysts and aneurysms.

Spinal cord tumors

- Should be differentiated as:
  - intramedullary (arising within the substance of the spinal cord), or
  - extramedullary (arising outside the spinal cord).
- Extramedullary tumors may be further classified as:
  - extradural (in the vertebral bodies or epidural space, or
  - intradural (in the leptomeninges or roots).
- Both extra- and intramedullary tumors may be primary CNS or metastatic in origin.
- Symptomatology may be secondary to invasion, disruption, and/or compression of spinal tracts.

> • Presentation is typically heralded by spastic weakness, sensory level, bowel/bladder dysfunction, posterior column dysfunction, and back or radicular pain.

1 Primary extramedullary tumors
  1.1 **Meningioma**: (up to 65% of primary extramedullary adult spine tumors)
  1.2 **Neurofibroma**: (25% of extramedullary adult)
  1.3 Neuroblastoma: more common in children
  1.4 Sarcoma: more common in children
  1.5 Vascular tumors
  1.6 Chordoma
2 Metastatic extramedullary tumors: very common in adults, rare in children
  2.1 **Carcinoma of breast, lung, prostate, and kidney**
    ▪ May be discrete mass or meningeal carcinomatosis.
  2.2 Lymphoma
  2.3 **Myeloma**
3 Primary intramedullary tumors
  3.1 **Ependymoma**: (60% of primary intramedullary adult spine tumors)
    ▪ 40% of ependymomas involve the filum terminale.
  3.2 **Astrocytoma**: (25% of intramedullary adult)
    ▪ Astrocytomas are up to 90% of primary intramedullary tumors in the pediatric population.
  3.3 Oligodendroglioma 15%
  3.4 *Hemangioblastoma* 8%
    ▪ ~1/3 of spinal hemangioblastomas occur in association with von Hippel-Lindau syndrome.
  3.5 Lipoma
  3.6 Epidermoid/dermoid (inclusion cysts)
4 Metastatic intramedullary tumors
  4.1 Most common: **lung carcinoma** (49% of intramedullary metastases); breast carcinoma (15%), colon carcinoma (7%)
  4.2 Less common: lymphoma (9%), head and neck carcinoma (6%), renal cell carcinoma (6%)

Spinal cord: intra- vs. extramedullary tumors

> • Primary spinal cord tumors are rare.
> • The most common primary spinal cord tumors are extramedullary meningiomas and neurofibromas and intramedullary astrocytomas and ependymomas.

- Metastatic tumors are typically extradural and extramedullary and commonly include lung, breast, prostate, melanoma, and lymphoma.

Signs & symptoms	Intramedullary	Extramedullary
Radicular pain	Less common	Common
Sensory loss	Dissociative	Lateralized
Parasthesias	Early	Late
Dermatomes	Segmental	Caudal
Sensory level	Ascending	Level stops at lesion
Trophic changes	Common	Less common
Urinary incontinence	Early	Late (except conus lesions)
Focal tenderness	Less common	Common

Adopted from Haymaker W., *Bing's Local Diagnosis in Neurological Diseases*, 15th edition, 1969.

Spinal cord: primary intramedullary tumors

- Intramedullary tumors are those which arise from spinal cord parenchyma.
- Refer to spinal cord tumors gray-box discussion for additional details.

Neoplasm	% total	Peak age of presentation
Ependymoma	60–65	2nd–6th decade
Astrocytoma	25–35	All ages
Oligodendroglioma	15	
Hemangioblastoma	1–8	3rd–5th decade
Glioblastoma	1.5	
Lipoma	Rare	
Epidermoid/dermoid cyst	Rare	

Spinal cord: tumors by age and location

- Intramedullary infers within the spinal cord.
- Extramedullary infers outside the spinal cord.
- Intra- and extramedullary tumors may be primary CNS or metastatic.
- Intradural infers within or enclosed by the dura mater.

- Extradural infers on the outer side of and unconnected to the dura mater.
- Intradural tumors may be intra- or extramedullary.
- Symptoms are generally spastic paraparesis and back pain. Sensory deficits (sensory level) and sphincter dysfunction may also occur. Small children may present with a refusal to stand/walk as an initial symptom.
- Treatment includes steroids, followed by surgical resection and radiation.

Classification	% in pediatric population	Types in pediatric population	% in adult population	Types in adult population
Intradural / intramedullary	22–40	**Astrocytoma** **Ependymoma** Lipoma Epidermoid Dermoid Teratoma Vascular tumors	10–20	**Ependymoma** **Astrocytoma** **Metastasis** Oligodendroglioma Lipoma Epidermoid Dermoid Teratoma Vascular tumors
Intradural / extramedullary	10	**Sarcoma** **Neurofibroma** Chondroma Epidermoid	60	**Neurofibroma** **Meningioma** Ependymoma Sarcoma Vascular tumors Chordoma Epidermoid
Extradural	40–59	**Neuroblastoma** **Sarcoma** **Neurofibroma**	20	**Meningeal carcinomatosis** **Metastasis** (lung, breast, prostate, lymphoma, myeloma) Neurofibroma

Associated syndromes

Paraneoplastic syndromes

- Characterized as syndromes resulting from the remote effects of cancer, as distinguished from mass effect, metastases, and nutritional deficiencies.
- Presumed to be due to autoimmune antibody-mediated pathology with shared epitopes between tumor and nervous tissue.
- Symptoms typically evolve in a subacute fashion.
- Small cell lung and ovarian cancers account for most syndromes.
- Diagnosis supported by CSF pleocytosis with elevated protein and IgG.

Antibody	Neoplasm	Neurologic signs and symptoms
Anti-Hu (ANNA-1)	Small cell lung carcinoma, neuroblastoma	Encephalomyelitis, sensory polyneuropathy
Anti-Yo (PCA-1)	Gynecological, breast	Cerebellar degeneration
Anti-Ri (adult)	Small cell lung carcinoma, gynecological, breast	Cerebellar ataxia, opsoclonus
Anti-Ri (pediatric)	Neuroblastoma	Opsoclonus-myoclonus
Anti-Ma1	Many	Cerebellar degeneration, brainstem dysfunction
Anti-Ma2	Testicular	Limbic encephalitis
Anti-Tr	Hodgkin lymphoma	Cerebellar degeneration
Anti-CV2 (CRMP-5)	Small cell lung carcinoma, thymoma	Cerebellar degeneration, encephalomyelitis, peripheral neuropathy
Anti-voltage-gated calcium channel (VGCC)	Small cell lung carcinoma	Lambert-Eaton syndrome
Anti-amphiphysin	Breast, small cell lung carcinoma	Stiff-person syndrome, encephalomyelitis
Anti-PCA-2	Small cell lung carcinoma	Cerebellar degeneration, encephalomyelitis, Lambert-Eaton syndrome
ANNA-3	Lung cancer	Sensory neuropathy, encephalomyelitis

Leptomeningeal carcinomatosis

- There are a myriad of presentations. Altered mental status is common, as are seizures, multiple cranial and root signs, and headache.
- The onset may be fulminant (as in leukemia), or subacute, with stuttering multifocal deficits and deterioration of cognitive function.
- The first CSF tap has a 50% yield of positive cytology. By the third tap, the yield goes up to 85%.
- Gadolinium-enhanced MRI is the neuroimaging of choice.
- Unfortunately, the prognosis is poor, especially in metastasis from solid tumors.

1 **Leukemia**
   - The most common in children.
   - 70% of patients with leukemia have leptomeningeal carcinomatosis. That explains why the treatment includes prophylaxis CNS radiotherapy.
2 **Adenocarcinoma**
   - **Breast cancer**: the most common among solid tumors and in adults.
   - **Lung carcinoma**: the second most common.
   - Gastrointestinal carcinoma.
3 Others
   - Non-Hodgkin lymphoma.
   - Melanoma.
   - Untreated, certain primary CNS tumors also have a high risk of leptomeningeal metastasis.

Neoplasms causing endocrinopathies

- Typically, the result of neoplasm in the pituitary-hypothalamic axis. Some neoplasms exert endocrine effects by invading the hypothalamic region.
- Tumors may be either suprasellar or in the pituitary sella.
- Symptoms may be the result of excess hormone secretion, hypopituitarism, or both.
- Suprasellar extension may cause compression of the optic chiasm, resulting in the classic presentation of bilateral heteronymous temporal hemianopia.

1 Primary suprasellar tumors
   - 1.1 **Suprasellar glioma**
   - 1.2 **Craniopharyngioma**
   - 1.3 **Germ cell tumor**
   - 1.4 Meningioma
   - 1.5 Hamartoma
2 **Pituitary adenomas**
   - 2.1 Prolactinoma (25–30%)
   - 2.2 Growth hormone secreting (15–30%)
   - 2.3 ACTH secreting (15%)
   - 2.4 FSH/LH secreting (4%)
   - 2.5 TSH secreting (<1%)
3 **Metastases**
   - 3.1 Suprasellar
   - 3.2 Pituitary

Neurological complications of cancer therapies

- All cytotoxic agents utilized in chemotherapy have demonstrated neurotoxicity when coming in direct contact with the CNS.
- Few agents readily cross the blood-brain barrier (BBB).
- Often, patients are treated with multiple agents, making elucidation of the offending agent difficult.
- Anticancer therapeutic modalities may have additive and/or synergistic neurotoxities.

Therapeutic modality	Known neurotoxicity	Neurotoxic synergism
Methotrexate	Encephalopathy, myelopathy (intra-thecal administration)	Radiation*
Cytosine arabinoside	Cerebellopathy	
5-fluorouracil	Cerebellopathy	
Cisplatin	**Sensory peripheral neuropathy**, focal and diffuse cortical pathology, optic neuritis, cranial nerve VIII pathology	
Vincristine	**Motor > sensory peripheral neuropathy**, encephalopathy (rare, though extremely neurotoxic when crossing BBB)	
Procarbazine	Mild encephalopathy, ataxia	
L-asparaginase	Altered mental status	
Etoposide (VP-16)	Altered mental status	
Hexamethylmelamine	Ataxia	
Mitotane	Ataxia	
Tamoxifen	Reversible cerebellar dysfunction	
Taxol/taxotere	**Sensory > motor peripheral neuropathy**	
Suramin	Guillain-Barré-like syndrome	
Diffuse brain radiation	Headache, nausea, somnolence, late-onset leukoencephalopathy (6 months to years) with cognitive decline, gait disorders, and urinary incontinence, optic atrophy, cataracts	Focal radiation, methotrexate
Focal radiation	Focal radiation-induced leukoencephalopathy, myelopathy (early- and late-delayed), brachial and lumbosacral plexopathies, focal peripheral neuropathies	Diffuse radiation, methotrexate

* Do not give methotrexate following radiation therapy.

Chapter 11
Pediatric Neurology

Paroxysmal disorders and seizures

Paroxysmal disorders

Paroxysmal disorders in infants/toddlers

- Often present as 'spells' or 'seizures' that resolve by the time the child reaches medical attention.
- History is of utmost importance, as examination is often normal.
- Accurate description of the paroxysmal event is critical, including any preceding activities, triggering events/factors, duration of episode, change in color, eye movements, focal motor activity, means of resolution, post-ictal behaviors, and frequency.
- Parental or care giver report is essential. Videotapes or digital video clips can be very helpful.
- EEG is important to identify if spells are epileptic in nature.

1 **Seizures** (see Pediatric seizure syndromes, pp. 350–1)
    1.1 **Seizure with fever**
        ▪ **Simple febrile seizure**
        ▪ ***Central nervous system infection: sepsis/meningitis/encephalitis***
        ▪ *Epilepsy triggered by fever*: difficult to distinguish from febrile seizure.
    1.2 **Seizure without fever**: may be provoked or unprovoked. Seizures may be provoked by electrolyte abnormalities, hypoglycemia, intoxication, etc.

2 **Breath-holding or apnea**

    2.1 *Neonatal apnea*: due to prematurity, rarely seizure

    2.2 **Cyanotic syncope/breath holding spells**

- Occurs in up to 5% of all infants. Often family history is positive.
- Almost always provoked by anger, frustration, fear; child crying at on-set.
- Breathing stops in expiration, followed by cyanosis, then unconsciousness.
- Onset before age 3 years; ceases by age 4–8 years. Benign.

    2.3 *Pallid syncope*

- Provoked by sudden, unexpected painful event.
- Crying rare, becoming white and limp, then unconsciousness.
- Due to reflex asystole. Benign. Outgrown by age 4–8 years.

3 Migraine: unusual in infancy

    3.1 Cyclic vomiting

    3.2 Paroxysmal vertigo or torticollis

4 Movement disorder: (see Pediatric paroxysmal movement disorders, p. 349)

5 Stereotypy: repeated purposeless movements that may be simple or complex

Paroxysmal disorders in children

- As in infants/toddlers, these often present as 'spells' or 'seizures' that resolve by the time the child reaches medical attention.
- History remains of utmost importance, as examination is often normal.
- Accurate description of the paroxysm is critical, including any preceding activities, triggering events/factors, duration of episode, motor activity, means of resolution, post-ictal behaviors, and frequency.
- An eyewitness report, videotape, or digital video clips can be very helpful.
- Febrile seizures become increasingly rare over the age of 4–5 years.

1 **Seizures** (see Pediatric seizure syndromes, pp. 350–2)

    1.1 **Seizure with fever**

        1.1.1 **Simple febrile seizure**

        1.1.2 Complex febrile seizure

        1.1.3 *Central nervous system infection: meningitis/encephalitis*

        1.1.4 *Epilepsy triggered by fever*

    1.2 Seizure without fever

        1.2.1 **Absence seizure**

        1.2.2 **Complex partial seizure**

        1.2.3 Myoclonic seizure

        1.2.4 Benign age-specific syndromes

1.2.5 Seizure provoked by other systemic abnormality – electrolyte disturbance, hypoglycemia, intoxication, etc.

2 **Migraine and migraine variants**
- Primary symptoms do not necessarily require headache. Family history of migraine (although not necessarily of specific variant) often present.
- Migraine is a clinical diagnosis. Alternative, more dangerous diagnoses should be ruled out if the clinical picture warrants.
    2.1 Acute confusional migraine: ages 6–16 years, episodic confusion, spells last hours. DDx: non-convulsive status epilepticus, toxin ingestion.
    2.2 Basilar migraine: adolescents, episodic ataxia, other brainstem symptoms (vertigo, tinnitus, alternating hemiparesis, paresthesias), often followed by throbbing headache.
    2.3 Benign paroxysmal vertigo/ataxia: infants/toddlers, episodic vertigo, pallor, nystagmus, fright, spells last only minutes. Consciousness unimpaired.
    2.4 Cyclic vomiting: infants, episodic vomiting. DDx: gastroenteritis, reflux, malrotation.
    2.5 Other variants: retinal, opthalmoplegic, transient global amnesia.

3 **Syncope**: sometimes associated with brief stiffening/trembling after loss of consciousness and falling to ground. Characterized by brief duration of unconsciousness (few seconds) and rapid recovery (few minutes).
    3.1 **Vasovagal**: reflex peripheral vasodilation resulting in loss of consciousness.
        - Triggered by emotional experience; prodrome of faintness/dizziness.
        - Pallor, skin cold/clammy. Duration only seconds, recovery rapid.
    3.2 *Cardiac arrhythmia*: consider if syncope occurs while lying/sitting. May have family history.
    3.3 *Orthostatic hypotension*: occurs shortly after rising to standing position.
    3.4 Hyperventilation syndrome: triggered by emotional upset, patient begins deep hyperventilation, then finger/lip paresthesias, headache, may lose consciousness.

4 Movement disorder (see Pediatric paroxysmal movement disorders, p. 349)

5 Sleep disorder
    5.1 Narcolepsy, cataplexy: daytime sleepiness, sleep attacks with paralysis during waking hours; cataplexy is loss of tone induced by emotional experience.
    5.2 Night terrors: partial arousal from non-REM sleep, 2 hours after sleep starts. Onset usually <6 years old. Recurrent episodes of wakening in terrified state. Frequency 1+/week. Usually stop by 8 years. 50% are also sleepwalkers
    5.3 Parasomnias

6 **Staring spells/daydreaming**: common. EEG normal.
7 Pseudoseizures/psychogenic seizures

Pediatric paroxysmal movement disorders

- The paroxysmal movement disorders are frequently misdiagnosed as epilepsy, although anti-epileptic medications are also effective in these conditions. The normality of ictal EEG is a major differentiating characteristic.

1 **Tic disorders** (see Chapter 6: Movement Disorders)
2 Benign paroxysmal torticollis of infancy
   - Attacks tend to occur frequently at onset (before 3 months of age).
   - Most episodes are accompanied by irritability, pallor, vomiting, ataxia, and then infant may remain quiet in the abnormal posture, which can last from minutes to days. Laterocollis, retrocollis, or torticollis is a major feature, although trunk or limb involvement can also occur. Work-up is normal.
   - Attacks usually disappear before the age of 5 years.
   - The etiology is unclear, although vestibular dysfunction is probable.
3 Paroxysmal tonic upgaze deviation in infancy
   - The onset is usually within the first months of life.
   - Characterized by prolonged episodes lasting hours of sustained or intermittent upward gaze deviation, occurrence of downbeating nystagmus on attempts to look downward, normal horizontal eye movements, disappearance with sleep, and aggravation during daytime. Work-up normal.
   - Spontaneous remission occurs in a few years.
4 Paroxysmal dyskinesias
   - Refers to sudden episodes of chorea, ballism, or dystonia precipitated by ingestion of alcohol, coffee, exercise, or stress.
   - Various types have been described (see Chapter 6: Movement Disorders).
5 Hyperekplexia: startle disease (see Chapter 6: Movement Disorders).
6 Episodic ataxia: often responsive to acetazolamide (see Chapter 6: Movement Disorders).
7 Stereotypy (see Chapter 6: Movement Disorders).
8 Secondary paroxysmal dyskinesias
   - Secondary paroxysmal dyskinesias may not be correlated with any specific focal lesion in the CNS. Cases have also been reported to involve basal ganglia, cerebral cortex, brainstem, or spinal cord.

Seizure syndromes by age

Pediatric seizure syndromes

- Seizures are a common occurrence in childhood.
- The etiology and appearance of seizures differs based on age of presentation.
- A first nonfebrile seizure merits work-up, including laboratory, neuro exam, EEG, and imaging, if indicated.
- Provoking factors should be sought, including toxic and metabolic abnormalities (hypoglycemia, electrolyte disturbances, drug ingestions, etc.).
- Work-up for a simple febrile seizure may be abbreviated, unless there is an initial suspicion of meningitis/encephalitis, in which case lumbar puncture should be performed. Children with CNS infection will generally have altered mentation.
- There are more self-limited, benign types of seizures in children than in adults (i.e. febrile seizures, benign Rolandic epilepsy with centrotemporal spikes, etc.).
- There are also more catastrophic epilepsy syndromes in children, and these are associated with intractability and developmental impairment.

1 Neonatal seizure semiology/syndromes
   - EEG is often necessary to definitely diagnose neonatal seizures.
   - Work-up must include evaluation for *infection/sepsis/meningitis*.
   - *For additional causes see Neonatal seizures: etiology, p. 357.*
   - 1.1 Tonic seizures with or without apnea: particularly in premies
   - 1.2 Tonic eye deviation
   - 1.3 Focal clonic jerks
   - 1.4 Multifocal clonic jerking
   - 1.5 Myoclonic jerks
   - 1.6 Benign familial neonatal seizures: AD
     - Rare; family history may not be evident until relatives interviewed.
     - Diagnosis of exclusion, does NOT preclude work-up for other causes.
   - 1.7 Ohtahara syndrome
     - Rare catastrophic epilepsy syndrome of neonates. High mortality.
     - Associated with burst suppression on EEG; poor prognosis.
2 Infant/toddler seizure semiology/syndromes
   - *Infection/sepsis/meningitis* is still a major concern when seizures occur in infancy.
   - *For additional causes see Infantile seizures: etiology, p. 357*
   - 2.1 Infantile spasms (see Infantile spasms DDx, p. 353).
   - 2.2 **Febrile seizures**

- Occur in 4% of all children. Not caused by CNS infection.
- **Simple febrile seizure**: single, brief, generalized seizure in association with a fever. Awake, alert shortly afterwards.
  - Many are familial, probably AD.
  - 1/3 will have a recurrent febrile seizure. Half of these will have a third.
- Cease after age 5–6 years. Risk of later epilepsy is minimal (2%).
- Complex febrile seizure: prolonged, focal, and/or multiple seizures in association with fever. Slightly higher risk of later epilepsy.
- Pre-existing neurological or developmental abnormalities and family history of epilepsy increase risk for later (nonfebrile) seizures.

2.3 Benign familial infantile convulsions: AD.
- Onset as early as 3 months.
- Easily controlled with medications; remit spontaneously.

2.4 Complex partial seizures

2.5 Benign infantile myoclonus: normal EEG during episode.

2.6 Myoclonic epilepsy: may be benign or severe.

3 Childhood/adolescent seizure semiology/syndromes

3.1 Febrile seizures: may occur up to age 6 years (see above).

3.2 Benign occipital epilepsy of childhood.
- Clinical characteristics: visual seizure semiology (visual hallucinations with flashing lights/spots, blindness, illusions, or loss of consciousness). Focal clonic activity, eye deviation, headache, and nausea may occur.
- EEG shows occipital spike waves, may be photosensitive.
- Generally outgrown by age 12 years. Family history of seizures is common.

3.3 Benign Rolandic epilepsy of childhood.
- Clinical characteristics: simple partial seizures, usually involving the face, causing paresthesias or focal clonic activity. Usually nocturnal. Can spread from face to upper extremity to generalize.
- EEG shows centrotemporal spikes.
- Generally outgrown by age 14 years. Family history of seizures is common.

3.4 **Childhood/juvenile absence epilepsy**
- Clinical characteristics: absence seizures manifest as brief staring spells or episodes of behavioral arrest. May present with poor attention in school or 'daydreaming'. Tonic-clonic seizures can occur. Seizures may be provoked by hyperventilation.
- EEG pathognomonic: generalized 3 Hz spike and wave.

3.5 Autosomal dominant nocturnal frontal lobe epilepsy
- Onset often in childhood. Familial seizure syndrome with 70% penetrance.

- Bizarre seizures during sleep. Gasping, psychic phenomena, shivering, thrashing, clonic jerks, semi-awareness, eyes may open, grabbing onto things.

3.6 **Complex partial seizures**: similar to adults – may have aura, impaired consciousness, automatisms, confusion, tonic arm extension (see Chapter 4: Paroxysmal Disorders).

3.7 Juvenile myoclonic epilepsy
- Presents with absence seizures in childhood; myoclonic seizures in adolescence, and generalized tonic-clonic seizures in adolescence and young adulthood.
- Myoclonic seizures are brief, bilateral, and may cause falls. Usually consciousness is preserved. Tend to occur upon awakening.

3.8 Progressive myoclonus epilepsies
- Clinical characteristics: myoclonus, seizures (tonic-clonic, tonic, or myoclonic), progressive dementia, and ataxia.

3.9 *Lennox-Gastaut syndrome* (see Lennox-Gastaut syndrome DDx, pp. 354–5).

3.10 Rasmussen syndrome (see Epilepsia partialis continua DDx, pp. 355–6).

3.11 Acquired epileptiform aphasia/Landau-Kleffner syndrome
- Onset usually in childhood.
- Loss of previously acquired language milestones, may be associated with continuous spike wave discharges during sleep (CSWS).

Neonatal jitteriness vs. myoclonus vs. seizure

- Jitteriness/tremor can be seen in a substantial portion of normal neonates, and should be distinguished from neonatal seizures.
- Jitteriness can also be seen in newborns with perinatal asphyxia (with or without concomitant seizures), hypoglycemia, maternal drug addiction, and occasionally with metabolic disorders.
- Neonatal seizures can take a myriad of clinical forms. If there is any doubt, an EEG is indicated.
- Work-up for sepsis/infection is necessary in any neonate suspected of having a seizure.

	Jitteriness	Benign nocturnal myoclonus	Seizure
Rhythmic movement	Rapid, approx. 5–6/second	Variable, often very brief	Slower, 1–3 jerks/second
Associated with sleep	No	Always	Maybe
Stimulus-responsive	Often	No	Very rare
Reduced by restraint or repositioning	Often	No	No
Associated signs	Excessive startle reflex	None	Apnea, tonic eye deviation, tonic stiffening of body
Associated risk factors	Often occurs in normal neonates; also perinatal asphyxia, hypoglycemia, maternal drug use, metabolic disorders	Occurs in normal infants	Associated with multiple etiologies, including perinatal asphyxia, fetal distress, cerebral dysgenesis, infection, hypoglycemia, maternal drug use, metabolic disorders, intracranial hemorrhage, etc.
Abnormal EEG	No	No	Often

Infantile spasms

- Age-specific seizure syndrome; onset typically at 3–8 months.
- Clinical characteristics: flexor or extensor spasms, usually upon awakening, not stimulus-dependent. Typical appearance is a sudden muscular contraction with neck flexion, arm extension and leg flexion, associated with a cry.
- May occur in clusters up to 50–100 times per day.
- Often classified as symptomatic (resulting from a diagnosable underlying problem) or cryptogenic (occurring in previously normal infants and in whom no etiological diagnosis can be made).
- EEG generally shows hypsarrhythmia, a chaotic, high amplitude pattern of random multifocal spikes, and slow wave discharges that are not repetitive. In sleep, this pattern may more closely resemble burst-suppression.

DDx of infantile episodic spasm-like movements
1 Infantile spasms.
2 Sandifer syndrome: gastroesophageal reflux causing intermittent extension/posturing.

3 Colic.

4 Benign infantile myoclonus: EEG is normal.

5 Exaggerated Moro response: by 5 months of age, the reflex Moro response is absent or reduced in the majority of infants.

Etiological DDx of infantile spasms

1 **Pre- and perinatal insults (25–30%)**
    1.1 Maternal infection/chorioamonitis
    1.2 Prematurity
    1.3 Perinatal asphyxia
    1.4 Birth trauma
    1.5 Perinatal hypoglycemia

2 **Cerebral dysgenesis (30+%)**: better neuroimaging results in greater detection
    2.1 **Focal cortical dysplasia**
    2.2 Hemimegalencephaly
    2.3 Ulegyria, pachygyria, polymicrogyria, lissencephaly, schizencephaly

3 **Tuberous sclerosis (20–25%)**

4 *Inborn errors of metabolism*
    4.1 Pyridoxine deficiency or dependency
    4.2 Nonketotic hyperglycinemia
    4.3 Maple syrup urine disease
    4.4 Phenylketonuria

5 Aicardi syndrome: agenesis of the corpus callosum and eye involvement

6 Neurofibromatosis

7 Infection
    7.1 Cytomegalovirus

8 Cryptogenic (<15%)

Lennox-Gastaut syndrome

- Catastrophic epilepsy syndrome of childhood.
- Age of onset typically 3–6 years.
- Clinical characteristics: multiple seizure types (atypical absence, atonic, tonic, myoclonic, generalized tonic-clonic), slow spike and wave on EEG, and mental retardation. Generally intractable to medication.
- EEG shows pattern of slow (1.5–2.5 Hz) spike and wave or multiple independent spike discharges (MISD).
- About 2/3 are symptomatic and 1/3 idiopathic.
- 20–30% of children with Lennox-Gastaut have a prior history of infantile spasms.

1 **Pre- or perinatal insult**
   1.1 Maternal infection/chorioamonitis
   1.2 Prematurity
   1.3 Perinatal asphyxia
   1.4 Birth trauma
2 **Neurocutaneous syndromes**
   2.1 **Tuberous sclerosis**
   2.2 Neurofibromatosis
   2.3 Hypomelanosis of Ito
3 Prior meningitis/encephalitis
4 Cerebral dysgenesis (less common than in infantile spasms)
5 Congenital infections
6 *Brain tumors*
7 *Intracranial hemorrhage*
   7.1 Intraventricular hemorrhage
   7.2 Subdural hematoma
8 **Idiopathic** (approx. 30%)

Epilepsia partialis continua (EPC)

- Focal motor status epilepticus, usually involving the face or upper extremity; consciousness is preserved.
- Post-ictal weakness is often noted.
- Must rule out a focal lesion.

1 **Rasmussen syndrome**
   - Clinical characteristics: childhood onset, infection <1 month prior to onset. Generally EPC involving face or upper limb, with normal mental state.
   - Progresses relentlessly, intractable to medication. Has been successfully treated using early hemispherectomy.
   - Untreated results in atrophy and degeneration in hemisphere contralateral to clinical EPC and disastrous cognitive impairment.
2 **Tumor**
3 **Focal cortical dysplasia**
4 **Cerebrovascular disease/stroke**
5 Neurocutaneous syndromes
   5.1 Tuberous sclerosis
   5.2 Sturge-Weber syndrome
6 *Infection*
   6.1 Tick-borne encephalitis
   6.2 Measles encephalitis

Progressive myoclonus epilepsy

- Onset is typically in late childhood or adolescence.
- The syndromes consist of myoclonic seizures, tonic-clonic seizures, and progressive deterioration in neurological function, especially ataxia and dementia.
- Myoclonus is multifocal and may be precipitated by stimuli such as action, light, sound, or touch.

1 Unverricht-Lundborg disease
- mutation in the gene encoding a cysteine protease inhibitor
- onset in early adolescence

2 Lafora body disease
- mutation in gene encoding intracellular tyrosine phosphatase
- onset in early adolescence
- dementia prominent
- eosinophilic inclusion bodies in skin, brain, and liver

3 Neuronal ceroid lipofuscinosis
- dementia
- visual loss
- inclusion bodies in nerve and skin

4 Sialidosis
- α-N-acetylneuraminidase deficiency
- macular cherry red spot

5 Mitochondrial encephalopathy with ragged red fibers (MERRF)
- mitochondrial genome mutation
- myopathy
- optic atrophy
- neuropathy

6 Subacute sclerosing panencephalitis (SSPE)
- in nonimmunized persons, onset around 8 years
- personality change may be first symptom

- ◆ myoclonic seizures and progressive dementia
- ◆ EEG shows periodic spike wave bursts synchronous with the myoclonus.

Seizure etiology by age

- • Treatment of seizures is directed at acutely suppressing uncontrolled seizure activity and at treating the underlying cause. Hence, even the less common diagnoses considered here are still considered *important* as they are treatable.
- • Older children with seizures classified as idiopathic are becoming fewer, as improved neuroimaging and potential genetic testing results in more etiological diagnoses.

Neonatal seizures: etiology
1 ***Intraventricular hemorrhage*** (in premie)
2 ***Hypoxia-ischemia*** (40–46%)
3 ***Infection (meningitis/sepsis)*** (17–20%)
4 *Birth trauma/intracerebral hemorrhage/subdural hematoma* (7%)
5 *Cerebral infarction* (6%)
6 Cerebral dysgenesis (4%+)
7 *Hypoglycemia* (5%)
8 *Inborn error of metabolism* (4%)
9 *Subarachnoid hemorrhage* (2%)
10 *Hypocalcemia*
11 *Venous sinus thrombosis*
12 *Drug withdrawal*

Infantile seizures: etiology
1 **Febrile seizure**
2 Infection (meningitis/sepsis)
3 Cerebral dysgenesis
4 *Cerebral infarction*
5 *Inborn error of metabolism*
6 *Drug/toxin ingestion*
7 *Non-accidental trauma/intracranial hemorrhage*
8 *Metabolic* (hypoglycemia, hypocalcemia, hyponatremia, etc.)

Childhood/adolescent seizures: etiology
1 **Idiopathic** (may include genetic, undiagnosed congenital) (69%)
2 Perinatal causes (birth trauma, hypoxia-ischemia, etc.) (7%)
3 *Trauma* (4%)
4 Congenital/cerebral dysgenesis (3%+)

5 *Infection (meningitis/encephalitis)* (3%)
6 *Toxic: drug ingestion, etc./metabolic: hypoglycemia, etc.* (2%)
7 *CNS neoplasm* (<1%)
8 Mesial temporal sclerosis
9 Miscellaneous/multiple (12%)

Developmental disorders

Developmental delay

- Defined as a static, nonprogressive, significant delay in ≥2 of the following domains: gross/fine motor, language, cognition, social/personal, and activities of daily living.
- Referred to as mental retardation in children over 5 years of age.
- Up to 5–10% of children have some developmental disability, 1–3% of all children have global developmental delay.
- Important to distinguish from developmental REGRESSION, which is a loss of previously achieved milestones.
- Important to distinguish from a predominantly language delay or a predominant motor delay, both of which have narrower, more specific differential diagnoses.

1 Predominantly language delay
   1.1 **Hearing impairment**
   1.2 **Autism**: developmental disorder, usually becomes evident near 1–2 years of age (see Developmental regression in toddlers/children).
       ■ Etiology is likely multifactorial, with a genetic component.
       ■ Characterized by impaired socialization, poor language development, repetitive behaviors, and a desire for sameness.
       ■ Some demonstrate a relative insensitivity to pain.
   1.3 Landau-Kleffner syndrome, acquired epileptiform aphasia (usually regression).
       ■ Acquired language regression.
       ■ Epileptiform activity, including status epilepticus, on EEG during sleep.
   1.4 Bilateral perisylvian syndrome
2 Predominantly motor delay
   2.1 **Cerebral palsy**
       ■ Nonprogressive motor and cerebral impairment due to brain injury acquired during development (almost always prenatal or perinatal).

- Associated with intrauterine infection, birth asphyxia, cerebral infarction, cerebral dysgenesis. In most cases, specific etiology undetermined.
- Patterns of motor impairment include: hemiplegia, spastic diplegia, quadriplegia, extrapyramidal, and rarely cerebellar/ataxic.
- Variable degree of cognitive impairment.
- (Greatest impairment) quadriplegia >> spastic diplegia > hemiplegia > extrapyramidal or ataxic (less impairment).

2.2 Myopathy: congenital, metabolic (tend to slowly progress).

2.3 Neuropathy: genetic, metabolic (tend to progress).

3 Global developmental delay (GDD)

3.1 **Perinatal or prenatal insult/disorder**
- Perinatal asphyxia, infection, premature birth, intracranial hemorrhage, hydrocephalus, etc.

3.2 **Chromosomal/genetic abnormality**: particularly suspect if dysmorphic features or congenital abnormalities in other organs present.

3.2.1 **Fragile X syndrome**: FMR1 gene. Most common GDD in males.
- Triplet repeat expansion at Xq27.
- Characterized by long facies, enlarged ears, macro-orchidism, moderate mental retardation, occasionally autistic behavior.

3.2.2 **Rett syndrome**: MECP2 gene. Major etiology in females.
- Mutation at Xq28, only manifest in females. Onset at 1 year of age.
- Clinical signs include acquired microcephaly, developmental arrest/regression, hypotonia, ataxia, seizures, autistic behavior.
- Other findings include breathing irregularities with hyperpnea and loss of purposeful hand movements (constant hand wringing movements).

3.2.3 **Down syndrome**: Trisomy 21.
- Characteristics: hypotonia, round/flat (Mongoloid) facies, Brushfield spots, flat nape of neck.
- Associated congenital cardiac disease.

3.3 **Cerebral malformation**: particularly suspect if dysmorphic features present.
- Dysgenesis, cortical dysplasia, agenesis of the corpus callosum, etc.

3.4 **Neurocutaneous syndromes**

3.4.1 Neurofibromatosis: learning disability/cognitive impairment

3.4.1.1 NF1
- Neuro signs: neurofibromas, optic glioma
- Cutaneous signs: multiple café au lait spots, axillary/inguinal freckling
- Other: Lisch nodules, bony lesions, family history

3.4.1.2 NF2: bilateral acoustic neuromas

3.4.2 Tuberous sclerosis

- □ Neuro signs: developmental delay, intractable seizures, cortical tubers, subependymal hamartomas, retinal tumors.
- □ Cutaneous signs: ash leaf spots, café au lait spots, Shagreen patch, adenoma sebaceum.
- □ Other: cardiac rhabdomyomas, renal tumors, cysts (renal, bone, lung).

3.5 *Lead encephalopathy*: association of elevated serum lead levels with cognitive impairment even in absence of other clinical signs.

3.6 Intrauterine infection (TORCH infections)

3.6.1 Toxoplasmosis

- □ May present acutely ill as neonate: fever, rash, organomegaly, jaundice, thrombocytopenia. Acute neuro symptoms of encephalopathy, seizures, increased intracranial pressure.
- □ May present with GDD after asymptomatic infancy. Characteristics include hydrocephalus, chorioretinitis, intracranial calcifications.
- □ Check for IgM, IgG antibodies.

3.6.2 Rubella encephalopathy: rare

- □ Neuro signs: lethargy, hypotonia, seizures.
- □ Other characteristics include intrauterine growth retardation, cataracts, chorioretinitis, congenital heart disease, deafness, organomegaly, jaundice, anemia, thrombocytopenia, rash.

3.6.3 Cytomegalovirus

- □ Neuro signs: microcephaly, intracranial calcifications.
- □ Other signs: rash, chorioretinitis, jaundice, organomegaly.
- □ Check for CMV virus or antibodies.

3.6.4 Herpes virus

- □ Neonatal presentation is usually diffuse, acute illness with encephalitis and seizures. May have systemic involvement, vesicular rash.
- □ Check CSF: elevated WBC (mostly lymphs), HSV PCR. Also EEG.

3.7 Progressive encephalopathy: see Developmental regression.

Developmental regression

- The differential diagnosis for developmental regression in children is very large. It is useful to break down the differential by the following parameters:
  - age of presentation,

- involvement of CNS only or including other organ systems,
- involvement of CNS only or including peripheral NS involvement,
- primarily gray matter or white matter disease.
- Involvement of CNS + other organ systems suggests lysosomal, peroxisomal, or mitochondrial disease.
- Involvement of CNS + PNS suggests lysosomal or mitochondrial disorders.
- Involvement of gray matter more often presents with seizures, dementia, and personality change.
- Involvement of white matter more often presents with spasticity, focal neurological deficits, and blindness.
- Regression can occur in several clinical scenarios. These scenarios can be helpful in narrowing the differential:
  1 Acute, rapid deterioration
  2 Acute intermittent attacks with cumulative regression
  3 Gradual, more chronic loss of milestones.
- Chronic nonprogressive conditions (such as cerebral palsy) may seem to evolve as the affected child develops, and must be distinguished from true regression.

Developmental regression in infants

- No single entity is predominant in this age range, and specific differential diagnosis is based on clinical characteristics of the patient's presentation.
- Rare but potentially treatable disorders that result in acute episodes of regression/neurological dysfunction include disorders of amino acid metabolism.
- Other potentially treatable conditions include progressive hydrocephalus, hypothyroidism, and AIDS.
- It is still important to diagnose the many rare but untreatable conditions including lysosomal disorders, mitochondrial disorders, and the predominantly white or gray matter disorders. Knowledge of a specific diagnosis may assist in prognosis, genetic counseling, participation in clinical research trials, and long-term care.

1 Primarily gray matter disorders
   1.1 **Autism** (see Developmental regression in toddlers/children, p. 364)
   1.2 **Rett syndrome** (see Developmental regression in toddlers/children, pp. 364–5)
   1.3 Early-infantile neuronal ceroid lipofuscinosis (Santavuori-Haltia): AR
      ■ Visual impairment and myoclonus are prominent.

- Dx: skin, leukocyte, or conjunctival biopsy.
  1.4 Menkes disease: AR, deficiency of copper transport
  - Characteristics: kinky hair, intractable myoclonic seizures.
  - Dx: low serum copper, ceruloplasmin.
  1.5 Infantile neuroaxonal dystrophy: AR
  - Initially motor regression and hypotonia.
  - Followed by spasticity, optic atrophy, movement disorder, dementia.
  - Dx: nerve or conjunctival biopsy.
  1.6 Lesch Nyhan disease: XL, low hypoxanthine guanine phosphoribosyl-transferase.
    - Initially hypotonia, motor delay. Then increasing rigidity, torticollis.
    - By 2 years of age, facial grimacing, choreiform movement disorder.
    - After 2 years of age, compulsive self-mutilation, aggressive behavior.
    - Dx: elevated uric acid; fibroblast culture.

2 *Progressive hydrocephalus*
  - Clinical characteristics: enlarged head circumference, full anterior fontanelle, lethargy, vomiting, 'sunset sign': white sclera visible above pupils.
  - Results from congenital malformations, tumors, hemorrhage, infections.
  - Dx: head CT scan. Treat with VP shunting.

3 *Amino/organic acid metabolic disorders* (may present with acute encephalopathy, or intermittent attacks followed by stepwise decline): when considering these diagnoses, check serum amino acids/urine organic acids while symptomatic.
  3.1 Homocystinuria: AR, impaired metabolism of homocystine
    - Developmental delay, thromboembolism, lens dislocation, osteoporosis.
  3.2 Maple syrup urine disease: AR, impaired branched chain amino acid metabolism
    - Acute presentation: encephalopathy, seizures, spasticity, hypoglycemia.
    - Intermittent presentation: episodes of ataxia, encephalopathy, seizures.
    - Cerebral edema, urine odor sickly sweet.
  3.3 Phenylketonuria: AR, impaired phenylalanine metabolism
    - Projectile vomiting, irritability, delayed development.
    - Dx: usually detected on newborn screening.
  3.4 Urea cycle disorders: AR, except ornithine transcarbamoylase deficiency: XL
    - Variable, but intermittent encephalopathy, vomiting, seizures, high ammonia.
  3.5 Organic acidurias: usually AR
    - Variable, but may present as acute encephalopathy, vomiting, hypotonia.
    - Isovaleric acidemia, glutaric aciduria type II – sweaty feet odor.
  3.6 Lowe syndrome (oculocerebrorenal syndrome): XL
    - Congenital glaucoma or cataract, myopathy, renal acidosis, neuropathy.

4 *Hypothyroidism*
  - Suspect in infants not born in US, or who somehow missed newborn screening.
  - Clinical characteristics: wide open posterior fontanelle, constipation, jaundice, poor thermoregulation, umbilical hernia, macroglossia.
  - Treat with thyroxine. Delay in diagnosis and treatment results in lower IQ.
5 Lysosomal disorders: many have Hurler phenotype, organomegaly, developmental regression. Check urine for mucopolysaccharides; fibroblast culture for enzymes.
  5.1 GM1 gangliosidosis: AR, Hurler phenotype, cherry red spot.
  5.2 GM2 gangliosidosis (Tay-Sachs, Sandhoff): AR, cherry red spot; Sandhoff: hepatosplenomegaly.
  5.3 Gaucher disease: AR, head retraction, poor suck, ocular palsies, splenomegaly.
  5.4 I-cell disease: AR, Hurler phenotype, heart failure.
  5.5 Mucopolysaccharidoses: AR, hepatosplenomegaly.
     5.5.1 Type I Hurler: Hurler phenotype, corneal opacity, skeletal abnormalities.
     5.5.2 Type III Sanfilippo: Hurler not prominent; delayed cognitive impairment.
  5.6 Neimann Pick disease: AR, cherry red spot, delayed splenomegaly.
6 Mitochondrial disorders – may show elevated lactate/pyruvate.
  6.1 Mitochondrial myopathy, encephalopathy, lactic acidosis, and stroke (MELAS).
  6.2 Leigh disease: seizures, ocular palsies, respiratory irregularities, hypotonia.
  6.3 Other – Alpers disease, MERRF, Kearns-Sayre (see Developmental regression in toddlers/children, p. 366).
7 Primarily white matter disorders
  7.1 Galactosemia: AR, vomiting, hepatomegaly, cerebral edema; newborn screen.
  7.2 Canavan disease: AR, macrocephaly, optic atrophy.
  7.3 Alexander disease: sporadic, macrocephaly, seizures.
  7.4 Krabbe disease: AR, opisthotonus, hyporeflexia, seizures, blindness.
  7.5 Neonatal adrenoleukodystrophy (also a peroxisomal disorder): XL, hyperreflexia, spasticity, blindness, seizures.
  7.6 Pelizaeus-Merzbacher disease: XL, spasmus nutans/nystagmus, choreoathetosis.
  7.7 Metachromatic leukodystrophy: AR, peripheral neuropathy.
8 Peroxisomal disorders
  8.1 Zellweger syndrome: dysmorphic features, hypotonia, arthrogryposis. Also biliary cirrhosis, polycystic kidneys, retinal degeneration, cerebral malformations.

8.2 Infantile refsum disease: blindness, deafness, different from later onset form.

9 AIDS encephalopathy
- Clinical characteristics: microcephaly, regression, dementia, spasticity.
- May also have ataxia, movement disorders, myoclonus, seizures.
- Additionally, may develop complications of CNS opportunistic infections.

AR = autosomal recessive inheritance, AD = autosomal dominant, XL = X-linked.

Developmental regression in toddlers/children

- Autism is a major diagnosis of developmental delay or regression in children between the ages of 18 and 26 months; less severely affected individuals may manifest with more limited behavioral deficits at a later age.
- Rett syndrome is a major cause of progressive intellectual decline and acquired microcephaly in females, usually starting around 12 months of age.
- Developmental regression in childhood is often associated with disorders connected with abnormal accumulation of products of cellular metabolism (lysosomal disorders, neuronal ceroid lipofuscinosis) or chronic impairment of energy metabolism (mitochondrial disorders).
- Acute metabolic errors are less likely to present in this age range, although some aminoacidopathies can cause intermittent attacks with gradual regression over time.
- Intractable or poorly controlled seizures associated with developmental regression may be a manifestation of a particular etiology or may be idiopathic.
- Furthermore, diagnosing untreatable conditions remains important for the purposes of genetic counseling and planning future care.

1 Primarily gray matter disorders
  1.1 **Autism**
  - Clinical characteristics: impaired or regressed language development, profound disturbance of socialization, stereotypic behavior. May demonstrate insensitivity to pain, rigid behavioral patterns, seizures.
  - Etiology is unknown, although genetic component suspected.
  - Broad range of autistic spectrum disorders includes milder, more specific learning and socialization disabilities that may manifest later in life.
  - Spectrum of disorders covers (most to least severe): classic autism, pervasive developmental disorder-NOS and Asperger syndrome.

1.2 **Rett syndrome**
- Clinical characteristics: girls only, acquired microcephaly, hypotonia, loss of language, nonpurposeful hand movements/hand wringing, episodic hyperpnea, bruxism, seizures. May have autistic behavior.
- Gradual neurological deterioration, but can survive into adulthood.

1.3 Neuronal ceroid lipofuscinosis: AR.
- Additional signs include retinopathy, blindness, myoclonic jerks, seizures.
- Dx: skin or conjunctival biopsies show lipofuscin inclusions.

1.4 Huntington disease: AD, trinucleotide repeat disorder.
- 10% of HD presents at <20 years old; 5% presents at <14 years old.
- Rigidity is a more prominent manifestation than chorea or hyperkinesis.
- Cognitive/behavioral disturbance, ataxia (20%), seizures (50%).
- Progression of symptoms is more rapid than adult-onset cases.

1.5 Xeroderma pigmentosum: AR.
- In addition to dementia, other signs include photosensitive dermatitis, acquired microcephaly, deafness, spinocerebellar degeneration.
- Defective DNA repair mechanisms.

2 *Intractable epilepsy/seizures*: as a component of an underlying degenerative disorder (neuronal ceroid lipofucsinosis), neurocutaneous syndrome (tuberous sclerosis), or may be idiopathic (e.g. Lennox-Gastaut, Landau-Kleffner, untreated childhood absence seizures).

3 *Progressive hydrocephalus*: usually presents with headache, nausea, and vomiting, but can manifest primarily as regression/mental decline in a previously impaired child.

4 *Amino/organic acid metabolic disorders*: see Developmental regression in infants, p. 362.
    4.1 Urea cycle disorders: mostly AR, except ornithine transcarbamoylase (OTC) deficiency (XL). These disorders more typically present in neonates. However, incomplete enzyme deficiencies may have intermittent attacks of encephalopathy, seizures and ataxia with gradual progressive intellectual decline. This is particularly so in female carriers of OTC deficiency.
    4.2 Other aminoacidopathies: maple syrup urine disease, phenylketonuria

5 Infectious disease
    5.1 AIDS encephalopathy: see Developmental regression in infants, p. 364)
    5.2 Subacute sclerosing panencephalitis: see Chapter 5: Neuropsychiatry and Dementia)
    5.3 Congenital syphilis: may present >2 years with mental regression and:
- Hutchinson triad – sensorineural deafness, interstitial keratitis, peg-shaped upper incisors,
- In newborn period: condylomata lata, rash, periostitis/osteochondritis.
- Treat with penicillin. Test for co-infection with HIV.

6 Lysosomal disorders
  6.1 Gaucher disease (type III): AR, seizures, enzyme replacement may help.
  6.2 Krabbe disease (late onset): AR, blindness, spasticity. No neuropathy.
  6.3 GM2 gangliosidosis: AR, gait ataxia, spasticity, seizures.
  6.4 Mucopolysaccharidoses
    6.4.1 Type II (Hunter): XL, Hurler phenotype without corneal clouding, ivory colored upper back/shoulder cutaneous lesion, entrapment neuropathy.
    6.4.2 Type VII (Sly): AR, incomplete Hurler phenotype without corneal clouding.
  6.5 Neimann Pick disease (type C): AR, organomegaly, ataxia, oculomotor apraxia. Also, slower onset, delayed variants present in older ages/adults.
  6.6 Glycoprotein degradation disorders
7 Mitochondrial disorders
  7.1 Myoclonus epilepsy with ragged red fibers (MERRF): myoclonic seizures, ataxia, deafness, short stature, endocrinopathy, associated myopathy.
  7.2 MELAS: deafness, attacks of headaches, seizures, lactic acidosis, and stroke-like focal neurological deficits.
  7.3 Alpers disease: seizures, occasional hemiplegia or blindness.
  7.4 Kearns-Sayre syndrome (KSS): external ophthalmoplegia.
8 Primarily white matter disorders
  8.1 Adrenoleukodystrophy: XL, behavioral deterioration, visual/hearing loss, late seizures, late adrenal insufficiency.
  8.2 Alexander disease: sporadic, macrocephaly, spasticity, seizures.
  8.3 Cerebrotendinous xanthomatosis: AR, teenage cataracts and tendinous xanthomas, developmental regression may be very slow.
  8.4 Metachromatic leukodystrophy: AR, gait ataxia, eventual seizures, and neuropathy.

Risk factors for developmental language disorder

- A developmental language disorder (DLD) is diagnosed when a child with normal intelligence and hearing fails to develop language in an age-appropriate fashion.
- Most children have good receptive language and are starting to put words together by the age of 2 years, along with a 50–100 word vocabulary.
- Lack of well-developed expressive language by the age of 3 years is definitely abnormal.
- The prevalence is probably 1–2.5% in preschool children.

Risk factors as defined by the National Collaborative Perinatal Project include:
1 Low birth weight
2 Prematurity
3 Parental mental retardation
4 Family history of developmental language disorder

Motor dysfunction

- Defined as a reduction in muscle tone. May be due to central or peripheral causes.
- Exam findings include: head lag, poor posture in horizontal or vertical suspension, variably reduced deep tendon reflexes.
- Look for bulbar involvement.
- Earliest presentation is infantile or congenital hypotonia.
- Later presentation may include motor regression.
- Hypotonia and weakness may progress acutely/subacutely to require ventilatory support – particularly in cases of spinal cord injury, botulism, myasthenia, Guillain-Barré syndrome or congenital myopathy. Spinal muscular atrophy and metabolic disorders/myopathies may also require respiratory support but progress more slowly.

Infantile hypotonia
1 Cerebral hypotonia: diagnose by clinical history or imaging
   - Associated with reduced mental status, seizures, persistent primitive reflexes, other organ malformations. May later develop hypertonia – fisted hands, legs scissoring.
   1.1 **Nonprogressive encephalopathy**
      1.1.1 **Cerebral malformation**: associated with dysmorphic features, abnormal head size/shape.
      1.1.2 **Perinatal asphyxia**
      1.1.3 **Other acquired cerebral disorders: infection, hemorrhage, trauma.**
   1.2 **Chromosomal disorders**
      1.2.1 Prader-Willi syndrome
         □ Deletion of maternal chromosome 15q11–13
         □ Poor feeding, hypogonadism, developmental delay; later hyperphagia.
      1.2.2 Trisomy 21: dysmorphic features, developmental delay, seizures, congenital cardiac anomalies.
   1.3 Metabolic disorders

       1.3.1 Peroxisomal disorders

            1.3.1.1 Zellweger syndrome: AR, dysmorphic features, arthrogryposis, cerebrohepatorenal syndrome, infantile seizures.

            1.3.1.2 Neonatal adrenoleukodystrophy: AR, dysmorphic features, seizures, hepatomegaly, retinal degeneration.

       1.3.2 Oculocerebrorenal syndrome (Lowe syndrome): XL, congenital cataracts, glaucoma, renal impairment.

       1.3.3 Familial dysautonomia (Riley-Day syndrome): AR or sporadic, poor feeding, autonomic symptoms, pain insensitivity, cyclic vomiting.

       1.3.4 Acid maltase deficiency: see metabolic myopathies, p. 369.

       1.3.5 Infantile GM1 gangliosidosis: AR, weakness, developmental regression, cherry red spot.

     1.4 **'Benign' congenital hypotonia**: initial hypotonia that resolves.

2 Spinal cord disorders

     2.1 *Birth injuries*: vaginal delivery, associated with severe traction or twisting, may have respiratory failure due to brainstem or high cervical injury. Sensory level may be difficult to detect.

     2.2 Perinatal asphyxia with hypoxic-ischemic myelopathy.

3 Neuromuscular junction disorders

     3.1 Infantile botulism

- Caused by toxin from *C. botulinum*. Associated with honey ingestion.
- Constipation, proximal > distal weakness, preserved alertness, sluggish pupils, dysphagia, weak cry.
- May cause progressive respiratory failure and/or SIDS.
- Repetitive stimulation EMG shows incremental response.
- Antitoxin treatment has been shown to shorten hospitalization.

     3.2 *Myasthenia (congenital or neonatal)*

       3.2.1 Congenital: multiple distinct syndromes; mothers without myasthenia

           □ Genetic (mostly AR), acetylcholine receptor seronegative.

           □ Respiratory and feeding difficulty, ptosis, arthrogryposis, some with ophthalmoplegia.

           □ Response to edrophonium; decremental response on EMG.

           □ Prone to later episodes of weakness during intercurrent illness.

       3.2.2 Neonatal: 10–20% of infants born to myasthenic mothers

           □ Passive transfer of maternal acetylcholine receptor antibodies.

           □ Poor feeding, fatigability, arthrogryposis, weak cry.

           □ Complete recovery in weeks or months.

4 Polyneuropathies

     4.1 *Guillain-Barré syndrome*: can occur in infants, see Chapter 8: Peripheral Neurology

     4.2 Congenital hypomyelinating neuropathy

4.3 Hereditary motor-sensory neuropathies (HMSN III).

5 Muscle disorders

  5.1 Congenital myopathy: diagnosed by muscle biopsy.

- Common signs: weakness, arthrogryposis, contractures, scoliosis, hip dislocation, some with respiratory or swallowing weakness, ophthalmoplegia.

    5.1.1 Central core disease: AD, mutation in ryanodine receptor

    5.1.2 Congenital fiber-type disproportion myopathy: several types

    5.1.3 Myotubular myopathy: acute form XL, chronic AR or AD

    5.1.4 Nemaline rod myopathy: AR or AD

  5.2 Congenital myotonic dystrophy

- AD triplet repeat disease, maternal carrier.
- Respiratory distress, facial diplegia, arthrogryposis, feeding difficulties, cardiomyopathy.
- Later develop progressive weakness, mental retardation, temporal wasting, cataracts, frontal balding, endocrinopathies including testicular atrophy.

  5.3 Congenital muscular dystrophy

  5.4 Metabolic myopathies

    5.4.1 Acid maltase deficiency: AR, cardiomyopathy/congestive heart failure.

    5.4.2 Cytochrome c oxidase deficiency: lactic acidosis, high CK.

    5.4.3 Phosphofructokinase deficiency: normally presents with cramps following exertion in children; neonatal form AR more severe.

    5.4.4 Phosphorylase deficiency (McArdle disease): normally presents with exercise intolerance in children; neonatal form rare, AR.

6 Spinal muscular atrophy

  6.1 Acute infantile (SMA I)

- Onset <6 months. Reduced fetal movement.
- AR, located on Chr 5q, deletion(s) in survival motor neuron (SMN) gene.
- Weakness, proximal > distal, areflexia, respiratory distress. No arthrogryposis.
- Eventually atrophy, fasciculations, aspiration.
- Diagnosed by genetic testing. Progressive, but survival quite variable.

  6.2 Chronic infantile (SMA II)

- Onset between 3 and 18 months. Fetal movements normal. Normal at birth.
- AR, located on Chr 5q, deletion(s) in SMN gene.
- Usually survive to adulthood, but are wheelchair-bound.
- Diagnosed by genetic testing.

Common causes of persistent toe walking in children

- Some children begin walking with their heels off the ground and never attain a normal heel-toe gait.
- The tendency toward toe walking increases with time.
- The most common cause is an idiopathic shortening of the ankle tendon in which there may be a familial trait.
- Other differential diagnoses are listed below. However, these are unlikely if neurological examination and development are normal.
- In the absence of family history, MRI imaging of the lumbosacral spine may be considered to exclude the congenital lesions in this region before concluding that the etiology is idiopathic.

1 **Idiopathic shortening of the ankle tendon**
   - The most common cause of persistent toe walking in children.
   - Family history of toe walking may be present.
2 Structural lesions in the lumbosacral plexus or spinal cord
   - Should strongly be considered if there is abnormal neurological examination suggesting the localization in this region.
   - For example, tethered cord.
3 Muscular dystrophy
   - Usually accompanied by other physical findings.
4 Infantile autism
5 Cerebral palsy

Ataxia

Dizziness/vertigo in children

- The most common causes of vertigo and dizziness in childhood are similar to those in the adult; peripheral vestibulopathy, infections, and trauma.
- Migraine is a significant cause of episodic vertigo and dizziness in childhood and should be considered even if headache is absent.
- Benign paroxysmal vertigo in childhood; a variant of migraine, can be differentiated from temporal lobe seizures with a vestibular component by the preservation of consciousness during an attack.

1 **Infections**
   1.1 Bacterial otitis media/labyrinthitis

- Acute: nausea, vomiting, vertigo, and ipsilateral hearing loss.
- Chronic otitis: as acute, but persistent.
- Cholesteatoma: debris-filled sac due to recurrent/chronic otitis, may erode tissue/bone. May produce perilymph fistula (classic symptom is vertigo induced by sneezing, coughing or external ear pressure).

1.2 Bacterial meningitis: consider with fever, altered mental status, meningismus. May occur due to seeding from a parameningeal ear/mastoid infection.

1.3 Vestibular neuritis (viral): isolated vertigo, begins improving within 48 hours. Less common in children than adults.

2 **Drugs/intoxications**

2.1 Anticonvulsants: rarely vertigo, but often dizziness/ataxia. No hearing loss.

2.2 Neuroleptics: same as above.

2.3 Antibiotics: may cause specific vestibular toxicity, with or without hearing impairment.

3 **Motion sickness**

- Caused by mismatch between visual and vestibular inputs.
- Small children in back of vehicles with small windows are more susceptible.

4 Migraine: should be considered even if headache is absent. Benign paroxysmal vertigo is considered by many to be a migraine variant.

5 *Trauma*

- Almost half of children complain of dizziness/headache within 3 days of a closed head injury.
- Some experience vestibular concussion, distinguished by persistent vertigo/nausea triggered by head movement. Should be evaluated for basilar skull fracture.

6 *Epilepsy*: vertiginous aura may precede a complex partial seizure. Children often stop activity, appear frightened, and may complain of nausea.

7 Others: rare
- Brainstem lesions
- Congenital anomalies of the inner ear
- Ménière disease

Ataxia in children

- Ataxia may be the presenting symptom of a myriad of underlying diagnoses in children.
- It is helpful to distinguish between:
  1 acute episodic and
  2 chronic/progressive presentations.

<u>Acute ataxia</u> (minutes/hours/days)

1 **Drug/toxin ingestion**: major cause of acute ataxia in children
2 Post-infectious/immune-mediated
    2.1 **Acute post-infectious cerebellitis**: major cause of acute ataxia in children
    2.2 *Miller-Fisher syndrome*
        ▪ Guillain-Barré variant; watch respiratory status.
        ▪ Signs: ophthalmoplegia, ataxia, areflexia.
    2.3 Multiple sclerosis
3 **Migraine**: common cause, even without headache, episodic
    3.1 Benign paroxysmal vertigo
    3.2 Basilar migraine
4 Traumatic
    4.1 **Post-concussive**: recovers spontaneously over days/weeks
    4.2 *Intracranial hematoma*
    4.3 *Vertebrobasilar occlusion/dissection*
5 *Brain tumor*: tumors usually present slowly, but can be acute as described here.
    5.1 *Hemorrhage into tumor*
    5.2 *Hydrocephalus due to obstruction by tumor*
        ▪ Accompanied by symptoms of increased intracranial pressure such as headache, nausea, vomiting, altered mentation.
    5.3 *Neuroblastoma paraneoplastic syndrome (opsoclonus/myoclonus)*
        ▪ Signs: ataxia, chaotic eye movements (opsoclonus), alteration in mental status, myoclonus.
        ▪ Opsoclonus persists in sleep.
        ▪ Neuroblastoma equally likely to be in chest or abdomen.
6 *Infection* (brainstem encephalitis, presumed viral)
7 Genetic disorders: episodic ataxia is a component of many metabolic disorders.
    7.1 Episodic ataxias: some responsive to acetazolamide.
    7.2 Hartnup disease: episodic ataxia and encephalopathy; pellagra-like skin rash.
    7.3 Maple syrup urine disease (intermittent variant): episodic ataxia and encephalopathy.
    7.4 Pyruvate dehydrogenase deficiency: episodic lactic acidosis, ataxia, hypotonia, and encephalopathy.
8 Cerebrovascular disorders
    8.1 *Cerebellar hemorrhage*
    8.2 *Kawasaki disease*: systemic vasculitis with fever, conjunctival congestion, reddened oropharynx/lips, limb edema, rash, lymphadenopathy. May also have arthralgias, carditis and aseptic meningitis.
    8.3 *Cerebellar infarction*: rare in children
9 Epilepsy (pseudoataxia)
10 Conversion disorder

Chronic ataxia (days/weeks/months)

1 **Cerebral palsy/developmental delay** (see Developmental delay, pp. 358–9)
2 **Congenital malformation**
    2.1 Basilar impression
    2.2 Congenital cerebellar hemisphere hypoplasia
    2.3 Congenital cerebellar vermian hypo/aplasia
    2.4 Chiari I malformation: can also cause headache.
3 *Brain tumor*: in addition to ataxia, may also produce signs/symptoms of hydrocephalus and increased intracranial pressure (headache, nausea, vomiting).
    3.1 Cerebellar astrocytoma
    3.2 Cerebellar hemangioblastoma (von Hippel-Lindau)
    3.3 Ependymoma
    3.4 Medulloblastoma
4 Genetic disorders
    4.1 Autosomal dominant spinocerebellar ataxias (SCAs) – many variations, usual onset 3rd–5th decade (see Chapter 12: Neurogenetics)
    4.2 Autosomal recessive ataxias
        4.2.1 **Friedreich ataxia**: most common inherited ataxia.
            ▪ Characteristics: progressive ataxia, dysarthria, areflexia, upgoing toes, impaired proprioception, scoliosis.
            ▪ Also associated with pes cavus, cardiomyopathy, and diabetes.
            ▪ Caused by unstable triplet repeat in frataxin gene.
        4.2.2 Hypobetalipoproteinemia: may lead to vitamin E deficiency; supplementation helps.
        4.2.3 Abetalipoproteinemia (Bassen-Kornzweig, acanthocytosis): secondary vitamin E deficiency may corrected with supplementation.
        4.2.4 **Ataxia-telangiectasia**: most common inherited ataxia in infancy.
            ▪ Characteristics: progressive ataxia, telangiectasias (initially conjunctival), recurrent sinopulmonary infections (due to IgA deficiency).
            ▪ Increased risk of lymphoma and leukemia.
        4.2.5 Hartnup disease: see Acute ataxia, p. 372.
        4.2.6 GM2 gangliosidosis (juvenile): tremor, ataxia, dysarthria.
        4.2.7 Maple syrup urine disease: see Acute ataxia, p. 372; may be recurrent.
        4.2.8 Metachromatic leukodystrophy (juvenile): ataxia, seizures, dementia.
        4.2.9 Marinesco-Sjögren syndrome: progressive ataxia, congenital cataracts, mental retardation.
        4.2.10 Pyruvate dehydrogenase deficiency: see Acute ataxia, p. 372.
        4.2.11 Progressive myoclonus epilepsies (see pp. 356–7).

□ Characteristics: myoclonus, progressive ataxia, seizures, variable dementia.

4.2.12 Refsum disease

□ Characteristics: ataxia, polyneuropathy, retinitis pigmentosum.

□ Also icthyosis, hearing loss, cataracts, cardiomyopathy, pes cavus.

4.3 X-linked ataxias

4.3.1 Adrenoleukodystrophy: white matter degeneration on MRI imaging.

4.3.2 Leber optic neuropathy: mitochrondrial disorder; visual loss, ataxia.

Headache in children

- Differential diagnosis for pediatric headache can be approached by the presentation or by the headache pattern.
- Headaches generally fall into one of the following four patterns:
  1 Acute, new-onset,
  2 Acute, episodic or recurrent,
  3 Subacute or chronic, progressive, and
  4 Chronic, fluctuating or constant.
- Acute, new-onset headaches will more likely present urgently (emergency department or urgent care clinic).
- Acute, episodic, or recurrent headaches can present both at emergency departments, and urgent care clinics (or even at a regular clinic).
- Subacute or chronic progressive headache raises concern for mass lesion/abscess/tumor, particularly if associated with nausea, vomiting, persistent unilateral localization, or neurological deficit. More likely to be seen in clinic, but can present acutely if associated with worsening vomiting, increasing pain, seizure, or new neurological deficit.
- Chronic headaches may fluctuate or be fairly constant. These generally present in a clinic setting.
- Signs/symptoms of a mass lesion associated with headache include:
  - Persistently focal/unilateral headache
  - Focal neurological exam finding(s) – hemiparesis, visual field cut, etc.
  - Focal seizure
- Signs/symptoms of elevated ICP associated with headache include:
  - Persistent nausea or vomiting
  - Nocturnal awakening or exacerbation of headache/nausea/vomiting
  - Altered or depressed mental status
  - Papilledema
- Infants with elevated ICP may present with poor feeding, irritability, vomiting, and altered mental status.

- Exam findings consistent with chronically elevated ICP include enlarging head circumference, open full fontanelle, split sutures, and the 'sunset sign' (sclera visible above pupils; impaired upgaze).
- The diagnosis of elevated ICP due to child abuse may be obscured at presentation, with many nonspecific symptoms suggesting alternate diagnoses – rule out sepsis, colic, gastroenteritis. Be vigilant!
- If bruising, retinal hemorrhages or old fractures are noted on evaluation. Consideration must be given to child abuse and intracranial hemorrhage.

Acute headache presentation (more likely at emergency department or urgent care clinic)

1 **Fever, extracranial infection** (28.5–44.1%)
2 **Post-traumatic/post-concussion** (6.6–20%)
   - Persistent post-concussive headaches preclude return to contact sports.
   - Worsening post-concussive headaches, particularly with other signs such as nausea, vomiting, change in mental status, etc. raise concern for increased intracranial pressure (ICP).
   - Rarely associated with intracranial lesion.
3 **Sinusitis** (16%): sinus tenderness, chronic rhinitis, fever.
4 **Migraine** (8.5–15.6%)
   - Clinical characteristics include episodic: throbbing/pulsatile pain, visual scotoma, nausea, vomiting, dizziness, photophobia, phonophobia.
   - Migraine duration tends to be shorter in children (<1 hour) than in adults.
   - Migraine very likely for recurrent/episodic headaches if child is normal between attacks.
   - Family history is common.
5 *Aseptic meningitis* (2.3–5.2%)
   - Associated with fever; in children >18 months, meningismus may be present.
   - Lumbar puncture (LP) shows lymphocytic pleocytosis.
6 Tension-type (1.5–4.5%)
   - Clinical characteristics include: diffuse, pressure-like pain, nonlocalizing.
   - Usually more chronic in presentation.
7 *Seizure* (3%), post-ictal
8 *Brain tumor* (1.5%): very rare to present acutely.
9 Hypertension (1.5%)
10 Others (in no particular order)
   10.1 *Drugs/toxins*: associated mental status change, ataxia.
   10.2 *Intracranial hemorrhage*: elevated ICP signs.
   10.3 *Hydrocephalus*, VP shunt malfunction: elevated ICP signs.

10.4 *Bacterial meningitis*: fever, meningismus, elevated ICP signs.

10.5 *Metabolic* (hypoglycemia, porphyria).

10.6 Cluster: rare in children.

10.7 Post-LP headache: positional, worse when upright.

10.8 Neuralgia: rare in children.

10.9 Vascular (phenochromocytoma): rare in children.

Overall 'serious diagnoses' (6.6–6.9%): mostly viral/aseptic meningitis; also reported intracranial hemorrhage, VP shunt malfunction, skull fracture/trauma.

Chronic headache presentation (more likely at clinic)

- Many of the less frequent but potentially dangerous etiologies can be clinically ruled out by careful history and physical examination.
- In a setting of steadily worsening symptoms, focal signs, or signs associated with elevated ICP, neuroimaging is necessary.

1 **Migraine** (54–55%): see Acute presentation, p. 375, for clinical characteristics.
   - Not consistently unilateral; may be unilateral or bilateral for a given attack.
2 **Tension-type** (22–36%): see Acute headache presentation, p. 375, for clinical characteristics
   - Much more common presenting as a chronic headache; may be constant or may fluctuate over time.
   - Usually diffuse or bilateral; nonlocalizing.
3 Others (less frequent etiologies, not in any particular order)
   3.1 *Head trauma/post-concussive*: acutely, most resolve in minutes/hours.
      - Chronic post-traumatic headaches may be part of post-concussive syndrome, which typically resolves with time (days/weeks).
      - As evidence of incomplete post-concussive recovery, persistent headache precludes return to contact sports until at least 1 week after resolution.
   3.2 *Epileptic/postictal*: may cause recurrent headaches; sometimes seizure is not witnessed.
   3.3 *Vascular (hypertension, intracranial bleed, AVM, pheochromocytoma)*: elevated ICP signs.
   3.4 *Brain tumor*: elevated ICP signs, may have focal signs, progressive.
   3.5 *Infection/abscess*: fever, stiff neck, elevated ICP signs, may have focal signs.
   3.6 *Hydrocephalus*: elevated ICP signs.
   3.7 *Pseudotumor cerebri*: visual field defects, elevated ICP signs.
   3.8 *Drugs/toxins* (CO, MSG, nitrates, alcohol, analgesic/narcotic abuse, caffeine withdrawal).

3.9   Sinusitis: associated sinus tenderness, rhinitis.

3.10 Chronic daily headache (0.2–0.9%): nonlocalizing headache present more than 15 days/month or 4–5 days/week, normal neurological examination.

3.11 Ocular (glaucoma, astigmatism).

3.12 *Metabolic* (hypoxia, altitude, sleep apnea, hypoglycemia, porphyria).

3.13 Post-LP headache: positional, worse when upright.

3.14 Cluster: rare in children.

3.15 Analgesia overuse/'rebound': rare in children.

3.16 Neuralgia: rare in children.

4 Psychological: diagnosis of exclusion.

Neoplasms (see Chapter 10: Neuro-oncology)

Visual disturbances

- Many of the same diseases that affect vision in adults also affect children, but some are specific to young people or present during early growth and development.

Visual loss in children: neurological causes

1 Optic nerve hypoplasia
- Optic nerve hypoplasia is a congenital and nonprogressive condition that may reflect a primary defect in differentiation of the retinal ganglion cell axons.
- May be unilateral or bilateral with variable visual acuity ranging from 20/20 to light perception. A pericapillary ring of pigmentation is often present; called double ring sign.
- Usually sporadic but can be associated with fetal alcohol syndrome, maternal diabetes, maternal ingestion of anticonvulsants, and various endocrinologic abnormalities.

2 Leber congenital amaurosis
- This condition is broadly defined as a syndrome of bilaterally poor vision beginning in early childhood that is associated with a depressed or absent electroretinogram.
- This disease is not related to Leber hereditary optic neuropathy.
- 30% of cases have neurologic abnormalities including poor coordination, spastic paraparesis, or hydrocephalus.

3 Albinism
  - Albinism is a genetically determined abnormality in melanin synthesis that is associated with congenital nystagmus, foveal hypoplasia, and impaired visual acuity.
  - The ocular fundus can be totally devoid of pigment or have a blond appearance. The degree of visual impairment is usually inversely related to the degree of ocular pigmentation.
4 Compressive lesions
  - Craniopharyngiomas
  - Optic nerve or chiasmatic gliomas – associated with neurofibromatosis.
5 Hereditary optic atrophies

Nystagmus in infants

- Nystagmus in infants can be difficult to detect. Although the onset may be at birth but it can be detected later.
- The common forms are spasmus nutans and congenital nystagmus. The common distinguishing features are provided in the table below.
- Spasmus nutans is a self-limited disorder of infants, characterized by a slow cephalic tremor associated with pendular horizontal and rarely vertical nystagmus that is often monocular. Abnormal head positions are frequently present.
- Optic nerve and chiasmatic gliomas can simulate spasmus nutans. Therefore, neuroimaging should always be obtained in such cases.

Features	Spasmus nutans	Congenital nystagmus
Age of onset	4 months–3 years	Birth
Family history	Negative	Positive or negative
Nystagmus	Asymmetric (30% unilateral)	Bilateral and symmetric
Head movement	Usually previous to nystagmus	Simultaneous with nystagmus
Natural history	Disappears in 36 months	Usually persists

Other

Guidelines for the determination of brain death in children

- The guidelines for determination of brain death in children are similar to adults, although they have some unique features, dealing specifically with the age group from full-term newborn to the 5-year-old.

- These features are mainly focused on longer periods of recommended observation relative to the patient's age as outlined below.

1 Coma and apnea must co-exist.
2 Absence of brainstem function
   2.1 Pupils unreactive to light (midposition or dilated).
   2.2 Absence of spontaneous eye movement, or in response to oculocephalic and oculovestibular testing.
   2.3 Absence of movement of bulbar musculature, including facial and oropharyngeal muscles (corneal, gag, cough, sucking, and rooting reflexes).
   2.4 Respiratory movements are absent with patient off the respirator.
   2.5 Apnea testing using 'standardized methods' can be performed.
3 Absence of hypotension for age or hypothermia.
4 Flaccid muscle tone, absence of spontaneous movements (excluding spinal reflexes).
5 Examination consistent with brain death throughout the period of testing and observation.
6 Observation and testing according to age
   6.1 7 days to 2 months: two examinations and EEGs separated by 48 hours.
   6.2 2 months to 1 year: two examinations and EEGs separated by 24 hours.
   6.3 Older than 1 year: when an irreversible cause exists, laboratory testing is not required and an observation period of at least 12 hours is recommended. A more prolonged period of at least 24 hours of observation is recommended if it is difficult to assess the extent and reversibility of brain damage (e.g. following an hypoxic-ischemic event). The observation period may be reduced if an EEG demonstrates electrocerebral silence, or the cerebral radionuclide and angiographic study does not visualize cerebral arteries.

(Ref: Guidelines for the determination of brain death in children. *Pediatrics* 1987; 80: 298–300.)

Macrocephaly

- Macrocephaly means enlargement of the head >2 standard deviations from normal.
- Statistically, most enlarged heads in children are due to either non-pathological familial large head size or less commonly, hydrocephalus.
- There are certain conditions with a large head without significantly enlarged ventricles that occur in the setting of serious neurological abnormalities. Most neurodegenerative conditions of children cause small heads.

1 **Benign familial macrocephaly**: large parental head size, child with normal development
2 *Hydrocephalus*
   - Features include frontal protuberance, bossing, sunset sign (a tendency for the eyes to turn down so that the sclera is visible between the upper eyelids and iris), thinning and/or prominence of scalp veins, and separation of cranial sutures.
   2.1 Obstructive/noncommunicating hydrocephalus
       2.1.1 Congenital malformation: aqueductal stenosis, Dandy-Walker, Klippel-Feil syndrome, Chiari II.
       2.1.2 *Brain tumors*: rare; particularly posterior fossa tumors (medulloblastoma, cerebellar, or brainstem astrocytoma, ependymoma, choroid plexus papilloma), and pineal region tumors.
       2.1.3 *Vein of Galen malformation*: may present with neonatal heart failure.
   2.2 Communicating hydrocephalus
       - Secondary to subarachnoid hemorrhage or meningitis.
       - Meningeal malignancy.
3 **Benign enlargement of subarachnoid space**: also known as benign subdural effusions, etc.
   - More often in males, associated with large paternal head size.
   - Distinguished by soft fontanelle, large head, normal development.
   - Normal ventricular size on CT scan.
4 *Subdural hematoma*
   - Signs include bulging fontanelle, vomiting, altered mental status.
   - Unusual bruising, retinal hemorrhages, or fractures may point to child abuse.
5 Megalencephaly (large brain size)
   5.1 Achondroplasia: AD, most are new mutations. True, often alarming, megalencephaly. Usually normal cognitive development.
   5.2 Sotos syndrome: variable inheritance, megalencephaly with gigantism.
   5.3 Hemimegalencephaly: unilateral cerebral enlargement, associated with poor development and intractable seizures/infantile spasms.
   5.4 Neurocutaneous disorders: hypomelanosis of Ito, incontinentia pigmenti, neurofibromatosis, tuberous sclerosis, epidermal nevus syndrome (see Chapter 12: Neurogenetics – Neurocutaneous syndromes).
   5.5 Metabolic megalencephaly
       5.5.1 Alexander disease (see Developmental regression in toddlers/children, p. 366)
       5.5.2 Canavan disease (see Developmental regression in infants, p. 363)
       5.5.3 Glutaric aciduria type I: normal development with macrocephaly until experiencing an encephalopathic event around age 2–3. After this, spasticity and movement disorders may be prominent, with variable cognition.

5.5.4 Storage disorders: gangliosidoses (Tay-Sachs, etc.), Krabbe, maple syrup urine disease, metachromatic leukodystrophy, mucopolysaccharidoses (see Developmental regression, pp. 364 and 366).

6 Hydranencephaly
  • Means hydrocephalus plus destruction or failure of development of parts of the cerebrum, often associated with enlargement of the skull.
  • The fluid-filled region of the cranium is seen when transilluminated.

7 Conditions with a thickened skull: include anemia, cleidocranial dysostosis, osteogenesis imperfecta, osteopetrosis, rickets, etc.

Nightmares vs. night terrors

• Individuals, especially children, sometimes have isolated episodes of sudden arousal from sleep in a condition of terror and confusion.
• Common disorders include nightmare and night terror. The important clues for differentiation are provided below. Other differential diagnoses include sleepwalking disorder, other parasomnias, hypnagogic hallucinations in narcolepsy, substance-induced sleep disorders, and nocturnal seizures.
• Normal neurological exam

Nightmare	Night terror
Repeated, clinically significant awakening from sleep with a detailed recall of disturbing dreams	Abrupt, recurrent, and clinically significant awakening from sleep, accompanied by panic and autonomic arousal
Individuals rapidly become alert and oriented after awakening from nightmares	**Individuals are usually unresponsive to the environment and have subsequent amnesia for the episode**
Polysomnographic recording shows sudden awakening from REM sleep at the time the individual reports nightmares	**Polysomnographic recording shows sudden partial awakening from NON-REM sleep**
Often begins in childhood and resolves quickly	Onset is usually middle childhood and resolves during late childhood or early adolescence
Reassurance only. No therapy or medications are required	Reassurance is helpful. Diazepam or clonidine have been used to treat, but are not necessary

Chapter 12
Neurogenetics

When to suspect genetic disease

1 Positive family history. This should be explored in detail, as many patients will initially deny any known history of hereditary disease.
2 Unusual morphologic features, especially:
   - facial dysmorphology
   - atypical body habitus
3 Absence of obvious alternative etiologies (such as ischemia, infection, and trauma).
4 Clinical constellation with known neurogenetic association, such as:
   - ataxia
   - neuropathy
   - ophthalmoplegia
   - muscle weakness
   - progressive myoclonic seizures
   - developmental regression in children
5 Neurologic disease with additional organ system involvement, such as:
   - cardiomyopathy
   - hepatosplenomegaly
   - cutaneous manifestations
   - renal disease

Patterns of inheritance

Patterns of inheritance	Risk to offspring	Gender bias	Transmission
Autosomal dominant	50%	Males and females equally affected	Multiple affected generations and multiple individuals in one generation: includes father to son transmission.
Autosomal recessive	25%	Males and females equally affected	May 'skip' a generation. Carriers may be asymptomatic
X-linked recessive	50% risk to males or female carriers	Males	Multiple affected generations and multiple individuals in one generation: father to son transmission is not seen
Mitochondrial	All children at risk	Males and females equally affected	Variable expression and disease severity, maternal transmission only

Autosomal Dominant

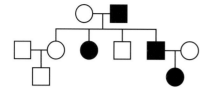

Autosomal Recessive

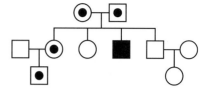

X-Linked

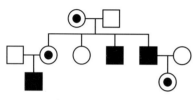

Mitochondrial

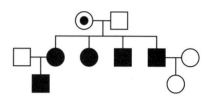

Patterns of inheritance

Examples of autosomal dominant disorders

- Autosomal dominant nocturnal frontal lobe epilepsy
- Benign familial neonatal seizures
- Bethlem myopathy
- Central core myopathy
- Charcot-Marie-Tooth disease (HMSN I)
- Childhood absence epilepsy
- Dentatorubro-pallidoluysian atrophy
- Dopa-responsive dystonia
- Essential tremor
- Familial amyloid polyneuropathy
- Familial episodic ataxia
- Familial hyperkalemic periodic paralysis
- Familial hypokalemic periodic paralysis
- Familial paroxysmal choreoathetosis
- Fascioscapulohumeral dystrophy
- Hereditary neuralgic amyotrophy
- Hereditary neuropathy with pressure palsies
- Huntington disease
- Hyperekplexia
- Juvenile myoclonic epilepsy
- Myotonic dystrophy
- Neurofibromatosis 1
- Spinocerebellar ataxias (many types)
- Tuberous sclerosis
- Von Hippel Lindau disease

Examples of autosomal recessive disorders (many others)

- Ataxia telangiectasia
- Canavan disease
- Cerebrotendinous xanthomatosis
- Dejerine-Sottas disease (HMSN III)
- Friedreich ataxia
- Galactosemia
- Gaucher disease
- Homocystinuria
- Isovaleric acidemia
- Krabbe disease
- Maple syrup urine disease
- Metachromatic leukodystrophy
- Mucopolysaccharidosis type I (Hurler)
- Mucopolysaccharidosis type III
- Neuronal ceroid lipofuscinosis, infantile
- Niemann-Pick disease
- Phenylketonuria
- Propionic academia
- Refsum disease, infantile
- Sandhoff disease
- Spinal muscular atrophy type I (Werdnig-Hoffman)
- Tay-Sachs disease
- Most congenital metabolic disorders

Examples of X-linked disorders

- Adrenoleukodystrophy, juvenile
- Becker muscular dystrophy
- Duchenne muscular dystrophy
- Emery-Dreifuss muscular dystrophy
- Fragile X syndrome
- Lesch-Nyhan disease
- Menkes disease
- Mucopolysaccharidosis type II (Hunter, X-linked recessive)
- Rett syndrome (X-linked dominant, lethal in males?)
- Ornithine transcarbamylase deficiency
- X-linked hydrocephalus

Examples of chromosomal autosomal disorders

- Angelman syndrome (deletion of part of long arm of maternal 15q)
- Cri-du-chat syndrome (deletion of short arm of 5p)
- Down syndrome (trisomy 21)

- Prader-Willi syndrome (deletion of part of long arm of paternal 15q)
- Trisomy 13
- Trisomy 18

Examples of sex chromosome disorders
- Klinefelter syndrome (XXY)
- XYY karyotype
- Turner syndrome (45,X)

Mitochondrial encephalomyopathies

- Mitochondrial DNA (mtDNA) is nearly exclusively maternally inherited.
- mtDNA is a closed, circular DNA molecule consisting of ~16,000 nucleotides coding for 37 genes.
- Every cell contains multiple mitochondria with multiple copies of DNA, a condition known as polyplasmy.
- Mitochondrial diseases demonstrate a threshold effect, whereby disease onset and severity are a function of the balance between the proportion of mutant and wild-type mtDNAs.
- May involve multiple tissues with high energy requirements – such as brain, retina, muscle, cochlea, etc.

Disorder	Disease features
Mitochondrial encephalomyopathy, lactic acidosis, and stroke-like episodes (MELAS)	Seizures, developmental delay, growth retardation, headaches, and stroke-like episodes with focal neurologic deficits
Myoclonic epilepsy and ragged red fibers (MERRF)	Myoclonus, ataxia, seizures, myopathy, and peripheral neuropathy
Leber hereditary optic neuropathy (LHON)	Optic disc swelling with visual field loss progressing to involve central vision
Neurogenic weakness, ataxia, and retinitis pigmentosa syndrome (NARP)	Developmental delay, seizures, dementia, ataxia, sensory neuropathy, proximal weakness, and retinitis pigmentosa
Maternally inherited Leigh syndrome (MILS)	Dementia, spasticity, optic atrophy
Chronic progressive external ophthalmoplegia (CPEO)	Ptosis, extra-occular ophthalmoplegia, proximal limb myopathy
Kearns-Sayre syndrome (KSS)	A CPEO-plus syndrome which includes the above as well as onset prior to age 20 years, heart block, ataxia, and pigmentary retinopathy

Diseases due to trinucleotide repeat expansions

- Unstable expansion of trinucleotide repeats is the mechanism underlying disorders featuring anticipation, the tendency for subsequent generations to be affected at an earlier age and with increased severity.
- The molecular mechanisms of disease are poorly understood as the triplet expansions are known to be located in coding sequences (Huntington disease), non-coding sequences (Friedreich ataxia), 5'-untranslated regions (fragile X syndrome), and 3'-untranslated regions (myotonic dystrophy).
- CAG repeat expansions that encode polyglutamines appear to result in protein misfolding, a recuring theme in many of these disorders.
- DNA molecular diagnostic tests are available. However, estimating disease onset and severity within an individual is not accurately predicted by absolute repeat number. Therefore, great care must be taken to ensure accurate information is provided when using molecular data in genetic counseling, particularly in asymptomatic individuals.

Disorder	Gene and locus	Protein	Repeat sequence and location	Disease features	Inheritance
Fragile X syndrome 1/1,500 males	FMR1 Xq27.3	FMRP	CGG 5'-UTR	Mental retardation, elongated facies, large ears, macroorchidism	X-linked
Friedreich ataxia 1/50,000	X25 9q13–21.1	Frataxin	GAA 1st intron	Ataxia, dysarthria, extensor plantar response, areflexia	AR
Huntington disease 1/20,000 Caucasians 1/100,000 African Americans	IT15 4p16.3	Huntington	CAG coding	Personality change, motor abnormalities, extrapyramidal signs, dysarthria	AlzD
Myotonic dystrophy 1/7500	DMPK 19q13.3	Myotonic dystrophy protein kinase	CTG 3'-UTR	Ptosis, facial atrophy, proximal weakness, cardiac conduction abnormalities	AlzD
Dentatorubro-pallidoluysian atrophy	DRPLA 12p13.31	Atrophin-1	CAG coding	Ataxia, personality changes, chorea, tonic-clonic seizures, dementia	AlzD
Spinobulbar muscular atrophy (Kennedy disease)	AR Xq13.21	Androgen receptor	CAG coding	Lower motor neuron disease, feminization	X-linked

Continued

Disorder	Gene and locus	Protein	Repeat sequence and location	Disease features	Inheritance
Spinocerebellar ataxia type 6	CACNA1A 19p13	α_{1A} subunit of voltage-gated Ca channel	CAG coding	Ataxia, cerebellar symptoms	AlzD
Spinocerebellar ataxia type 3 (Machdo-Joseph disease)	SCA3/MJD1 14q32.1	Ataxin-3	CAG coding	Ataxia, peripheral sensorimotor neuropathy, pyramidal, and extrapyramidal signs	AlzD
Spinocerebellar ataxia type 2	SCA2 12q24.1	Ataxin-2	CAG coding	Ataxia, areflexia, dementia, slow saccades	AlzD
Spinocerebellar ataxia type 1	SCA1 6p23	Ataxin-1	CAG coding	Ataxia, pyramidal signs, vibratory loss, dysphagia	AlzD
Spinocerebellar ataxia type 7	SCA7 3p12–13	Ataxin-7	CAG coding	Ataxia, retinal degeneration	AlzD
Spinocerebellar ataxia type 8	SCA8 13q21	KLH1	CTG 5'-UTR	Ataxia, cerebellar signs	AlzD
Spinocerebellar ataxia type 10	SCA10 22q13	Ataxin-10	ATTCT 9th intron	Ataxia, cerebellar signs with epilepsy	AlzD
Spinocerebellar ataxia type 12	PPP2R2B 5q31–33	PP2A regulatory protein	CAG 5'-UTR	Ataxia, upper extremity and head tremor, cerebellar signs, hyperreflexia, dementia	AlzD
Spinocerebellar ataxia type 17	SCA17 6q27	TATA binding protein	CAG coding	Ataxia, hyperreflexia, plantar responses, seizures, cognitive decline	AlzD
Oculopharyngeal dystrophy	PABP2 14q11	Poly-A binding protein	GCG coding	Ptosis, diplopia, dysphagia, proximal weakness	AlzD
Fragile XE mental retardation	FMR2 Xq28	FMR2	GCC 5'-UTR	Mental retardation	X-linked
Myotonic dystrophy type 2	ZNF9 3q13–24	Zinc finger protein 9	CTG 1st intron	Ptosis, facial atrophy, proximal weakness, cardiac conduction abnormalities	AlzD

Heritable human prion diseases

- Poorly understood pathogenesis mediated by prion protein.
- Multiple mutations characterized.
- All show autosomal dominant inheritance.
- Amyloid plaques and spongiform changes seen histologically.
  Caused by mutations in the human prion protein gene, PRNP (unknown function), located on chromosome 20pter-12.

Disorder	Disease features
Creutzfeldt-Jakob disease	Rapidly progressive (over weeks/months) dementia with cerebellar dysfunction, myoclonus, and combinations of pyramidal and extrapyramidal pathology. Characteristic EEG evolution to either 1–2 Hz triphasic spikes or 'burst suppression'
Gerstmann-Sträussler-Scheinker syndrome	Predominant ataxia with dysphagia, dysarthria, hyporeflexia, and dementia. Slower course (months/years). Familial
Fatal familial insomnia	Predominant intractable insomnia, endocrine dysfunction, and dysautonomia with progressive dementia, rigidity, and dystonia. Slower course (months/years). Familial

Clinical syndromes

Hereditary/genetic ataxias

- The hereditary ataxias collectively share many clinical features, including gait ataxia, limb dysmetria, intention tremor, and dysphagia. Most of these pathological features arise by virtue of cerebellar dysfunction.
- Though there is great overlap amongst the hereditary ataxias, some carry defining features such as bulbar involvement, peripheral neuropathies, oculomotor palsies, and dementia.
- Typically present around the third decade, though onset varies from 1st to 7th decade.
- Slow, though relentless, progression over the course of approximately 15 years.
- Important to rule out other more common causes of ataxia when making diagnosis.
- Molecular diagnostic testing available for disease confirmation in many hereditary ataxias.
- See Chapter 6: Movement Disorders and Diseases due to trinucleotide repeat expansions, pp. 387–8.

Hereditary/genetic epilepsy syndromes

- Family history is not uncommon in epilepsy syndromes. Improved genetic testing is delineating a genetic etiology to many previously idiopathic seizure syndromes.
- Some genetic syndromes are associated primarily with epilepsy, with few additional neurological or behavioral symptoms. Mutations in ion channels are increasingly being identified as the etiology for these syndromes.
- Many genetic syndromes have seizures and developmental delay as components of multisystem dysfunction due to abnormal metabolism or storage. Mutations in metabolic enzymes are often responsible for these disorders.
- Structural chromosomal abnormalities are also associated with seizures and developmental delay. Dysmorphic features and structural abnormalities of the brain and other organs occur more commonly in these patients.
- Improved neuroimaging techniques can detect subtle cerebral dysgenesis in epilepsy patients that might have previously been classified as idiopathic.

Disorder	Location	Gene/protein	Disease features	Inheritance
Angelman syndrome	15q11–13 maternal deletion	UBE3A/ E6-AP ubiquitin-protein ligase	Seizures, mental retardation, 'happy puppet syndrome'	Maternally inherited deletion
Autosomal dominant nocturnal frontal lobe epilepsy	20q13, 15q14? 1?	CHRNA4/α4 subunit AChR Unknown CHRNB2/-2 subunit AChR	Nocturnal seizures, onset 10 years, normal development	AlzD
Benign childhood epilepsy with centro-temporal spikes	1? 15q14?	Unknown CHRNA7/-7 subunit AChR?	Simple partial orofacial seizures, onset 3–13 years, associated with sleep or awakening	AlzD
Benign familial infantile convulsions	19q 16p12-q12?	Unknown	Partial seizures, onset 4–7 months, normal development	AlzD
Benign familial neonatal convulsions	20q13, 8q24	KCNQ2 or KCNQ3/KQT-like K+ channel	Multifocal clonic seizures that self-resolve, onset 1st postnatal week, normal development	AlzD

Disorder	Location	Gene/protein	Disease features	Inheritance
Bilateral periventricular nodular heterotopia	Xq28	Unknown	Lethal in males, seizures and normal development in females	XL
Childhood absence epilepsy	20q? 8q24?	CHRNA4/-4 subunit AChR? Unknown	Absence seizures, onset 3–12 years, 3 Hz spike wave on EEG, normal development	AlzD
Down syndrome	Trisomy 21	Unknown	Mental retardation, seizures, hypotonia, characteristic facies	Triploidy
Familial temporal lobe epilepsy	10q?	Unknown	Complex partial seizures, some febrile seizures	AlzD
Febrile seizures with temporal lobe epilepsy	8q?	Unknown	Febrile and complex partial seizures	AlzD
Febrile seizures alone	19p13	FEB2/?	Febrile seizures alone	AlzD
Fragile X syndrome	Xq27.3	FMR-1/frataxin	Mental retardation, seizures, large ears, hypotonia, macrocephaly, macroorchidism	XL
Generalized epilepsy with febrile seizures plus (GEFS+)	19q? 2q?	SCN1A, 1B, 2A/ sodium channel subunits	Febrile seizures, later afebrile seizures	AlzD
Incontinentia pigmenti	X	Unknown	Pigmented skin lesions, mental retardation, polymicrogyria	XL
Juvenile absence epilepsy	8q24? 21q22?	GRIK1?/GluR5? GABRA1/ $GABA_A$R subunit	Absence seizures, onset 8–17 years, >3 Hz spike wave, normal development	AlzD
Juvenile myoclonic epilepsy	6p? 15q14? 15q11–13?	EJM1? CHRNA7/-7 subunit AchR $GABA_A$/GABAR	Generalized seizures (tonic-clonic, myoclonic, absence), onset puberty, 4–6 Hz spike wave, normal development	AlzD

Continued

Disorder	Location	Gene/protein	Disease features	Inheritance
Lissencephaly and band heterotopia	Xq22	XSCLH or LIS/double cortin	Lissencephaly (lethal in males), band heterotopia (in females)	XL
MERRF	mt DNA	tRNA^{Lys}/tRNA^{Lys}	Myoclonic epilepsy, myopathy	Mitochondiral
Miller-Dieker syndrome	17q13 hemizygous deletion	LIS-1/homologue of G-protein subunit	Lissencephaly, severe seizures and developmental delay	?
Neuronal ceroid lipofuscinosis, type 1	1q32	PPT/palmitoyl protein thioesterase	Progressive myoclonic seizures, dementia, retinal degeneration	AR
Neurofibromatosis 1	17q12–22	neurofibromin	Macrocephaly, café-au-lait, axillary freckles, seizures	AlzD
Nonketotic hyperglycinemia	?	Unknown	Hypotonia, neonatal seizures, opisthotonus, myoclonus, apnea	AR
Partial epilepsy with auditory features	10q	LGI1/?	Partial seizures with ictal auditory disturbances, onset 8–19 years, normal development	AlzD
Primary reading epilepsy	?	Unknown	Simple partial jaw seizures, triggered by reading	AlzD
Progressive epilepsy with mental retardation	8p	Unknown	Progressive seizures, onset 5–10 years, mental retardation	AR
Pyridoxine dependency	?	Unknown	Neonatal seizures/status epilepticus	AR
Tuberous sclerosis	9q343.3 16p13.3	TSC1/Hamartin TSC2/Tuberin	Ash leaf spot, other skin lesions, mental retardation, seizures, visceral tumors, brain tumors	AlzD
Unverricht-Lundborg	21q22.3	EPM1/cystatin B	Generalized tonic-clonic seizures, myoclonus, onset 8–13 years, mild dementia	AR

Alzheimer disease genetics

- The most important risk factor for AlzD is age, with family history as the second most important risk factor.
- Familial AlzD is characterized by multiple affected individuals in which the disease segregates in a manner consistent with fully penetrant autosomal dominant inheritance. They probably comprise 5% or less of all cases with AlzD.
- Familial AlzD is divided into early and late onset categories with 60–65 years as the dividing line. Thus far, familial AlzD has been shown to be caused by three different genes.
- Recently, apolipoprotein E (APOE) has been considered as an important genetic susceptibility risk factor for the development of sporadic AlzD. Individuals who are homozygous and carry two APOE-4 alleles have an increased probability (>90%) of developing AlzD by the age of 85 and do so about 10 years earlier than individuals carrying the -2 or -3 allelic variants.

Gene	Chromosome	Age at onset	% of AlzD
Amyloid precursor protein (APP)	21	45–60	< 1
Presenilin-1 (PS-1)	14	30–60	1–5
Presenilin-2 (PS-2)	1	50–65	< 1
Apolipoprotein E (APOE-4 alleles)	19	60+	50–60

Hereditary/genetic movement disorders

- Some movement disorders are clearly hereditary, and family history should be sought as a clue to the underlying diagnosis. Incomplete penetrance may obscure autosomal dominantly inherited disorders.
- Particularly for paroxysmal movement disorders, family history may be incomplete or unknown by the patient.
- Many of the hereditary movement disorders demonstrate variable but nonspecific symptoms of basal ganglia involvement, including dystonia, Parkinsonism, choreoathetosis, tics, and dyskinesias.
- Neuroimaging abnormalities may also be seen in the basal ganglia (e.g. Fahr disease with calcification, Hallervorden-Spatz with iron deposition, Wilson disease with copper deposition).

For hereditary ataxias, see p. 389 and Chapter 6: Movement Disorders.

Disorder	Gene/location	Clinical features	Inheritance
Essential (familial) tremor	3q13 2p	Limb or head tremor, normal development	AlzD
Huntington disease	4p16.3	Choreoathetosis, dementia, psychosis	AlzD
Tics/Tourette syndrome	Unknown	Tics, ADHD, obsessive compulsive behavior	AlzD
Benign familial chorea	Unknown	Mild continuous childhood chorea, normal development	AlzD
Chorea-acanthocytosis	9q21	Tics, self-mutilating orofacial dyskinesia, dystonia, dementia, normal lipid profile	AR
Dementia-Parkinsonism-amyotrophy complex	17q21–23	Parkinsonism, dementia, weakness, spasticity	AlzD
Dopa-responsive dystonia	14q11-q24.3	Dystonia, Parkinsonism, diurnal worsening of symptoms	AlzD
DRPLA	12p12	Chorea, myoclonus, ataxia, seizures, dementia	AlzD
Fahr disease	14q	Dementia, choreoathetosis, focal dystonia, Parkinsonism, calcification of basal ganglia	AlzD
Familial CJD	20p terminal p12	Dementia, ataxia, myoclonus	AlzD
Glutaric aciduria	19p13.2	Megalencephaly, dystonia, choreoathetosis	AR
Hallervorden-Spatz or PKAN	20p12.3-p13	Dystonia, retinitis pigmentosum, dementia	AR
Hereditary hyperekplexia	5q	Exaggerated startle response	AlzD
Idiopathic torsion dystonia	9q32-q34	Dystonia, initially focal, but later generalized	AlzD
Juvenile myoclonic epilepsy	6p	Seizures (tonic-clonic, myoclonic and/or absence), myoclonus	AlzD
LHON	mito 3460, mito 11778, mito 14484l	Optic neuropathy, dystonia	Maternal
Lubag disease	Xq13	Dystonia, parkinsonism	X-linked
MERRF	tRNA gene	Encephalomyopathy	Maternal

Disorder	Gene/location	Clinical features	Inheritance
McLeod syndrome	Xp21	Areflexia, dystonia, chorea, cardiomyopathy, muscular dystrophy, dementia, seizures, tics, normal lipid profile	X-linked
NARP	mito 8993	Neuropathy, ataxia, retinitis pigmentosa	Maternal
Paroxysmal kinesigenic choreoathetosis	16p11.2-q12.1	Episodic choreoathetosis or dystonia, triggered by movement	AlzD
Paroxysmal nonkinesigenic choreoathetosis	2q	Episodic choreoathetosis or dystonia, not triggered by movement	AlzD
Unverricht-Lundborg disease	21q22.3	Progressive myoclonic epilepsy	AlzD
Wilson disease	13q14.3	Tremor, dementia, hepatic failure	AR

CJD – Creutzfeldt-Jakob disease, DRPLA – dentatorubral pallidoluysian atrophy, LHON – Leber hereditary optic neuropathy, NARP – neuropathy, ataxia, retinitis pigmentosa, MERRF – mitochondrial encephalopathy with ragged red fibers, PKAN – pantothenate kinase-associated neurodegeneration, SCA – spinocerebellar ataxia.

Ref: Modified from Fahn S., Greene P.E., Ford B., Bressman S.B. *Handbook of Movement Disorders.*

Hereditary/genetic myopathies

- The muscular dystrophies are primarily genetic myopathies resulting from disturbances in structural proteins. Many of the actual gene defects are known, as is the pathophysiology in some cases.
- Clinically, patients present with weakness and atrophy.
- The childhood dystrophies may present with failure to achieve milestones.
- In most instances there is a slow and progressive decline in function.
- Patterns of weakness vary and may be predominantly distal, proximal, or involve specific muscle groups such as extraocular muscles.

Disorder	Gene and locus	Protein	Disease features	Inheritance pattern
Duchenne MD 1/3,300 male births	DMD Xp21	Dystrophin (absent)	Severe, progressive proximal muscle weakness, loss of ambulation by age 10, cardiomyopathy, mental retardation	X-linked

Continued

Disorder	Gene and locus	Protein	Disease features	Inheritance pattern
Myotonic dystrophy 1/7500 live births	DMPK 19q13.3	Myotonic dystrophy protein kinase	Ptosis, facial atrophy, proximal weakness, cardiac conduction abnormalities, cataracts, testicular atrophy, diabetes mellitus	AlzD
Becker MD 1/20,000 male births	BMD Xp21	Dystrophin (reduced)	Similar to DMD, though less severe and later onset, ambulation after age 10	X-linked
Facioscapulohumeral MD 1/320,000 live births, higher in Dutch ancestry	FSHD 4q35	Unknown	Facial weakness as well as shoulder girdle and mild leg weakness	AlzD
Emery-Dreifuss MD	EDMD Xq28	Emerin	Similar to BMD, though less severe; joint contractures and cardiac conduction defects	X-linked
Fukyama type MD	FCMD 9q31–33	Fukutin	Hypotonia, atrophy, weakness, intellectual delay with seizures and cortical dysplasia	AR
Limb-girdle 1A MD, prevalence of ALL LGMD 1/100,000	LGMD 1A 5q22–34	Unknown	Progressive weakness of shoulder and pelvic girdle muscles	AlzD
Limb-girdle 1B MD	LGMD 1B 1q11–21	Unknown	Same as LGMD 1A	AlzD
Limb-girdle 1C MD	LGMD 1C 3p25	Caveolin-3	Same as LGMD 1A	AlzD
Limb-girdle 2A MD	LGMD 2A 15q15.1	Calpain 3	Same as LGMD 1A	AR
Limb-girdle 2B MD	LGMD 2B 2p13	Dysferlin	Same as LGMD 1A	AR
Limb-girdle 2C MD	LGMD 2C 13q12	γ-sarcoglycan	Same as LGMD 1A	AR
Limb-girdle 2D MD	LGMD 2D 17q21	α-sarcoglycan	Same as LGMD 1A	AR

Disorder	Gene and locus	Protein	Disease features	Inheritance pattern
Limb-girdle 2E MD	LGMD 2E 4q12	β-sarcoglycan	Same as LGMD 1A	AR
Limb-girdle 2F MD	LGMD 2F 5q31	δ-sarcoglycan	Same as LGMD 1A	AR
Limb-girdle 2G MD	LGMD 2G	Unknown	Same as LGMD 1A	AR
Miyoshi distal myopathy	2p13	Dysferlin	Plantar flexion weakness with gastrocnemius atrophy	AR
Epidermolysis bullosa simplex with MD	MD-EBS 8q24	Plectin	Proximal muscle weakness with blistering disorder	AR
Scapuloperoneal MD	SPMD 12q21	Unknown	Foot drop and shoulder girdle weakness	AlzD
Oculopharyngeal MD	OPMD 14q11.2-q13	Poly(A)binding protein	Ptosis, dysphagia, diplopia, shoulder girdle weakness	AlzD
Bethlem myopathy 1	21q22	α1(VI) collagen	Flexion contractures with mild proximal muscle weakness and atrophy	AlzD
Bethlem myopathy 2	21q22	α2(VI) collagen	Same as Bethlem myopathy 1	AlzD
Bethlem myopathy 3	2q37	α3(VI) collagen	Same as Bethlem myopathy 1	AlzD
Hyperkalemic periodic paralysis	17q23.1-q25.3	Sodium channel subunit, SCN4A	Episodic paralysis, often after exertion, myotonia	AlzD
Paramyotonia congenita	17q23.1-q25.3	Sodium channel α subunit, SCN4A	Mytonia precipitated by cold or exertion	AlzD
Myotonia congenita (Thomsen disease or Becker disease)	7q32	Voltage-gated chloride channel, CLCN1	Myotonia, muscle stiffness, muscular hypertrophy	AlzD (Thomsen) AR (Becker)

MD – Muscular dystrophy, DMD – Duchenne MD, BMD – Becker MD.

Neurocutaneous syndromes

- The hereditary phakomatoses derive their name from the shared features of either cutaneous or neurological abnormalities, or both.
- Most share autosomal dominant transmission, high penetrance, and variable phenotypic expression.
- Many carry a predisposition to the formation of various tumors.

Disorder	Gene and locus	Protein	Disease features	Inheritance
Neurofibromatosis type 1 (NF1) 1/3,500	NF1 17q11.2	Neuro-fibromin	Café-au-lait spots, lisch nodules, neurofibromas, bony abnormalities, learning disabilities, epilepsy, vascular malformations, benign and malignant tumors	AlzD
Tuberous sclerosis 1/10,000	Tuberous sclerosis complex 1 (TSC1) 9q34.1–34.2	Hamartin	Cortical tubers with developmental delay and epilepsy, facial sebaceous angiofibromas, periungual fibromas, shagreen patch, ash-leaf spots, subependymal giant cell astrocytoma, atrial myxoma, renal angiomyolipoma	AlzD
Tuberous sclerosis	TSC2 16p13.3	Tuberin	Same as TSC1	AlzD
Neurofibromatosis type 2 (NF2) 1/35,000	NF2 chrom22	Schwannomin (merlin)	Bilateral vestibular schwannomas, neurofibromas, retinal hamartomas, meningiomas, ependymomas	AlzD
Sturge-Weber syndrome	Unknown	Unknown	Facial port-wine stain, seizures, hemiparesis/plegia, glaucoma, mental retardation	Variable
Von Hippel-Lindau disease	VHL 3p25–26	pVHL	Retinal angioma, cerebellar hemangioma, spinal hemangioma, pheochromocytoma, pancreatic cysts	AlzD

Disorder	Gene and locus	Protein	Disease features	Inheritance
Incontinentia pigmenti	Xq28	Unknown	Erythematous and vesicular neonatal rash, seizures, bizarre polymorphic pigmentary skin patterns in infancy, mental retardation, hydrocephalus	X-linked, lethal in males
Hypomelanosis of Ito	Xp11	Unknown	Hypopigmented cutaneous whorls in infancy, hypotonia, pyramidal signs, mental retardation, seizures, ophthalmologic signs	AlzD or X-linked

Hereditary/genetic peripheral neuropathies

- Inherited disorders of peripheral nerves represent a fairly common group of heterogeneous neurologic diseases. These conditions roughly fall into one of three categories termed hereditary motor neuropathy, hereditary sensorimotor neuropathy, and hereditary sensory and autonomic neuropathy.
- Typically present with an insidious and indolent course, progressive over years to decades.
- Frequently, there is a poor appreciation on the part of the patient for a familial component.
- When considering a hereditary peripheral neuropathy, it is important to rule out other potential causes. Many etiologies are treatable (diabetes, B_{12} deficiency), and others are harbingers of serious systemic disease (paraneoplastic, heavy metal intoxication).

Disorder	Gene and locus	Protein	Disease features	Inheritance pattern
Charcot-Marie-Tooth (CMT) type 1A	PMP22 17p11.2–12	Peripheral myelin protein 22	Onset in 1st or 2nd decade, foot deformity with ambulation difficulties, distal weakness and atrophy, mild sensory loss, pes cavus	AlzD

Continued

Disorder	Gene and locus	Protein	Disease features	Inheritance pattern
CMT type 1B	P_0 1q22–23	Myelin protein zero	Similar to CMT type 1A	AlzD
CMT type 1C	Unknown	Unknown	Similar to CMT type 1A	AlzD
CMT type 2A	Unknown 1p35–36	Unknown	Similar to CMT type 1A with later onset, less severe symptoms, and lower occurrence of skeletal deformities	AlzD
CMT type 2B	Unknown 3q	Unknown	Similar to CMT type 2A	AlzD
CMT type 2C	Unknown	Unknown	Weakness of vocal cords, diaphragm, and intercostal muscles with respiratory failure	AlzD
CMT type 2D	Unknown 7p14	Unknown	Similar to CMT type 2A	AlzD
CMT type X	CX32 Xq13.1	Connexin 32	Demyelinating neuropathy, males more severely affected at earlier age	X-linked
CMT type 4A	Unknown 8q13–21	Unknown	Onset in childhood with progressive distal weakness and ambulation difficulties	AR
CMT type 4B	Unknown 11q23	Unknown	Similar to CMT type 4A	AR
CMT type 4B	Unknown 5q23–33	Unknown	Similar to CMT type 4A	AR
Dejerine-Sottas Disease (DSD) type A (CMT 3A)	PMP22 17p11.2–12	Peripheral myelin protein 22	Onset in childhood with severe disability, proximal weakness, areflexia	AlzD
DSD type B (CMT 3B)	P_0 1q22–23	Myelin protein zero	Similar to DSD type A	AlzD
Congenital hypomyelination	P_0 1q22–23	Myelin protein zero	Similar to DSD type A with severe, congenital onset	AlzD

Disorder	Gene and locus	Protein	Disease features	Inheritance pattern
Hereditary neuropathy with pressure palsies (HNPP) type A	PMP22 17p11.2–12	Peripheral myelin protein 22	Onset typically 2nd to 3rd decade with recurrent isolated mononeuropathies frequently provoked by compression, traction, or minor trauma, usually with complete resolution	AlzD
HNPP type B	Unknown	Unknown	Similar to HNPP type A	AlzD
Hereditary neuralgic amyotrophy	Unknown 17q23–25	Unknown	Onset in childhood with attacks of parasthesias, pain, and weakness involving the brachial plexus	AlzD
Hereditary sensory and autonomic neuropathy (HSAN) type I	Unknown 9q22.1–22.3	Unknown	Onset 2nd or later decade, protopathic sensory loss, variable neural hearing loss	AlzD
HSAN type II	Unknown	Unknown	Onset in infancy, distal multimodality sensory loss, bladder dysfunction, impotence	AR
HSAN type III	Unknown 9q31–33	Unknown	Onset at birth with prominent autonomic features including episodic vomiting, pulmonary infections, fever, episodic hypertension, sweating, cutaneous blotching, and defective lacrimation, also pain insensitivity and hyporeflexia	AR
HSAN type IV	NGF-trkA 1q21–22	Nerve growth factor tyrosine kinase	Congenital insensitivity to pain, impaired temperature regulation, anhidrosis, mild mental retardation	AR

Continued

Disorder	Gene and locus	Protein	Disease features	Inheritance pattern
Familial amyloid polyneuropathy (FAP) type I	TTR 18q11.2–12.1	Transthyretin	Onset in 3rd to 4th decade with distal sensory loss progressing to weakness and atrophy with impotence, postural hypotension, bladder dysfunction, anhidriosis, diarrhea, and liver failure	AlzD
FAP type II	TTR 18q11.2–12.1	Transthyretin	Onset 4th to 5th decade with carpal tunnel syndrome	AlzD
FAP type III	ApoA-1 11q23–24	Apolipoprotein-1	Similar to type I with renal involvement	AlzD
FAP type IV	Gelsolin Chrom9	Gelsolin actin-binding protein	Onset in 3rd decade with corneal clouding (lattice corneal dystrophy) and cranial nerve involvement	AlzD

Chapter 13

Neuroradiology

Types of neuroimaging

CT scanning

Current role of CT in neuroimaging

- Although magnetic resonance imaging (MRI) has better sensitivity than computed tomography (CT) for detecting intra-axial and extra-axial brain and spine lesions, CT still remains the quickest and the most efficient means of screening the patient with certain conditions, such as head trauma, and detecting calcifications and subarachnoid hemorrhage.
- CT scans account for 13% of the radiological examinations and 30% of the overall radiation exposure attributable to such examinations. Recently, CT brain scan with low mAs (low-dose CT with approximately 50% of a routine dose) has been evaluated to have acceptable diagnostic quality, comparable to a conventional CT scan. The low-dose CT brain scans may be well suited to minimize radiation doses for:

* use in younger patients, including those in neonatal intensive care units
* patients who undergo serial examinations over a short follow-up.

1 **Acute head trauma**
2 **Detecting subarachnoid hemorrhage**
   * CT is the most sensitive imaging study for the detection of subarachnoid hemorrhage and is the study of choice for initial evaluation of patients suspected of having this diagnosis.
3 **When MRI is contraindicated**
   * MRI cannot be performed in patients with:
      ▪ Pacemakers
      ▪ Non-MR-compatible vascular clips
      ▪ Metallic implants
      ▪ Deep brain stimulators
      ▪ Foreign bodies in the eyes or other vulnerable areas
      ▪ Severe claustrophobia
4 Fractures of orbit, temporal bones, face, and skull
5 Detection of calcification
   * The sensitivity of CT for calcification is critical in increasing diagnostic specificity, particularly for CNS tumors.
   * MRI is less sensitive than CT for the detection of calcification as calcium alone is weakly paramagnetic and hard to see on spin echo MRI.
6 Subtle bony irregularities
7 Bony spinal lesions or odontogenic lesions
8 Disease of the temporal bone
9 Sinusitis

(Ref: Grossman R.I., Yousem D.M. *Neuroradiology: The Requisites*. Mullins M.E., Lev M.H., Bove P., *et al.* Comparison of image quality between conventional and low-dose nonenhanced head CT. *AJNR* 2004; 25: 533–538.)

Scale for CT absorption

* The scale for CT absorption generally ranges from –1000 to +1000, with zero allocated to water and –1000 to air. The units are termed Hounsfield units (HU) after the discoverer of the technique.

- The values vary on different types of tissue. At values less than zero, one finds the structures that show less CT attenuation than water. In human beings, the structures with less CT attenuation than fat are relatively limited to air-containing materials. On the other hand, tissues with high protein concentration equate to higher HU values, for example, clotted blood, sinus secretions, or the lens of the eye.

Tissue	Hounsfield unit (HU)
Bone	1000
Liver	40–60
White matter	46
Gray matter	41
Muscle	10–40
Kidney	30
Cerebrospinal fluid	15
Water	**0**
Fat	−50 to −100
Air	−1000

Intracranial calcifications

- Intracranial calcifications appear punctate, curvilinear, or even mass-like.
- They may occur within brain parenchyma, associated with the dura, or as part of a larger mass lesion.
- The location and pattern of calcification provides clues as to its etiology.

1 **Physiological calcifications**
   - Pineal gland (20%)
   - Choroid plexus (usually bilateral)
   - Dura/falx
   - Habenula
2 Abnormal intracranial calcifications (**most diagnoses** fall into the range of **neoplastic or inflammatory conditions**)
   - 2.1 **Neoplastic conditions**
     - Most common in **oligodendrogliomas**. Also seen in astrocytomas, ependymomas, choroid plexus tumors, and craniopharyngiomas.
     - 10–18% of meningiomas are calcified (either psammomatous or dystrophic types).

- All types of gliomas may contain calcifications.

2.2 **Inflammatory conditions**
   - Granulomatous diseases, such as sarcoidosis.
   - Infectious causes, including tuberculosis, TORCH infections (TOxoplasmosis, Rubella, Cytomegalovirus, Herpes simplex virus), chronic abscesses, and cysticercosis.

2.3 Vascular lesions
   - Arterial calcifications are usually curvilinear, paired, and occur in the expected locations in the parasellar area.
   - Aneurysms uncommonly become calcified and are found in the region of circle of Willis.
   - Vascular malformations.

2.4 Others
   - Chronic subdural hematoma: curvilinear calcifications along the convexities.
   - Sturge-Weber syndrome: gyral calcification is a typical feature, trolley track (train track) calcification is uncommon and never present in neonates.
   - Tuberous sclerosis: calcification is located near the lateral ventricles.
   - Basal ganglia calcifications are seen in Fahr disease, hyperparathyroidism, and pseudohyperparathyroidism.

Stages of hemorrhage on MR and CT imaging

- Understanding the MR and CT characteristics of the various stages of hemorrhage is critically important in neurological emergencies.
- Hemoglobin is composed of four protein subunits, each containing one heme molecule consisting of a porphyrin and an iron atom, which serves as a binding site for oxygen. Oxyhemoglobin has no unpaired electrons and is diamagnetic.
- When a hemoglobin loses its O_2, it forms deoxyhemoglobin. As a consequence, the water molecules in deoxyhemoglobin are unable to bind to the heme iron as they do in methemoglobin, resulting in a low intensity on T2WI during acute hemorrhage.
- Normally, an enzyme within red blood cells rapidly reduces methemoglobin back to deoxyhemoglobin. However, in late subacute hemorrhage, this process deteriorates and oxidation to free methemoglobin takes place, resulting in high intensity on T2WI.
- Months after hemorrhage, the iron atoms from metabolized hemoglobin are deposited in hemosiderin. The susceptibility effect of the supraparamagnetic cores of hemosiderin produce hypointensity on T2WI.
- All stages of hemorrhage produce low signal intensity on MRI GRE sequences.

Stage	CT	T1WI	T2WI	Explanation
Hyperacute (4–6 hours)	High density	Iso- or low intensity	High intensity	Oxyhemoglobin
Acute (7–72 hours)	High density	Iso- or low intensity	Low intensity	Deoxyhemoglobin and high protein
Early subacute (4–7 days)	High density	High intensity	Low intensity	Intracellular methemoglobin and high protein
Late subacute (1–4 weeks)	Isodense	High intensity	High intensity with rim of low intensity	Free methemoglobin with rim of hemosiderin
Chronic (months to years)	Low density	Low intensity	Low intensity	Hemosiderin

MRI scanning

Magnetic resonance signal patterns

- Different pulse sequences have been developed that emphasize T1 and/or T2 relaxation effects.
- T1-weighted images (T1WI) are most useful for analyzing anatomical details and are employed in conjunction with gadolinium contrast agents, because enhancing lesions appear bright on T1WI.
- T2-weighted images (T2WI) are very sensitive to the presence of increased water and can visualize edema to great advantage. T2WI are also most sensitive to differences in susceptibility between tissues.
- Usually both T1WI and T2WI are used in routine brain, spine, and neck imaging. The combination of signal intensities on the two sequences often allows some tissue specificity.

	T1W	T2W
High intensity (bright)	• Calcification (calcium phosphate crystals) • Fat • Gadolinium • High protein • Melanin • Methemoglobin • Slow-flowing blood	• CSF • Edema • Extracellular methemoglobin

	T1W	T2W
Low intensity (dark)	• Air	• Air
	• Calcification	• Calcification
	• CSF	• Deoxyhemoglobin
	• Edema	• Flow (signal) void
	• Flow (signal) void	• High protein
	• Metals	• Intracellular methemoglobin
		• Metals

Stages of hemorrhage on MR and CT imaging (see pp. 407–8)

Bright lesions on diffusion-weighted MR images

- Although high signal intensity on diffusion-weighted images (DWI) and low apparent diffusion coefficient values (ADC) have a high sensitivity (94%) and specificity (100%) in the diagnosis of acute cerebral infarction, the same findings have been reported in other diverse conditions, such as hemorrhage, abscess, and tumors.
- The differential diagnosis of these conditions, for example, acute ischemic infarction versus acute cerebral hemorrhage, is critically important for the determination of appropriate treatment.

1 **Acute arterial infarction**
   - Acute ischemic lesions are characterized by high signal intensity on DWI and low ADC values. This is because the interruption of cerebral blood flow results in rapid (within minutes) breakdown of energy metabolism and ion exchange pumps. This leads to a massive shift of water from the extracellular into the intracellular compartment (cytotoxic edema), reducing the diffusibility of water and producing a typical 'bright spot' on DWI.
   - DWI and ADC maps show changes in ischemic brain tissue within hours after symptom onset, when no abnormalities are typically seen on conventional MRI. The signal intensity on DWI increases during the first week after symptom onset and relatively decreases thereafter. However, it remains hyperintense for a long period, up to 72 days. Therefore, DWI is not an ideal imaging protocol to estimate lesion age. The ADC values decline rapidly after the onset of ischemia and subsequently increase with the 'flip-flop' from dark to bright 7–10 days later.

2 Cerebral hemorrhage
   - The differential diagnosis of hyperacute ischemic stroke and hemorrhage may not be possible on DWI and ADC maps alone. Therefore, conjoint use of DWI, ADC maps, with T2W SE, T2W gradient-echo and T2W echo-planar imaging,

especially during the therapeutic window for thrombolysis (3 hours), is necessary in differentiation of hyperacute stroke from hyperacute hemorrhage.

3 Gliomas
  - The signal intensity of gliomas on DWI is variable (hyper-, iso-, or hypointense).
  - Occasionally, gliomas are hyperintense on DWI and show reduced ADC values, suggesting reduced volume of extracellular space. In other cases, ADC values are not reduced because of T2 shine-through effect.
  - ADC values cannot be used in individual cases to differentiate glioma types reliably.

4 Lymphoma
  - Enhancing components of lymphomas are generally hyperintense on DWI and show low ADC values.

5 Cerebral abscess
  - The presence of central hyperintensity on DWI and low ADC values strongly suggest the presence of pus and abscess. Ring enhancement further supports the possibility of abscess, as ring enhancement in acute stroke is unusual.

6 Venous infarction
  - The differential diagnosis of arterial and venous stroke may be impossible with acute stroke MR protocols.
  - The diffusion findings in human cerebral venous infarction remain controversial, with different reports suggesting either low or high signal intensity on DWI together with low ADC values.

7 Creutzfeldt-Jakob disease (CJD)
  - In cases of sporadic CJD (sCJD), high signal intensities on DWI have been reported in the putamen, caudate nucleus, and cortex.
  - In variant CJD (vCJD), high signal intensities are seen in the pulvinar, putamen, and caudate nucleus on T2W and proton density-weighted SE and FLAIR images. The value of DWI in imaging vCJD has not been established.

8 Others: the following conditions have been reported to cause high DWI signal intensity and low ADC values.
  - Sustained seizure activity
  - Eclampsia
  - Central pontine myelinolysis
  - Malignant meningioma
  - Encephalitis

(Ref: Stadnik T.W., *et al. *Imaging tutorial: differential diagnosis of bright lesions on diffusion-weighted MR images. *Radiographics* 2003; 23: e7.)

Fat-containing lesions

- Fat signal characteristics on neuroimaging include low density on CT, high intensity on T1WI, and low intensity on conventional T2WI, that suppresses even further when fat suppression techniques are used.

1 **Lipoma**
  - Almost all of the lipomas seen within the CNS are not neoplasms but are developmental or congenital abnormalities associated with abnormal development of the meninx primitive, a derivative of neural crest.
  - Lipomas are particularly common in association with agenesis of the corpus callosum, and 60% are associated with some type of congenital anomaly of the associated neural elements.
  - Common intracranial sites for lipomas include pericallosal regions, the quadrigeminal plate cistern, the suprasellar region, and the cerebellopontine angle cistern.
2 Dermoids and teratomas
  - The high signal intensity of fat and signal void of calcification on T1WI suggests a diagnosis of dermoid or teratoma.
  - The pineal and suprasellar regions are the common sites for teratomas.
  - Ruptured dermoid should be considered when multiple fat particles are seen scattered on an MRI or when lipid is detected in the CSF. Usually, the lesions are very well defined.
3 Fatty degeneration of meningioma
4 Pantopaque

Functional neuroimaging

- There are several cerebral imaging techniques available in which the principal aim is to derive information about brain function. These techniques include positron emission tomography (PET), single photon emission computed tomography (SPECT), and functional magnetic resonance imaging (fMRI). ^{133}Xe-enhanced CT has also been of considerable historical importance.
- Although functional neuroimaging is currently utilized mainly as a research tool, there is an increasing number of clinical scenarios where conventional structural CT and/or MRI are normal, despite evidence of neural dysfunction. Below are some situations where functional neuroimaging has an important role in clinical decision making.
  - Differentiation of tumor recurrence from radionecrosis (PET/FDG)

- Contribution to presurgical assessment of patients with refractory epilepsy (PET/FDG, SPECT/flow tracers)
- Differentiation of juvenile Parkinson disease from dopa-responsive dystonia
- Identification of critical gyri/sulci before neurosurgical procedures (cortical mapping)
- Neurochemical monitoring of patients undergoing neurotransplantation procedure

Features	PET	SPECT	fMRI
Isotopes	Fluorine-18 Carbon-11 Oxygen-15	Technetium-99m Iodine-123	None
Time per image	2 min to 2 hours	Minutes to hours	0.01 seconds to a few minutes
Spatial resolution	About 5–6 mm	About 8 mm	0.75 mm upwards
Repeated studies	Very few (limited by radiation)	Very few (limited by radiation)	Possible
Able to study	• Metabolism • Blood flow • Receptor-ligand interactions	• Blood flow • Receptor-ligand interactions	• Blood flow • Venous drainage • Neural activation

Bony abnormalities

Basilar invagination

- Basilar invagination refers to upward protrusion of the odontoid process into the infratentorial space.
- Readers should be familiar with two lines:
  1 McGregor line, which extends from the posterior margin of the hard palate to the undersurface of the occiput, and
  2 Chamberlain line, which is from the hard palate to the midportion of the posterior margin of the foramen magnum. If the dens extends for more than 5 mm above these lines, basilar invagination is considered to be present.
- This condition is associated with syringohydromyelia (25–35%) and Chiari malformations.
- Basilar invagination should not be confused with platybasia, which is flattening of the base of the skull.

Causes are numerous and only common examples are provided below:
1 Paget disease of the skull
2 Rickets
3 Fibrous dysplasia
4 Osteomalacia
5 Achondroplasia
6 Osteogenesis imperfecta
7 Cleidocranial dysplasia

Craniosynostosis

- Craniosynostosis or craniostenosis refers to abnormal early fusion of the sutures of the skull. This leads to abnormal head shapes and a palpable ridge.
- This disorder, if severe and early in development, can result in abnormal growth of the brain.
  - The most common variety is sagittal suture premature closure. It produces a head that cannot grow side to side, so that the head looks long and thin (scaphocephalic).
  - Brachycephalic refers to a broad head with recessed lower forehead, which occurs if both coronal sutures are affected.
  - If only a unilateral coronal or lambdoid suture is affected, it is called plagiocephaly, with flattening on one side of the head.
  - Premature closure of the metopic suture results in trigonocephaly (triangular head with mid-forehead ridge).
  - Oxycephaly may appear like microcephaly, with closure of all skull vault sutures. This can result in elevated intracranial pressure, as well as severe impairment of brain growth and development.

1 Primary craniosynostosis: no causes are identified.
2 Secondary craniosynostosis
   2.1 Syndromes that are associated with craniosynostosis
- Crouzon disease
- Apert syndrome
- Carpenter syndrome

   2.2 Metabolic disorders
- Rickets
- Hypercalcemia
- Hyperthyroidism
- Hypervitaminosis D

   2.3 Hematological disorders
- Sickle cell anemia

- Thalassemia
2.4 Bone dysplasia
  - Hypophosphatasia
  - Achondroplasia
  - Hurler syndrome
  - Skull hyperostosis
2.5 Others
  - Secondary to shunt procedure
  - Microcephaly: microcephaly is a consequence of craniosynostosis, but is more often a consequence of abnormal or profoundly diminished brain growth.

Skull fracture

- There are several types of common skull fractures.
- It is important for the radiologist to comment on the extent of the depression as well as any associated brain injury, including contusion, shearing injury, or extracerebral collections.

1 **Depressed skull fracture**
  - Usually comminuted and can produce underlying brain damage.
2 **Comminuted skull fracture**
  - Usually associated with depressed skull fracture.
3 Linear skull fracture
  - Linear, nondepressed skull fracture alone has little clinical significance.
4 Diastatic skull fracture
  - 'Fracture' consisting of bony separation at a suture.

Wide skull sutures

- The size of suture width is different according to age. The sutures are usually splitable up to the age of 12–15 years and close completely by the age of 30 years.
- Suture widths that are considered abnormal:
  > 10 mm at birth
  > 3 mm at 2 years
  > 2 mm at 3 years

1 **Normal variant**
  - Probably the most common cause.

- More common in neonate with prematurity.

2 **Increased intracranial pressure**
- Seen only in children < 10 years.
- Coronal sutures are most commonly involved, followed by sagittal and lambdoid sutures.
- Common causes in children include intracranial tumors, subdural hematoma, and hydrocephalus.

3 Metabolic disorders
- Hypoparathyroidism
- Hypo- and hypervitaminosis A
- Lead intoxication

4 Congenital underossification
- Rickets
- Hypothyroidism
- Osteogenesis imperfecta
- Hypophosphatasia

5 Others: rare causes
- Infiltration of sutures by metastatic tumors.
- Recovery from chronic illness in childhood.

Atlantoaxial subluxation

- Atlantoaxial subluxation refers to displacement of atlas with respect to axis.
- Anterior subluxation is more common than the posterior subluxation. The degree of displacement is the distance between the dens and the anterior arch of C1.
- Pseudosubluxation occurs when there is ligamentous laxity allowing for movement of the vertebral bodies on each other, especially C2 on C3. It is more common in infants.

1 **Trauma**
- Usually associated with fractures and rupture of the transverse ligament.

2 Non-traumatic causes are seen when there are problems with transverse ligament or malformations of the odontoid process.
- 2.1 Arthritis, causing laxity of transverse ligament and erosion of dens
  - **Rheumatoid arthritis**
  - Ankylosing spondylitis
  - Psoriatric arthropathy
  - Reiter syndrome
  - Systemic lupus erythematosus
- 2.2 Infections and inflammation

- Pharyngitis/tonsillitis, especially in childhood
- Retropharyngeal abscess
- Adenitis
- Parotitis

2.3 Aplasia of the odontoid process
- Mucopolysaccharidoses (especially Morquio syndrome MPS IV)
- Klippel-Feil syndrome
- Several types of genetic chondrodysplasia
- Down syndrome (usually asymptomatic)

2.4 Others
- Marfan syndrome
- Neurofibromatosis
- Associated with syringomyelia/syringobulbia

Extra-axial pathology

Cavernous sinus lesions

- The cavernous sinuses are multiseptated, extradural venous spaces that lie on both sides of the sella turcica. They communicate with each other, the intracranial dural sinuses, and deep facial venous plexuses.
- The cavernous sinus contains several important structures.
  - Medially: carotid artery
  - Laterally: CN III, IV, V1, and V2
  - Transversely: CN VI
- The cavernous sinus drains into superior and inferior petrosal sinuses. It receives blood from the superior and inferior ophthalmic veins as well as the sphenoparietal sinus.

1 Tumors
1.1 Pituitary adenoma
- Indolent, non-aggressive lesions that slowly expand and erode the bony sella turcica and can extend into the cavernous sinus.
1.2 Cavernous sinus meningioma
1.3 Schwannoma
- The most common schwannoma to involve the cavernous sinus is a trigeminal schwannoma.
1.4 Metastases

2 Carotid-cavernous fistula (CCF)
- CCF is the most common traumatic AV fistula. It can occur following closed head injury or basal skull fracture.

- CCF is a direct communication between the intracavernous portion of the carotid artery and the venous cavernous sinus.
- Clinical presentation consists of:
  - pulsating exophthalmos
  - orbital bruits
  - ophthalmoparesis
  - conjunctival congestion/injection
- Carotid angiography is the investigation of choice.

3 Infections and inflammation of the cavernous sinus
  - Osteomyelitis can be a lethal complication of immunocompromised states, diabetes, mastoiditis, and paranasal sinus infections.

4 Others
  - Aneurysm of cavernous portion of internal carotid artery
  - Lymphoma
  - Chordoma
  - Lipoma

Clival masses

- The clivus is the part of the sphenoid bone forming the central portion of the base of the skull. In adults, the normal clivus consists of low- and high-intensity portions mixed in various proportions on T1W images.
- Enhancement of normal clival marrow sometimes occurs following contrast administration. However, it is usually mild and more common in young children (occasionally with marked enhancement).
- Chordoma and metastases represent the most common causes of destructive clival masses.

1 **Chordoma**
  - Chordomas are generally histologically benign and slow growing. However, there are more invasive types that tend to invade aggressively into the skull base and occasionally metastasize.
  - Presenting symptoms are usually cranial nerve palsies (most common oculomotor palsy, then CN VI, VII, VIII), as they tend to invade the skull base and cavernous sinus.
  - The tumors are usually bright on T2W images, with minimal enhancement, often associated with calcification.

2 **Metastases**
  - Any tumors that can metastasize to anterior and central skull base can also involve the clivus, usually from head and neck malignancies.

3 Nasopharyngeal carcinoma

- Squamous cell carcinoma accounts for 80% of nasopharyngeal tumors.
- It tends to spread directly into the skull base, as well as along muscles and their tendinous insertions. It can also extend intracranially along neural and vascular bundles via osseous foramina.

4 Chondrosarcoma – very rare tumor

Empty sella syndrome

- The sella region is an anatomically complex area composed of the bony sella turcica, pituitary gland, and adjacent structures (including optic nerves, chiasm, infundibulum, hypothalamus). It is bounded laterally by the cavernous sinus. The sphenoid sinus lies directly below the sella.
- The term 'empty sella' is probably a misnomer. It is a common anatomic variant in which the sella is partially filled with CSF. The infundibular stalk follows its normal course and inserts in the midline of the pituitary gland. The gland itself is thinned and flattened against the bony floor.
- Differential diagnosis of 'empty sella' on MRI should include cystic tumor and large herniated third ventricle or displaced infundibulum.

1 Primary empty sella syndrome
  - 10% incidence in adult populations with female predominance.
  - Patients are usually asymptomatic with no endocrine abnormalities. However, there is an increased risk of CSF rhinorrhea.
  - Probable causes include pituitary enlargement followed by regression during pregnancy, involution of a pituitary tumor, or related to congenital weakness of diaphragma sella.
2 Secondary (acquired) empty sella syndrome
  - Patients usually have visual impairment, headache, endocrine disturbances, and symptoms related to the original cause.
  - Common causes include postoperative change and pituitary gland infarction/ necrosis in pregnancy (Sheehan syndrome), and result in anterior pituitary hormone deficiency.

Pituitary stalk lesions

- Pituitary stalk tapers smoothly as it courses inferiorly from its hypothalamic origin to pituitary insertion. The normal stalk is 2–3.5 mm wide.
- Because it lacks a blood-brain barrier, the infundibulum normally enhances strongly and homogeneously following contrast administration.
- Increase in stalk size and contour alteration from its normal symmetric tapering shape are abnormal.

1 **Langerhan cell histiocytosis**
 - More commonly occurs in children, who present with diabetes insipidus.
 - MRI may show absent posterior pituitary 'bright spot', and a thickened, enhancing infundibular stalk with or without hypothalamic mass.

2 **Sarcoidosis**
 - More common in adults.
 - Neurosarcoidosis is relatively rare, affecting only 5% of all sarcoidosis cases.
 - Common locations for neurosarcoidosis include meninges, cranial nerves, hypothalamus, pituitary stalk, and pituitary gland.

3 **Tumors**
 - Germinoma is common in children.
 - Lymphoma and metastases are more common in adults.
 - Primary tumors of the infundibulum are very rare, including glioma (infundibuloma) and granular cell tumor (choristoma).

4 Others
 - Meningitis

Sellar mass

- MRI is the imaging modality of choice for a suspected sellar mass; pre- and post-gadolinium enhanced T1 in coronal and sagittal planes (thickness < 3 mm) with T2 and fat suppression sequences.
- Pituitary macroadenoma is the most likely primary sellar mass.
- However, always consider alternative etiologies, apart from pituitary tumor.

1 Neoplasms
  1.1 **Pituitary adenoma**
   - The most common sellar mass (micro defined as <10 mm; macro >10 mm).
   - Chromophobe adenoma is the most common pituitary tumor. There is frequent extension outside the sella. It is seldom hormone-producing.
   - Intrasellar tumors (microadenomas) are more likely to be hormone-producing.
   - Typical MRI features for macroadenomas are sellar enlargement, erosion, cavernous sinus invasion, and lobulated margins.
  1.2 Meningioma
   - 10–15% of meningiomas occur in the parasellar region.
   - An additional 20% arise from the sphenoidal ridge.
   - Meningiomas may be distinguished from pituitary adenomas by their suprasellar epicenter and broad dural base.
  1.3 Craniopharyngioma

- Usually arise from the suprasellar region but 50% extend to involve the sella.

1.4 Germ cell tumors
  - The majority are germinomas.
  - Usually centered in the suprasellar region but may arise from the sella.

1.5 Metastasis
  - Most commonly arising from a breast or bronchogenic primary.
  - Only 1% of patients with sellar mass.
  - Rarely becomes symptomatic (5–15%).
  - 'Dumb-bell' morphology on MRI.

2 Non-neoplastic lesions

2.1 **Rathke cleft cyst**
  - Most sellar epithelial cysts are remnants of derivatives of the Rathke cleft and arise in the region of the pars intermedia.
  - Usually asymptomatic and found in 13–22% at autopsy.

2.2 Enlarging arachnoid cysts
  - Indistinguishable from Rathke cleft cyst.

2.3 Lymphocytic hypophysitis
  - Inflammatory disorder of the pituitary gland, which is probably autoimmune in origin.

2.4 Granulomatous hypophysitis
  - Accounts for 1% of sellar masses.
  - Could be fungal, tuberculosis, sarcoidosis, Wegener granulomatosis, etc.

2.5 *Pituitary abscess*
  - Usually primary, but one-third are secondary from an existing adenoma surgical intervention.
  - Intrasellar extension of Gram-positive bacteria from the sphenoid sinus is the usual source of infection.

2.6 *Pituitary apoplexy*: actually a clinical syndrome, not specifically an imaging finding.
  - Acute pituitary vascular complication: usually hemorrhage, infarction, necrosis – acutely visualized radiographically as sellar mass.
  - Syndrome characterized by:
    - sudden, severe headache
    - nausea, vomiting, elevated ICP due to hydrocephalus
    - diplopia, oculomotor palsies
    - rapidly progressive visual loss, bitemporal hemianopsia
    - endocrine dysfunction
  - Multiple underlying associated diagnoses
    - adenoma: with hemorrhage or infarction
    - pregnancy: sometimes referred to as Sheehan syndrome

      ▫ trauma: vascular compromise with infarction of anterior lobe
      ▫ hypertension
      ▫ coagulopathy
      ▫ iatrogenic: bromocriptine therapy, post-LP, post-cerebral angiography, post-radiation

2.7 Others
    ▪ Histiocytic infiltration (very rare)
    ▪ Aneurysms
    ▪ Pituitary hyperplasia and hyperemia

(Ref: Connor S.E.J., Penney C.C. MRI in the differential diagnosis of a sellar mass. *Clin Radiol* 2003; 58: 20–31.)

Cranial intra-axial pathology

Cerebral hemispheres (cortex and white matter)

Thick and enhancing dura

Causes:
1 **Any infectious or inflammatory process involving leptomeninges**
2 **Subacute subarachnoid hemorrhage**
3 Leptomeningeal carcinomatosis
4 Intracranial hypotension
   • Most likely due to compensatory venous engorgement within the dura.

Selective cerebral atrophy and neurological conditions

- Volume loss in the cortex with secondary enlargement of adjacent sulci and cisterns can occur with aging. However, patients with primary neurodegenerative disorders usually have more marked sulcal enlargement. In addition, selective focal atrophy can occur with each specific disorder, correlating with the deficits seen.
- MRI is usually the preferred initial neuroimaging in patients suspected with neurodegenerative conditions. In addition to excluding the possibility of other treatable conditions, findings of selective cerebral atrophy may give a clue to the differential diagnosis. However, neuroimaging findings alone cannot replace a thorough history and physical examination.

Disorders	Imaging findings	Clinical features
Dementia of Alzheimer disease	Parietotemporal atrophy Hippocampal atrophy Increased hippocampal-choroidal fissure size	Speech and olfaction affected early Severe memory loss
Multi-infarct or vascular dementia	White matter and deep gray lacune Central pontine infarct	Stuttering course with discrete events Subcortical dementias
Pick disease	Marked frontal atrophy and mild temporal involvement	Personality change Disinhibition Abulia, apathy
Progressive supranuclear palsy (PSP)	Midbrain, collicular atrophy	Slow vertical saccades Ophthalmoparesis Parkinsonism with early postural instability
Corticobasal ganglionic degeneration (CBGD)	Diffuse cerebral atrophy, but parietal atrophy may be more involved	Apraxia Alien hand syndrome Asymmetrical Parkinsonism
Frontotemporal dementia (FTD)	Frontotemporal atrophy	Personality change Disinhibition May be associated with Parkinsonism Marked memory loss
Creutzfeldt-Jakob disease (CJD)	Frontal atrophy Abnormal intensity in basal ganglia	Rapidly progressive dementia Rigidity Myoclonus
Huntington disease (HD)	Caudate atrophy Diffuse cerebral atrophy	Generalized chorea Motor impersistence Neuropsychiatric symptoms Cognitive impairment

Corpus callosal lesions

- When there is a lesion involving the corpus callosum, glioblastoma and lymphoma should be considered high up in the differential diagnosis.
- Because of the compact nature of white matter fibers in corpus callosum, it is uncommon to see edema spread across this structure. In addition, blood supply is bilateral via anterior cerebral arteries. Therefore, infarcts involving the corpus callosum are very rare.
- Radiation injuries usually spare the corpus callosum.

1 Neoplastic lesions
   - Common tumors involving the corpus callosum include:
     - **Glioblastoma**
     - **Lymphoma**
     - Less commonly, metastasis
2 White matter lesions
   - **Multiple sclerosis**
   - Progressive multifocal leukoencephalopathy (PML)
   - Adrenoleukodystrophy (ALD)
   - Acute Marchiafava-Bignami disease
3 Acute shearing injuries
   - Referred to as diffuse axonal injury.
   - There is a propensity for shearing injuries in this location because of its relative fixed location spanning the interhemispheric fissure.

Multiple white matter lesions

- Multiple white matter lesions can be a normal finding. The importance is the character of the lesions and location, in conjunction with the clinical history. Most neurologists confront this problem when patients are referred with the possible diagnosis of multiple sclerosis. Do these lesions represent MS plaques?

1 **Multiple sclerosis**
   - **Characteristic features are:**
     - Ovoid
     - Peri-callosal locations
     - Periventricular locations
     - Perpendicular to the corpus callosum, Dawson fingers
     - Infratentorial lesions including brainstem, cerebellum, and spinal cord
     - At least some lesions >6 mm
   - Acute lesions (not necessarily symptomatic) may enhance with gadolinium.
2 **Ischemic white matter disease**, seen with chronic hypertension
   - Lacks the above features.
   - Further distinguishing it from MS, ischemic white matter disease is often associated with basal ganglia lacunes, and does not typically involve the corpus callosum or subcortical U-fibers.
   - Once it involves more than 25% of the white matter, it is called Binswanger disease.
3 **Could be normal, age-related white matter changes?**
   - They increase with age, +/- hypertension.

- Distinguished from MS in that these changes are generally NOT periventricular, infratentorial, or >6 mm in size.
4 Inflammation
    4.1 Infectious, e.g. Lyme disease, JC virus, Whipple disease.
    4.2 Non-infectious:
- Vasculitides, e.g. SLE, PAN, Sjögren syndrome: greater tendency to be in peripheral white matter than periventricular; also may have cortical involvement and evidence of arterial distribution infarction.
- Radiation-induced.
- Amyloid angiopathy.
5 Leukoencephalopathy
    5.1 Inherited (all rare, but have been known to occur on board examinations)
- Metachromatic leukodystrophy (MLD), most common in this group: diffuse white matter involvement, U-fibers spared, no contrast enhancement.
- Adrenoleukodystrophy (ALD): common patterns involve white matter in both occipital lobes and the splenium of the corpus callosum.
- Adrenomyeloneuropathy: like ALD, above, but with prominent spinal cord involvement.
- Alexander disease: macrocephaly, demyelination starts frontally.
- Canavan disease: macrocephaly, diffuse demyelination including U-fibers, also involvement of globus pallidus and thalamus.
    5.2 Acquired
- Acute disseminated encephalomyelitis (ADEM)

- MS and ADEM may be confused!!! Clues for differentiating include that ADEM is a monophasic type illness, unlike MS, which is usually relapsing-remitting. This can cause difficulties in distinguishing ADEM from a first attack of MS.
- In ADEM, clinical characteristics include acute fever, headache, more often in children, and occurrence following vaccination or infection.
- In ADEM, lesions are:
  - large and confluent
  - fewer in number than MS
  - variable in affecting the brainstem or cerebellum.

- Progressive multifocal leukoencephalopathy (PML): lesions in PML do not enhance.
- Drugs, e.g. cocaine, amphetamine.
6 *Embolism*: may have multiple lesions, potentially mimicking MS, but:

- Tend to occur at gray-white junction.
- Cause arterial branch occlusions with wedge-shaped infarctions.
- May be accompanied by small intralesional hemorrhages.

7 Metastases: features include
- Surrounding edema
- Irregular border
- May co-exist with hemorrhage.

8 Migraine
- Appears more often in peripheral rather than in periventricular white matter.
  - May see lesions involving cortex in complicated migraine.

Reversible posterior leukoencephalopathy syndrome (RPLS)

- MRI and CT imaging show edema located in the occipital, parietal lobes, and other posterior regions – these findings are seen in 85% of patients studied within 72 hours after the onset of symptoms.
- It is not certain why the posterior region is particularly affected. Possibly related to lack of sympathetic innervation in vertebrobasilar system.

Causes:

1 **Malignant hypertension**
- Renal failure and eclampsia can be contributory causes.

2 Toxins including chemotherapeutic and immunosuppressive agents
- Cyclosporine
- Methotrexate
- Cisplatin

3 Occipital lobe seizures

4 Others
- HIV disease
- Metabolic derangements including hypercalcemia

Other regions

Calcification of the basal ganglia

- Calcification of the basal ganglia is a frequent finding in multiple disorders and represents a heterogeneous syndrome rather than a specific disease entity.
- Calcification of the basal ganglia has been observed in patients with various neurological symptoms or signs without clear etiology, as either a familial or a sporadic condition. Calcifications can also involve subcortical frontal, parietal lobes or cerebellum. Age at disease onset is not uniform.

1 **Endocrine disorders**
- Any type of parathyroid disorders can result in basal ganglia calcifications including primary hypoparathyroidism, hyperparathyroidism, pseudohypoparathyroidism, and pseudopseudohypoparathyroidism.
- Hypothyroidism

2 **Intracranial infections**
- **TORCH** congenital infections (**TO**xoplasmosis, **R**ubella, **C**ytomegalovirus and **H**erpes simplex virus)
- Viral encephalitis
- Acquired immunodeficiency syndrome
- Cysticercosis

3 Perinatal hypoxia/ischemic encephalopathy

4 Familial idiopathic symmetric basal ganglia calcification

5 Genetic and metabolic disorders: usually rare conditions
- Tuberous sclerosis
- Pantothenate kinase-associated neurodegeneration
- Mitochondrial cytopathies
- Neurofibromatosis
- Phenylketonuria
- Albright syndrome
- Cockayne syndrome

6 Others
- Carbon monoxide intoxication: globus pallidus lesions
- Lead intoxication
- Radiation therapy
- Intrathecal methotrexate

Hyperintense basal ganglia lesions on T1WI

- The basal ganglia is a group of deep gray matter nuclei lying between the insula and midline. It comprises different structures including globus pallidus, putamen, caudate, subthalamic nucleus, and substantia nigra.
- The globus pallidus (GP) is the medial gray matter structure, lateral to the genu of the internal capsule. Lateral to the GP is the putamen. The caudate nucleus head lies just lateral to the frontal horns of the lateral ventricle and anterior to the GP. The tail of caudate nucleus ends near the amygdala.
- Various materials or tissues may result in hyperintense signal on T1WI, including fat, free methemoglobin, calcification, proteinaceous fluid, melanin, and gadolinium. These materials, if present in the basal ganglia, may cause the hyperintensity seen on T1WI.

1 **Hemorrhage**
   - The basal ganglia is the most common location for hypertensive intracranial hemorrhage.
   - In early subacute hemorrhage, the blood usually causes a high signal on T1WI and a low signal on T2WI.
   - In late subacute hemorrhage, there are hyperintense signals on both T1WI and T2WI.
2 Calcification
   - The causes may be idiopathic or related to metabolic disorders (see Calcification of the basal ganglia, pp. 425–6).
3 Metabolic disorders
   - 3.1 Parathyroid disorders
     - Hyperparathyroidism
     - Hypoparathyroidism
     - Pseudohypoparathyroidism
     - Pseudopseudohypoparathyroidism
   - 3.2 Chronic hyperalimentation therapy
   - 3.3 Hepatic encephalopathy
   - 3.4 Kernicterus
4 Neurodegenerative disorders
   - 4.1 Pantothenate kinase-associated neurodegeneration (Hallervorden-Spatz syndrome)
     - Autosomal recessive disorder, associated with abnormal involuntary movements, spasticity, and progressive dementia.
     - Characteristic accumulation of iron-containing compounds is present in the globus pallidus, red nuclei, and substantia nigra pathologically. This is seen as high signal intensity on T1WI and low intensity on T2WI. Additionally, cortical atrophy is often present.
5 Intoxication
   - 5.1 Carbon monoxide-bilateral GP lesions
   - 5.2 Manganese: bilateral GP hyperintensity
   - 5.3 Lead: late basal ganglia calcification
6 Neurofibromatosis type 1
7 Hyperglycemia: rarely associated with hemichorea or hemiballismus and high T1WI signal on MRI.

Choroid plexus lesions

   - Lesions in the choroid plexus often cause hydrocephalus and papilledema, due to overproduction of CSF (4–5 times the normal amount) or obstruction from tumor.

- Choroid plexus papilloma is the most common lesion in this location, comprising 3% of intracranial tumors in children less than 5 years old. In children, the papillomas tend to locate at the trigone and/or atria of the lateral ventricles, but in adults a fourth ventricular location is more common.

1 **Neoplastic lesions**: most common
   1.1 **Choroid plexus papilloma**: most common
      - 25% of lesions calcified.
      - The tumor is typically hyperdense on unenhanced CT imaging, with a frond-like appearance. It is of low signal on T1W and mixed intensity on T2W. It enhances dramatically with a heterogeneous appearance.
   1.2 Choroid plexus carcinoma
      - Much less common, but may be difficult to differentiate it from papilloma.
      - They are usually seen in the lateral ventricles, with a high tendency to disseminate along the CSF.
   1.3 Others, including meningioma or hemangioma
2 Congenital lesions
   2.1 Xanthogranuloma: fat density on imaging, located near the glomus of the trigone.
   2.2 Ependymal cysts.
3 Infections including cysticercosis, infectious cysts

Hydrocephalus vs. atrophy

- The differentiation between these two conditions is critically important, since the etiology, treatment, and prognosis are vastly different.
- Hydrocephalus reflects an expansion of the ventricular system from increased ventricular pressure, which is in most cases caused by abnormal CSF hydrostatic mechanics. Atrophy refers to the loss of brain tissue.
- Hydrocephalus is generally caused by overproduction of CSF, obstruction of CSF at the ventricular outlet level, or obstruction at the arachnoid villi leading to poor resorption of CSF.
- While there are usually treatments available for hydrocephalus, there is generally no effective treatment for atrophy. However, the appearance of increased CSF spaces suggesting atrophy occurs reversibly in several settings, including corticosteroid use, valproic acid use, dehydration, and alcoholism.
- Long-standing hydrocephalus can simulate atrophy on occasions, and the presence of hydrocephalus does not preclude concomitant atrophy.

Features	Hydrocephalus	Atrophy
Temporal horn	Enlarged	Normal except in Alzheimer disease
3rd ventricle	Convex	Concave
4th ventricle	Normal or enlarged	Normal except in cerebellar atrophy
Ventricular angle of frontal horn on axial scan	More acute	More obtuse
Corpus callosum	Thin, distended, rounded elevation with increased distance between corpus callosum and the fornix	Normal or atrophied. Normal distance between corpus callosum and the fornix
Transependymal CSF flow	Present acutely	Absent
Sulci	Flattened	Enlarged out of proportion to age
Flow void in aqueduct	Accentuated in normal-pressure hydrocephalus	Normal
Choroidal-hippocampal fissures	Normal to mildly enlarged	Markedly enlarged in Alzheimer disease
Mamillopontine distance	< 1 cm	> 1 cm

Pineal region masses

- The pineal region is an area that normally lies in the depression between the superior colliculi. The ventral lamina of the pineal stalk is continuous with the posterior commissure and the dorsal lamina with the habenula commissure. At its proximal ends, it forms the pineal recess of the third ventricle.
- The manifestation of pineal region masses depends on their location close to many critical structures; the adqueduct, the tectal plate, the midbrain, the vein of Galen. The pineal gland may regulate human response to diurnal daylight rhythms. Therefore, pineal region masses can cause hydrocephalus (by aqueductal obstruction), precocious puberty, and paresis of upward gaze (part of Parinaud syndrome).
- Pineal region tumors can best be differentiated on the basis of the sex of the patient.

1 In male patients
  1.1 **Germinoma**
     - The most common pineal tumor accounting for 40% of pineal region masses and 2/3 of pineal germ cell tumors.
     - **Nearly exclusively in males.**
     - It is a tumor of young adulthood, rarely seen in patients older than 30 years.

- The characteristic appearance is of a hyperdense mass on CT imaging, which enhances markedly with calcification occurring in 80% of cases.
- Germinomas are very radiosensitive and also respond well to chemotherapy. Serum marker is placental alkaline phosphatase.

1.2 Teratoma
- Teratoma may have fat, bone, calcification, cyst, or sebaceum.
- Secretes β-HCG or α-FP.

1.3 Embryonal cell carcinoma and endodermal sinus tumors

1.4 Glioma: occurring equally in males and females
- Usually located in tectal plate or causes hydrocephalus.

1.5 Pinealcytoma and pinealblastoma (see below)

2 In female patients

2.1 Pinealcytoma and pinealblastoma
- Accounting for 15% of pineal region masses.
- Occurs equally in males and females.
- Pinealblastoma occurs in a younger age group and is classified as PNET, but both have identical imaging appearances.
- Characteristically appears hyperdense on unenhanced CT and intermediate in signal intensity on T2WI. They enhance vividly.
- Both have high rates of subarachnoid seeding.

2.2 Glioma (see above)

Central pontine myelinolysis (CPM)

- Demyelinating disorder that affects the brainstem white matter, mostly central pons and occasionally cerebral hemispheres (then called 'extrapontine myelinolysis').
- Usually presents with a subacute progressive quadriparesis with lower cranial nerve involvement.
- Prognosis is poor. However, survival and recovery is possible.

Etiology:
1 **Rapid correction of hyponatremia:**
   - **Important cause but not the only etiology of CPM.**
   - **CPM can develop despite the absence of hyponatremia.**
2 Alcoholics with Wernicke encephalopathy
3 Liver transplants
4 Severe burns
5 Malnutrition
6 Severe electrolyte abnormalities, especially hypophosphatemia

Cerebellar atrophy/degeneration

- Cerebellar atrophy is not an uncommon finding on MRI scans. However, it is often difficult to decide whether the degree of cerebellar atrophy is significant. Age-related cerebellar atrophy is relatively common, although it is usually mild.
- The most dorsomedial vermian lobules, including declive, folium, and tuber, are commonly affected.
- Certain parts of cerebellum (e.g. vermian versus hemispheric), as well as surrounding structures that are affected, may give clues to an underlying etiology.

1 Toxic substances
   1.1 **Alcohol abuse**
      ■ **Probably the most common cause of cerebellar atrophy.**
      ■ The vermis is more commonly involved than other parts of the brain, although the whole cerebellum/cerebrum are affected.
   1.2 Long-term use of medications
      ■ Chronic phenytoin or phenobarbital may produce cerebellar atrophy.
      ■ Clinical signs are sometimes evident, including nystagmus, ataxia, and slurred speech.
2 Hereditary/neurodegenerative conditions
   2.1 Olivopontocerebellar atrophy
      ■ Causing cerebellar and brainstem atrophy.
      ■ Pons and inferior olives are small, as are the cerebellar peduncles.
   2.2 Hereditary ataxia
      ■ Different types of autosomal dominant cerebellar ataxia (ADCA) are associated with marked cerebellar atrophy.
      ■ Superior vermis usually affected, more than the rest of the cerebellum.
   2.3 Friedreich ataxia (FRDA)
      ■ Probably the most common inherited ataxia.
      ■ Autosomal recessive condition, associated with ataxia, kyphoscoliosis, dysarthria, cardiomyopathy, and peripheral neuropathy.
      ■ MRI typically shows atrophy of cervicomedullary junction and upper part of cervical cord. Cerebellar atrophy can also be seen, but is milder and less common.
   2.4 Other rare inherited conditions
      ■ Ataxia-telangiectasia
      ■ Ataxic form of Creutzfeldt-Jakob disease

3 Paraneoplastic cerebellar degeneration
  ◆ Cerebellar degeneration precedes the discovery of primary tumor in 60% of
    cases.
  ◆ Exact mechanism unclear, but probably related to autoantibodies (e.g. anti-
    Yo) from ovarian, gastrointestinal, breast, lung tumors.
4 Others
  ◆ Infections, e.g. rubella, cytomegalovirus
  ◆ Post-radiation changes
  ◆ Vertebrobasilar insufficiency

Spinal pathology

Enlarged spinal cord

- MRI has had a great impact on the diagnosis of spinal disorders.
- Enlarged spinal cord is a common radiological finding on spinal MR
  imaging and usually reminds clinicians to suspect tumors. However, not
  all enlarged cords are due to neoplasms. Inflammatory and demyelinating
  disorders may enlarge the spinal cord, especially in young patients.

1 **Spinal cord tumors**
  ◆ Specific diagnosis of tumors is not usually possible on MR imaging. Rather, it
    identifies that the cord is abnormal.
  ◆ Most common cause of spinal cord enlargement in the elderly.
    1.1 **Ependymoma**
      ▪ 50–60% of all spinal cord tumors.
      ▪ Associated with syringomyelia, cysts, subclinical repeated hemorrhag-
        es, neurofibromatosis type 2.
      ▪ Lesions are focal, well-circumscribed, histologically benign, and can be
        resectable, although they tend to recur.
    1.2 Astrocytoma
      ▪ 30–40% of all spinal cord tumors.
      ▪ Lesions are large, malignant, infiltrating, and involving the full diameter
        of the spinal cord, with the thoracic and cervical regions more often af-
        fected. They are not usually resectable.
    1.3 Hemangioblastoma
      ▪ Hemangioblastomas may involve cervical and thoracic spinal cord, and
        are composed of a dense network of capillary and sinus channels.
      ▪ 1/3 of cases are associated with von Hippel-Lindau disease.

2 **Demyelination/inflammation**
- Spinal cord lesions are common in multiple sclerosis (MS). This diagnosis should be considered in young patients whose MR reveals an enlarged cord without or with enhancement and high intensity on T2W and PDW images.
- 20% of patients with spinal cord MS may have a normal brain MR. However, the presence of brain lesions would further support the diagnosis of MS.
- Other causes include sarcoidosis and systemic lupus erythematosus.

3 Vascular lesions

   3.1 Acute infarction
- Preferentially affecting thoracic or thoracolumbar regions because of tenuous blood supply.
- This possibility should be considered in patients with acute onset of spinal cord, conus medullaris, and cauda equina symptoms with what appears to be an enlarged cord or tumor-like lesion on MRI.
- Commonly associated with descending aorta problems (artery of Adamkiewicz) during aortic surgery, dissecting aneurysm, atheroma, pregnancy, or sickle cell disease.

   3.2 Arteriovenous malformations
- MR imaging usually demonstrates a high signal on T2W images in the cord with little enhancement. The veins along the posterior surface of the cord may be prominent and enhanced. The cord itself may or may not be enlarged.

   3.3 Cavernous angioma – rare

4 Others
- Infections
- Syringohydromyelia
- Necrotizing myelopathy

Sacral masses or lesions

- The most common cause of sacral mass by far is tumor. The presence of a destructive lesion as well as internal ossification favors the diagnosis of aggressive, malignant tumors.

1 **Metastatic tumors**
- Commonly from breast, prostate, kidney and colon.

2 **Sacrococcygeal teratoma**
- Developmental in origin.
- Most common presacral mass in children.
- Histology ranges from mature teratomas to anaplastic carcinoma.

3 **Sacral chordoma**
  - Common locations of chordoma include sacrococcygeal region (50%), clivus, and C1–2.
  - Accounts for 40% of all sacral tumors.
  - The tumor is destructive, lytic, and is often associated with calcification.
  - Differential diagnosis includes chondrosarcoma.
4 Multiple myeloma
  - The rate of sacral involvement by plasmacytoma or multiple myeloma is 2–4%.
  - Solitary osseous plasmacytomas usually have longer survival periods following radiation therapy.
5 Others
  - Giant cell tumor (most common benign sacral tumor)
  - Osteomyelitis
  - Neurofibroma
  - Aneurysmal bone cyst

Specific diseases/differentials

Chiari malformations

- Chiari malformation is a disorder of primary neurulation, mostly neural tube closure defects and early CNS anomalies, typically occurring around 3–4 weeks' gestation.
- The spectrum of congenital anomalies labeled the Chiari malformations spans a wide range. Symptomatic patients with Chiari malformations are seen with ataxia, vertical nystagmus, headache, cranial nerve VI through XII abnormalities, and signs of syringomyelia.
- The different features of Chiari I and II are discussed in the table below. Chiari III malformations are associated with herniation of posterior fossa contents into an occipital or high cervical encephalocele with other features of Chiari II malformations. Chiari IV malformations are very rare and are associated with severe hypoplastic cerebellum, small brainstem, and large posterior fossa CSF spaces.

Features	Chiari I malformations	Chiari II malformations
Major abnormalities	Peg-like, pointed tonsils displaced into upper cervical canal, >5 mm below foramen magnum	Cerebellar tonsils, vermis, fourth ventricle, and brainstem are herniated through the foramen magnum, and the egress fourth ventricle is obstructed

Features	Chiari I malformations	Chiari II malformations
Associated anomalies		
Skull & dura	Normal	• Calvarial defects • Small posterior fossa • Fenestrated falx • Gaping foramen magnum
Brain	Normal	• Inferiorly displaced vermis • Medullary kink • Beaked tectum • Interdigitated gyri • Cerebellum creeps around brainstem
Ventricles	• Mild to moderate hydrocephalus (20–25%)	• Hydrocephalus (90%) • Elongated, tube-like fourth ventricle • Colpocephaly, scalloped, pointed walls of lateral ventricles
Spinal cord	• Syringomyelia (30–60%)	• **Myelomeningocele (nearly 100%)** • Syringohydromyelia (50–90%) • Diastematomyelia • Segmentation anomalies
Skeletal anomalies	• Basilar invagination (25–50%) • Klippel-Feil syndrome (5–10%) • Atlanto-occipital assimilation	None

Failed back syndrome

- Failed back syndrome refers to failure to improve or recurrence of low back pain in patients following lumbar disc surgery.
- The incidence of this syndrome varies between 5 and 40%.
- The diagnosis of scar versus residual/recurrent disc is critically important as the treatment is different. Surgery is not indicated for scar, but could be indicated if the disc causes radiculopathy.
- MRI with gadolinium enhancement is useful in this differentiation as diffuse enhancement occurs in the scar but not the disc.

1 Soft-tissue causes
    1.1 **Recurrent or residual disc herniation**
       • No enhancement on early T1W images.
    1.2 **Epidural fibrosis** (scarring)
       • Heterogeneous enhancement on early T1W images.
    1.3 Postoperative complications
       • Infections

- Hemorrhage
  - 1.4 Adhesive arachnoiditis
    - Thickened, irregular clumped nerve roots
2 Osseous causes (less common)
  - Central canal stenosis
  - Foramina stenosis
  - Spondylolisthesis
3 Iatrogenic causes
  - Direct nerve injury during surgery
  - Surgery at wrong level

Intracranial hemorrhage

Hypertensive hemorrhage vs. amyloid angiopathy

- Hypertension is the presumed cause of nontraumatic intraparenchymal hemorrhage in 70–90% of cases. The location of hypertensive hemorrhage varies.
- Cerebral amyloid angiopathy (CAA) results from deposition of amyloid in the media and adventitia of small and medium-sized vessels of the superficial layers of the cerebral cortex and leptomeninges, usually with sparing of the deep gray nuclei.
- CAA increases with advancing age and may be the most common cause of recurrent intracranial hemorrhage in elderly normotensive patients.

Neuroradiological features	Hypertensive hemorrhage	Hemorrhage from cerebral amyloid angiopathy
Common	Most common cause of intracranial hemorrhage (overall)	Less common, but probably the most common cause of recurrent hemorrhage in the elderly (10%)
Locations	• 60%: basal ganglia (esp. putamen), thalamus • 10–15%: brainstem (esp. pons) • 5–10%: cerebellum • 10–50%: can be lobar	• Usually lobar, involving frontal and parietal lobes • Rarely in the cerebellum, white matter, basal ganglia, or brainstem
Mutiple locations	Usually solitary	Clasically multiple
Pathogenesis	Unclear May be related to Charcot-Bouchard aneurysms (conflicting evidence!)	Amyloid depositions probably cause microaneurysms and fibrinoid degeneration. Loss of vessel elasticity due to amyloid deposits.

Neuroradiological features	Hypertensive hemorrhage	Hemorrhage from cerebral amyloid angiopathy
Neuroimaging findings	Follow hemorrhagic evolution pattern, (see hemorrhagic evolution for details)	Multiple areas of hemorrhages Gradient-echo imaging with emphasis on T2 effects are useful
Associations	• Coronary artery disease • Peripheral vascular disease	• Alzheimer disease (30–40%) • Down syndrome • Dementia pugilistica • Leukoencephalopathy • Spongiform encephalopathy (Not associated with systemic amyloidosis)

Non-neoplastic vs. neoplastic hemorrhage

- Distinguishing hemorrhagic intracranial neoplasms from non-neoplastic hematomas can be difficult, since there is considerable overlap between neuroimaging findings.
- The following are helpful differentiating features, although they should not be considered as pathognomonic for either etiology.
- In some cases where there is radiographic and clinical uncertainty, biopsy of lesions or close follow-up neuroimaging may be required.

Neuroradiological features	Neoplastic hemorrhage	Non-neoplastic hemorrhage
Edema	Prominent	Less prominent
Multiple lesions	Usually solitary, unless metastases	Supportive of vascular malformation in appropriate clinical setting
Hemosiderin rim	Incomplete	Usually complete
Heterogeneity	Heterogeneous and complex	More homogeneous
Hemorrhagic evolution	Delayed	Not delayed
Contrast enhancement	Enhancement in non-hemorrhagic areas	Varies depending on the nature of the lesion

Common intracranial tumors with hemorrhage

- The etiology of tumor-induced hemorrhage is unclear. However, many factors appear to contribute, including presence of a high-grade tumor, histologic type, presence of neovascularization, rapid tumor growth with necrosis, plasminogen activators, and direct vascular invasion.

- The overall incidence is approximately 1 to 15%. Virtually any tumor in any location can bleed, although some tumors are more likely to bleed than others.
- In general, the more malignant astrocytomas bleed, as do vascular tumors and necrotic tumors. Low-grade astrocytomas, mesenchymal cysts, and slowly growing tumors are less likely to bleed.
- Primary CNS lymphomas in immunocompetent patients rarely have necrosis or hemorrhage, in contrast to primary CNS lymphomas in HIV-infected patients, which tend to bleed.

1 **Anaplastic astrocytoma and glioblastoma**
   - Common cause of unexplained intracranial hemorrhage in normotensive, non-demented elderly patients.
2 **Pituitary adenoma**
   - The most common non-glial hemorrhagic primary intracranial tumor.
   - Other non-glial tumors rarely bleed.
3 **Metastatic tumors**
   - Hemorrhage occurs in up to 15% of brain metastases.
   - Common tumors include renal cell carcinoma, choriocarcinoma, melanoma, brochogenic carcinoma, and thyroid carcinoma.
   - Typical MR findings of hemorrhage into metastatic foci are:
     - Marked heterogeneity
     - Blood degradation products of different ages
     - Fluid-fluid levels
     - Located at gray-white interface
4 Oligodendroglioma
   - The most common non-astrocytic gliomas associated with hemorrhage.
5 Primitive neuroectodermal tumors and teratomas
   - More likely in young children.
6 Ependymoma
   - Especially in the spinal cord, can cause repeated hemorrhages resulting in superficial siderosis.

- Unless the metastatic deposit is hemorrhagic, calcified, hyperproteinaceous, or highly cellular (where it would be hyperdense on noncontrast CT), most metastases are low density on unenhanced CT imaging.
- Hemorrhagic metastases are usually seen as areas of high signal intensity on T1W and T2W MRI with a relative absence of hemosiderin deposition.

> • Hemorrhagic metastases must be differentiated from occult cerebrovascular malformations or non-neoplastic hematomas. In hemorrhagic metastases, the edema, mass effect, and enhancement tend to be larger and more persistent than occult hemorrhagic lesions in malformations.

Hemorrhagic metastases to the brain

1 **Breast and bronchogenic carcinoma**: the most common tumors to cause hemorrhagic metastases.
2 Mnemonic '**MR CT**'
   - **M** for melanoma
   - **R** for renal cell carcinoma and retinoblastoma
   - **C** for choriocarcinoma
   - **T** for thyroid carcinoma

(Ref: Modified from *Neuroradiology: The requisites.*)

Intracranial cysts

> • Intracranial cysts can be found incidentally or as space-occupying lesions producing focal deficits, signs of increased intracranial pressure, or hydrocephalus.
> • The etiology varies, commonly being congenital, infection-related, or part of the tumors.

1 Congenital lesions
   1.1 **Arachnoid cyst**
      - The most common congenital cystic abnormality in the brain.
      - It is a benign condition and rarely produces symptoms.
      - Thought to be due to accumulation of CSF between the layers of arachnoid membrane.
      - Common locations include the middle cranial fossa, parasellar cisterns, and the subarachnoid space over the convexities.
      - On MRI, the most common appearance is that of an extra-axial mass, which has a signal intensity identical to CSF on all pulse sequences.
   1.2 **Colloid cyst**
      - It probably arises congenitally as a result of encystment of ependyma.
      - Usually located in the anterior portion of the third ventricle near the foramen of Monro.

- Positional headaches or hydrocephalus may be the presenting complaints in 30–40-year-old patients.
- The lesion is usually hyperdense on CT imaging because of the high protein content.

  1.3 Rathke cleft cyst

- Rathke cleft cyst is an embryologic remnant of Rathke pouch, the endoderm that ascends from the oral cavity to the sellar region to form the pituitary anterior lobe and pars intermedia.
- The cyst is usually found incidentally showing high or low signal intensity on T1WI and high signal intensity on T2WI with hypodensity on CT and does not enhance with contrast.

2 Tumoral cyst

  2.1 Pineal cyst

- Pineal region tumors can have cystic components, especially germ cell tumors.

  2.2 Dermoid and epidermoid cyst

- Epidermoids have a single medium, but dermoids have multiple media, such as fat, cystic fluid, and soft tissue.

  2.3 Intratumoral cyst, e.g. in cystic astrocytoma.

3 Infections

  3.1 Cysticercosis

- Endemic in parts of Latin America, Mexico, Asia, and Africa.
- The parasite is acquired by ingestion of insufficiently cooked pork, containing the encysted larvae. Infestation to the CNS produces seizures as the most common neurological manifestation.
- Classically, the plain skull X-ray shows calcification in the brain parenchyma of 1–2 mm in diameter, representing the scolex, surrounded by a calcified sphere.

  3.2 Hydatid cyst, from Echinococcus infection.

4 Others

  4.1 Cyst of the cavum septum pellucidum

  4.2 Cava interpositum and vergae

5 Pseudocyst

  5.1 Porencephaly

- Porencephaly refers to an area of focal encephalomalacia that communicates with the ventricular system, causing what appears to be a focal dilated ventricle.
- The causes include trauma, infection, and perinatal ischemia.

Lymphoma vs. toxoplasmosis in AIDS

- The most common type of lymphoma to affect the brain is diffuse histiocytic lymphoma (primary cerebral lymphoma). It is mostly non-Hodgkin type.
- The classic teaching used to be that lymphoma was one of the lesions that is typically hyperdense on noncontrast CT and enhances to moderate degree. Such generalizations are no longer valid, since AIDS-related lymphoma causes a variety of appearances. AIDS-related lymphoma tends to present with multiple, smaller lesions and shows marked (and ring) enhancement with gadolinium, compared to lymphoma in immunocompetent patients.
- Primary lymphoma of the brain is usually supratentorial and located in deep gray nuclei or periventricular white matter. Coating of the ventricles and spread across the corpus callosum is suggestive of lymphoma.
- Toxoplasmosis remains the important differential diagnosis, especially in AIDS patients with lesions in deep gray nuclei. When radiological differentiation is not possible, empirical treatment with pyrimethamine should be considered. Patients with toxoplasmosis usually respond rapidly to the treatment, while patients with lymphoma do not.

Features	Lymphoma	Toxoplasmosis
Patient's immune status	Both immunodeficient and immunocompetent	Usually occurs in only immunodeficient patients
Multiple lesions	81%	61%
Size of lesions	75% of lesions are 1–3 cm	52% of lesions are < 1 cm 36% of lesions are 1–3 cm
Lesion locations	Periventricular and deep gray matter lesions, subependymal and spread across the corpus callosum	Often in deep gray matter. Less likely to be periventricular, subependymal or in corpus callosum
Homogeneous CT enhancement	Yes, in approximately 70%	Yes, in approximately 70%
Hyperdensity on non-enhanced CT	30% of lesions	Unlikely unless hemorrhage present
Hemorrhage	Very rare	May occur
T2W MRI	50% isointense	All hyperintense

Ref: Modified from Dinas T.S. Primary CNS lymphoma versus toxoplasmosis in AIDS. *Radiology* 1991; 179: 823–828.

Ring enhancing lesions

- When there is enhancement, it suggests that the process is subacute or chronic. Slowly progressive conditions should not enhance.
- In addition, enhancement is at the rim because the central area generally lacks a good blood supply and is necrotic. The process is usually focal or multifocal and unlikely to be diffuse.

1 **Infectious causes**: usually suggest hematogenous spread.
   - Pyogenic brain abscess.
   - Toxoplasmosis, especially in HIV.
   - Tuberculosis.
   - Fungal infection.
2 **Neoplastic**: the rim is usually thick, irregular and nodular.
   - Metastatic tumor (hematogenous metastases), more common than primary brain tumor.
   - Primary brain tumor, e.g. glioblastoma, primary CNS lymphoma.
3 Infarction
4 Granulomatous process
5 Demyelination
6 Subacute hematoma (suggests 6 days to 6 weeks old)

PS: in HIV patients, it is sometimes difficult to differentiate clinically and radiologically between toxoplasmosis and primary CNS lymphoma. Helpful clues are a greater predilection for basal ganglia (subcortical gray matter) and more surrounding edema in toxoplasmosis and less so in lymphoma. Occasionally, empirical treatment with pyrimethamine is indicated in cases with unclear diagnosis.

Chapter 14
Spinal Cord Disorders

Signs and symptoms

Distinguishing spinal cord from peripheral nerve pathology

- Spinal cord pathology is suggested when there is a triad of symptoms:
  - Sensory level (the hallmark of spinal cord disease)
  - Distal, symmetric, spastic weakness
  - Bowel and bladder dysfunction

- Spinal cord lesions do not disturb cortical and brainstem functions. The presence of aphasia, visual impairment, swallowing, or cognitive disturbances suggest that the lesion is above the level of the foramen magnum. The exception is Horner syndrome, in which the sympathetic fibers travel as low as T1-T2. The loss of pain and temperature in the face suggests brainstem involvement.
- Not uncommonly, distinguishing between spinal cord and radicular/peripheral nerve lesions can be difficult, especially if the signs are incomplete. Acute or profound spinal cord lesions or 'spinal shock,' can also abolish all spinal myotactic reflexes. The information below provides useful clues in differential localization.

Sign/symptom	Spinal cord	Peripheral nerve
Sensory loss	Discernable level	Dermatomal or individual nerve distribution
Weakness	Present	Present
Upper motor neuron signs (hyperreflexia, spasticity, upgoing Babinski sign)	Present	Absent
Bowel and bladder function disturbances	Present	Absent
Back pain and/or point spinal tenderness	May be present	Absent
Denervation changes, including atrophy, fasciculations	Absent	Present
Superficial reflexes	May be absent	Unchanged

Differential diagnosis and symptoms by location in cord

- Neurological symptoms and signs are very useful in localizing a spinal cord lesion.
- Compression or injury to the spinal cord at different levels may result in the symptom combinations listed below.
- *Acute spinal cord injury may result in FLACCID paralysis due to SPINAL SHOCK.*
- Acute traumatic spinal cord injury should be treated with high-dose corticosteroids.
- Exact incidence of disorders by rostral-caudal spinal cord location is uncertain.

- Once spinal localization is suspected, neuroimaging is performed to confirm the diagnosis. This imaging is generally performed *as an emergency/urgently*, due to risk of permanent damage to injured cord.
- Major concerns regarding mortality/morbidity due to spinal cord lesions depend upon localization:
  - Respiratory depression may occur with craniocervical and cervical cord lesions.
  - Autonomic instability may occur with cord lesions at the mid-thoracic level or above.
  - Urinary retention may occur with any spinal cord lesion, particularly conus or cauda lesions.
  - Motor paralysis may occur with any spinal cord lesion, but the pattern of motor involvement is dependent upon localization.

1 Craniocervical junction
  - Upper motor neuron weakness in all four extremities.
  - Downbeat nystagmus, other brainstem signs.
  - Respiratory failure.
  - Occipital or upper cervical pain.
    1.1 **Atlanto-occipital or atlanto-axial instability**: may be more likely in patients having congenital craniocervical anomalies.
      1.1.1 *Acute trauma: cervical/odontoid fracture, basilar skull fracture, etc.*
      1.1.2 **Chronic degenerative arthritis**
    1.2 *Neoplasm/tumor*
      1.2.1 Intramedullary: brainstem/cervical astrocytoma, ependymoma
      1.2.2 Extramedullary: meningioma at foramen magnum, schwannoma
      1.2.3 Metastases: may be intra- or extramedullary
    1.3 *Vascular*: aneurysm, malformation, ectatic vessel, ischemia
    1.4 *Infection*: abscess, cyst, etc.
    1.5 Chiari I malformation
    1.6 Syringomyelia/syringobulbia: may be associated with Chiari I
    1.7 Basilar impression, other congenital craniocervical anomalies
    1.8 Demyelination/multiple sclerosis: associated with vertigo, ophthalmoplegia, ataxia, motor dysfunction
    1.9 Bony disease: Paget, etc.
2 Cervical cord
  - Neck pain
  - May have lower motor neuron weakness in upper extremities
  - Upper motor neuron weakness in lower extremities

- Sensory loss in arms
- Bowel/bladder dysfunction
- May have respiratory failure (upper cervical lesions)
- May have Horner syndrome (cervico-thoracic lesions)
    - 2.1 ***Acute trauma: cervical fracture, dislocation, cord concussion, cord transection***
    - 2.2 **Chronic degenerative arthritis and spinal stenosis**
    - 2.3 *Neoplasm*
        - 2.3.1 Extramedullary: neurofibroma, schwannoma, meningioma, etc.
        - 2.3.2 Intramedullary: astrocytoma, less common ependymoma.
        - 2.3.3 Metastases: may be intra- or extramedullary; lung, breast, prostate, kidney, myeloproliferative, melanoma. May include 'drop mets': metastases from intracranial tumors that spread via CSF.
    - 2.4 *Vascular*: infarction, vascular malformation, dural arteriovenous fistula, etc.
    - 2.5 *Infection*: tuberculosis (Pott disease), spinal epidural abscess, osteomyelitis, etc.
    - 2.6 *Transverse myelitis*: viral, lupus, idiopathic
    - 2.7 *Cervical disc herniation/extrusion*
    - 2.8 Congenital craniocervical anomalies
    - 2.9 Demyelination/multiple sclerosis

3 **Thoracic cord**
- Back pain
- Usually normal strength and sensation in upper extremities
- Sensory level on trunk
- Upper motor neuron weakness in lower extremities
- Sympathetic nervous system involvement, Horner syndrome (cervico-thoracic lesions)
- Bowel/bladder dysfunction
    - 3.1 **Chronic degenerative arthritis and spinal stenosis**
    - 3.2 ***Neoplasm***: as in Cervical cord, above
    - 3.3 *Vascular*: as in Cervical cord, above
    - 3.4 *Infection*: as in Cervical cord, above
    - 3.5 *Transverse myelitis*: as in Cervical cord, above
    - 3.6 Demyelination/multiple sclerosis
    - 3.7 *Acute trauma/fracture*: trauma to the thoracic cord is less common

4 **Lumbar cord**
- Low back pain
- Normal upper extremities
- Upper motor neuron weakness in lower extremities
- Sensory findings on legs and 'saddle' distribution
- Bowel/bladder dysfunction
    - 4.1 **Chronic degenerative arthritis and spinal stenosis**
    - 4.2 *Lumbar disc herniation/extrusion*

    4.3 *Neoplasm*: as in Cervical cord, above

    4.4 *Vascular*: as in Cervical cord, above

    4.5 *Infection*: as in Cervical cord, above

    4.6 *Transverse myelitis*: as in Cervical cord, above

    4.7 Demyelination/multiple sclerosis

    4.8 *Acute trauma/fracture*: rare

5 **Conus medullaris**
- Normal upper extremities
- Early bowel/bladder dysfunction
- Sexual dysfunction
- Peri-anal sensory loss
- Variable, upper motor neuron lower extremity weakness
- Weakness more likely to be symmetric

    5.1 ***Lumbar disc rupture/extrusion***

    5.2 ***Neoplasm***: as in Cervical cord, above, with the following additions:

        5.2.1 Extramedullary: lipoma, teratoma

        5.2.2 Intramedullary: ependymoma, teratoma more common, astrocytoma less

        5.2.3 Metastases: 'drop mets' more common down here

        5.2.4 Meningeal carcinomatosis: breast, small cell lung

    5.3 **Lumbar spinal stenosis**: may be associated with spinal developmental anomalies

    5.4 *Infection*: spinal epidural abscess, etc.

    5.5 *Vascular*: as in Cervical cord, above

    5.6 *Spinal fracture*: for instance L1 burst fracture

    5.7 Arachnoiditis: bacterial, viral, intrathecal injections, post-myelography, etc.

6 **Cauda equina**
- Normal upper extremities
- Early severe radicular and perineal pain ('saddle' distribution)
- Lower motor neuron weakness of lower extremities
- Weakness can be asymmetric
- Bowel/bladder dysfunction

    6.1 ***Lumbar disc rupture/extrusion***

    6.2 ***Neoplasm***: as in Conus medullaris, above. No real intramedullary tumors; ependymomas, teratomas are extramedullary here

    6.3 **Lumbar spinal stenosis**: may be associated with spinal developmental anomalies

    6.4 *Infection*: spinal epidural abscess, etc.

    6.5 *Vascular*: as in Cervical cord, above

    6.6 *Spinal fracture*: as in Cervical cord, above

    6.7 Arachnoiditis: as in Conus medullaris, above

    6.8 Lumbar plexopathy mimicking cauda equina lesion: idiopathic, autoimmune, neoplastic, etc.

Distinguishing lesions of the conus medullaris vs. cauda equina

Finding (sign/symptom)	Conus syndrome	Cauda syndrome
Pain	Back pain, less severe pain	Early, severe radicular pain
Sensory loss	Peri-anal sensory loss	Radicular sensory loss (saddle anesthesia)
Weakness	Bilateral, upper motor neuron leg weakness	Asymmetric lower motor neuron leg weakness
Bowel/bladder dysfunction	Early urinary retention, early constipation, lax anal tone	Urinary retention, lax anal tone
Sexual impotence	Frequent	Occasional

Pain

Low back pain

- One of the most common presenting complaints in neurology.
- Lifetime prevalence in the range of 60–90%.
- Enormous social and economic impact due to disability and treatment costs.
- Frequently multifactorial; often escapes definitive diagnosis. There may be little or no association between signs, symptoms, and imaging results.
- Important to rule out serious neurological disease with the following 'red flags' and/or 'hard' neurological findings:
  - night pain: may suggest tumor
  - fever, along with history of bacterial infections and drug use: epidural abscess
  - leg pain: nerve root compression
  - bilateral lower extremity numbness/weakness with bladder and bowel dysfunction: cauda equina or conus lesions
  - history of carcinoma: metastasis
  - back pain in a child: tumor or tethered cord
  - minor trauma in osteoporotic patients: compression fracture
- In general, the majority of patients who present with acute low back pain have minor musculoskeletal disorders, and the majority with chronic low back pain have degenerative disorders. Causative etiologies hypothesized to include degenerative discs, osteoarthritis, ligamentous injury, and soft tissue injury/inflammation

1 **Mechanical etiologies** (97%)
    1.1 **Lumbar strain/sprain** (70%)

- The most common diagnosis made in cases of acute low back pain.
- Refers to stress to the musculoskeletal tissues without precise anatomical pathological localization.
- Pain is usually acute, in the midline lumbosacral area, precipitated by movement, and may or may not follow a minor injury.

1.2 Age-related degeneration of discs and facet joints (10%)
- Spinal stenosis may result from degenerative changes of bony spine and ligaments, or from congenital anomalies of the spine.
- Characteristic symptoms include low back pain, radiating to the buttocks, anterior thigh, and calves which is exacerbated by extension and relieved by flexion of the spine (neurogenic claudication). This pain, which is not relieved by rest, differentiates it from vascular claudication (see p. 451).

1.3 Disc herniation (4%)
- Pain is often sudden, precipitated by a lifting or twisting injury with severe radicular symptoms.
- The L5/S1 level is most often involved, causing entrapment of the S1 root.

1.4 Spondylolisthesis and spondylolysis (2%)
- These conditions are differentiated from spondylosis, which refers to general osteoarthritic changes of the spine and discs.
- Spondylolisthesis refers to an anterior or posterior slippage of one vertebra on another, while spondylolysis implies a fracture of the pars interarticularis of the arch.
- Symptoms are usually nonspecific, as persistent ill-defined low back pain.

1.5 Others
- Osteoporotic compression fracture (4%)
- Traumatic fracture (<1%)
- Congenital disease (<1%): however, often associated with degenerative changes.

2 *Visceral disease* (2%)
- Disease of pelvic organs
- Renal disease
- *Aortic aneurysm*: may be immediately life threatening
- Gastrointestinal disease

3 Non-mechanical etiologies (1%)
- *Neoplasm* (0.7)
- *Infection* (0.01%)
- Inflammatory arthritis
- Osteochondrosis
- Paget disease

Radiculopathy

- A radiculopathy is defined as a sensory or motor dysfunction resulting from pathology involving a spinal nerve root.
- Physical symptoms may include weakness, burning, tingling, and 'shooting' pain.
- Clinical diagnosis of a radiculopathy involves determination of the motor, sensory, and reflex abnormalities. Motor and reflex changes in radiculopathy are typically better localized than sensory abnormalities.
- Cervical radiculopathies are most commonly caused by spondylosis.
- Lumbar radiculopathies are most commonly caused by disc herniation.
- Radiculopathies are most commonly seen in the cervical and lumbo-sacral roots, with the following levels most commonly affected:
  1 cervical levels C5 (7%), C6 (18%), C7 (46%),
  2 lumbar levels L4 (10%), L5 (40%),
  3 sacral level S1 (50%).

1 **Disc herniation**
   - Most common cause of lumbar radiculopathies.
   - Lateral herniations tend to compress nerve roots as they exit the neural foramina.
   - Central herniations may compress multiple nerve roots/cauda equina.
   - Herniated discs may be managed medically.
   - Extruded disc fragments generally require surgical intervention.
2 **Chronic degenerative arthritis and spinal stenosis**
   - Most common cause of cervical radiculopathies
   - Cervical stenosis cause upper extremity radiculopathy and lower extremity myelopathy.
   - Lumbar stenosis may cause neurogenic claudication (see p. 451).
   - Many degenerative changes may be associated with congenital spinal anomalies.
3 Trauma: usually due to stretching of nerve roots. Multiple roots may be involved.
4 *Epidural abscess*
   - Other symptoms/signs include back pain, fever.
   - Risk factors include immunocompromised state, intravenous drug abuse, spinal surgery/instrumentation.
5 *Epidural metastases*
   - Most common neoplasms with epidural metastasis include lung, breast, prostate, kidney, and myeloproliferative malignancies.
6 Herpes zoster
   - Dermatomal pain, followed by dermatomal vesicular rash.
   - Spontaneous reactivation of latent varicella zoster infection.

7 Lyme disease
  - Polyradiculitis occurs weeks after tick bite and initial rash (erythema chroni-
    cum migrans).

Differentiating neurogenic from vascular claudication

- Neurogenic claudication is an exertional syndrome characterized by pain in
  the lower extremities following activity.
- Caused by narrowing of the spinal canal with resultant nerve root
  compression of the cauda equina.
- Believed to be a multifactorial illness that includes:
  - facet joint hypertrophy
  - intervertebral disc bulging/herniation
  - posterior osteophyte formation, and
  - ligamentum flavum hypertrophy.
- Nerve root compression results in reduced arterial blood supply as well as
  venous congestion.

Signs/symptoms	Neurogenic	Vascular
Pain relief following cessation of activity	5–20 minutes	Seconds to minutes
Back pain	Common	Rare
Numbness, weakness, parasthesias	Common	Rare
Position dependence	**Relieved by lumbar flexion (such as sitting), but not during rest or standing**	**Relieved by standing still or sitting (rest)**
Pulses	Normal	Reduced
Bruits	Rare	Common
Ambulating distance	Variable	Fixed

Syndromes

Spinal cord syndromes

- When the spinal cord is viewed in cross-section, it contains central gray
  matter, consisting of neuronal cell bodies, and peripheral white matter,
  which contains the ascending and descending pathways. It is important
  to consider the function and location of these tracts, as various spinal
  cord syndromes are caused by differential involvement of these fibers and
  pathways.

- Important ascending pathways include:
  1 Spinothalamic tract: carrying sensory information pertaining to pain and temperature, running contralateral in the anterolateral cord.
  2 Posterior columns: carrying sensory information pertaining to fine, discriminatory touch and proprioception, running ipsilateral in the posterior cord.
- Important descending pathways include:
  1 Corticospinal tract: conveying information from the motor cortex influencing lower motor neuron activity and mediating voluntary movement, running ipsilateral in the cord in both lateral (~85%) and anterior (~15%) tracts.
  2 Autonomic pathways running in the mediolateral cord.
- May be caused by traumatic, ischemic, metabolic, or structural pathologies.

1 **Brown-Séquard syndrome (cord hemisection)**
   - Ipsilateral upper motor neuron weakness, and loss of vibration and proprioception below the level of the lesion.
   - Ipsilateral loss of all sensation at the level of the lesion.
   - Contralateral loss of pain and temperature below the level of the lesion.
      1.1 ***Traumatic (usually penetrating) injury*** to one half of the spinal cord.
      1.2 Any process that affects one transverse half of the spinal cord.
          1.2.1 Eccentric tumor: neurofibroma, schwannoma, meningioma, etc.
2 **Anterior cord syndrome**
   - Bilateral lower motor neuron weakness at the level of the lesion.
   - Bilateral upper motor neuron weakness below the lesion from corticospinal tract involvement.
   - Bilateral loss of pain and temperature sensation below the level of the lesion from spinothalamic tract involvement.
   - Bowel/bladder dysfunction.
   - Sparing of vibration and position sensation.
      2.1 ***Infarction*** in the distribution of the anterior spinal artery.
      2.2 ***Anterior cord compression***
          2.2.1 Medial spinal (cervical) disc herniation
          2.2.2 Anterior extra-axial tumor
3 **Central cord syndrome**
   - 'Cape' anesthesia of pain and temperature involving shoulders and arms.
   - Upper extremities: lower motor neuron weakness; lower extremities: upper motor neuron weakness.
   - Urinary retention.
      3.1 **Syringomyelia**

3.2 **Intramedullary spinal tumor**: astrocytoma, ependymoma, more rarely hemangioblastomas, teratomas, dermoids. Intramedullary tumors may have associated cysts, leading to diagnostic confusion with syringomyelia.

3.3 *Traumatic cervical hyperextension*

3.4 *Intraspinal hemorrhage*

3.5 Pseudosyringomyelia: peripheral neuropathy with disproportionate involvement of pain and temperature fibers (Tangier disease, amyloid polyneuropathy). Rarely occurs in segmental distribution affecting arms but sparing legs.

4 **Posterior cord syndrome**

- Loss of vibratory and proprioceptive sensation
- Sensory ataxia
- Romberg sign
- Lhermitte sign

4.1 **Vitamin B$_{12}$ deficiency, pernicious anemia**

- Other associated findings include painful distal neuropathy, upper motor neuron signs, macrocytic anemia, and even dementia/cognitive impairment.
- Due to impaired B$_{12}$ absorption from atrophic gastritis (anti-parietal cell antibodies, reduced intrinsic factor), tropical sprue, gastric/ileal resection, jejunal diverticula, rarely due to inadequate dietary animal protein.

4.2 **Tabes dorsalis (syphilis)**

- Other associated findings include lancinating lightning-like pains, lower extremity areflexia, Argyll-Robertson pupils, muscle wasting, optic atrophy, ataxia, sphincter dysfunction.

4.3 N$_2$O inhalation-associated subacute combined degeneration.

4.4 Posterior cord compression: less common than anterior cord compression.

4.5 Posterior spinal artery infarction: rarely pure, due to collaterals.

4.6 AIDS-associated vascular myelopathy

4.7 Friedreich ataxia (see Chapter 6: Movement Disorders)

4.8 Vitamin E deficiency

5 Conus medullaris syndrome (see DDx by location, p. 447)

6 Cauda equina syndrome (see DDx by location, p. 447)

Acute paresis/plegia

- *Acute spinal cord injury may result in FLACCID paralysis due to SPINAL SHOCK.* Typical upper motor neuron signs (spasticity, hyperreflexia) may be absent in the acutely injured spinal cord. The presence of a sensory level, upgoing plantar responses, urinary retention, and spinous point tenderness are all clues pointing toward an acute spinal cord injury.

- Acute traumatic spinal cord injury should be treated with high-dose corticosteroids.
- 'Para-' refers to involvement of only the lower extremities, and thus spinal cord involvement below the cervical level. The prefix 'quadri-' reflects involvement of all four limbs, and thus pathology at the level of the cervical cord or craniocervical junction.
- When the onset is acute, it suggests vascular, traumatic, or possibly demyelinating/inflammatory etiologies and represents a NEUROLOGICAL EMERGENCY. There are also nonspinal causes of acute paralysis that should be included in the differential.
- Major immediate medical concerns include respiratory distress and inability to maintain airway. Associated acute problems may include autonomic instability and urinary retention. Reduced mobility may also result in increased risk of veno-occlusive disease, pulmonary embolism, and skin breakdown.

1 Traumatic: usually acute onset (seconds or minutes); excludes chronic compressive lesions.
  1.1 **Cord transection**
    1.1.1 Complete: total loss of sensation and movement below level of lesion.
    1.1.2 Incomplete: partial loss of sensation and movement below lesion (see Spinal cord syndromes, above).
      1.1.2.1 Brown-Séquard syndrome
      1.1.2.2 Central cervical cord syndrome
      1.1.2.3 Anterior or posterior cord syndrome
  1.2 **Disc herniation/extrusion**: may present with anterior cord syndrome.
  1.3 **Shock cord syndrome or spinal concussion**: may present with complete cord syndrome, even though the continuity of the spinal cord remains intact. Deficits, to a large degree, may be reversible.
  1.4 Monoparesis/plegia: upper extremity (usually birth injury)
    1.4.1 Erb-Duchenne palsy (resulting from avulsion injury of C5/6 nerve roots)
    1.4.2 Dejerine-Klumpke palsy (resulting from avulsion injury to C8/T1 nerve roots)
2 Vascular: ischemia, infarction, or hemorrhage – usually acute onset (minutes).
  2.1 *Anterior spinal artery infarct*: usually midthoracic.
    ▪ Most common etiology is aortic atherosclerotic disease.
    ▪ Other etiologies include: collagen vascular disease, vasculitis, embolism, aortic dissection, pregnancy, sickle cell disease, angiography, vascular

compression by tumor, aortic surgery, systemic hypotension following cardiac arrest, decompression sickness.

2.2 *Spinal cord hemorrhage*: rare. May be intramedullary, subarachnoid, subdural, or epidural.

- Intramedullary (hematomyelia) usually due to trauma.
- Other etiologies include: blood dyscrasias, anticoagulation, arteriovenous malformation, venous spinal cord infarction, hemorrhage into spinal tumor, vasculitis.

2.3 *Spinal dural arteriovenous malformation*

3 Inflammatory/autoimmune disorders: usually subacute onset (hours or days).

3.1 **Multiple sclerosis** (see Chapter 7: Infectious, Inflammatory, and Demyelinating disorders).

3.2 **Acute inflammatory demyelinating polyneuropathy (AIDP, Guillain-Barré)** (see Chapter 8: Peripheral Neurology).

3.3 **Acute transverse myelitis**: see Transverse myelitis, below.

3.4 *Myasthenia gravis*: (see Chapter 8: Peripheral Neurology).

- Usually presents as fluctuating/fatigable proximal/bulbar weakness without sensory symptoms.

3.5 Acute polymyositis

3.6 *Acute disseminated encephalomyelitis (ADEM)*: encephalopathy, fever.

3.7 Paraneoplastic myelopathy

4 *Infectious disorders*: usually subacute onset (hours or days) (see Chapter 8: Peripheral Neurology – Primary motor involvement, Acute weakness).

5 Hereditary metabolic disorders: may occur acutely (minutes or hours) (see Chapter 8: : Peripheral Neurology – Primary motor involvement, Acute weakness).

5.1 *Hypokalemic periodic paralysis* (calcium channel mutation)

5.2 *Hyperkalemic periodic paralysis* (sodium channel mutation)

5.3 *Acute intermittent porphyria*

6 Toxins/miscellaneous: usually subacute onset (hours or days) (see Chapter 8: Peripheral Neurology – Primary motor involvement, Acute weakness).

6.1 *Tick paralysis*: ascending paralysis, history of outdoor activity

6.2 Aminoglycosides

6.3 Organophosphates, other environmental toxins

Transverse myelitis

- Defined as an inflammation of the spinal cord, often producing weakness, numbness, and bowel and bladder dysfunction.
- Presents as the development of isolated spinal cord dysfunction *in the absence of a compressive lesion*.
- It typically has a dramatic presentation, with rapid onset of symptoms over several hours to a few days. However, it may present as an acute (days), subacute (2–6 weeks), or chronic (>6 weeks) process.

- Signs and symptoms may include preceding febrile illness (~30% of cases), weakness, paralysis, sensory deficit levels in mid-thoracic area, parasthesias, hyperreflexia, bowel and/or bladder incontinence, and back pain. The onset may be so abrupt that patients manifest clinically as spinal shock.
- Transverse myelitis typically affects the mid-thoracic region. Therefore, most patients have weakness and numbness that spare the arms. However, 20% of patients develop cervical myelitis.
- Transverse myelitis in a young patient should always raise the suspicion of multiple sclerosis.

Remember: you must first rule out acute compressive lesions such as tumors, hemorrhage, or trauma using neuroimaging. Imaging must be directed at the correct spinal location, based on examination.

1 Demyelinating and dysmyelinating disorders (see Chapter 7: Infectious, Inflammatory, and Demyelinating Disorders)
  1.1 **Multiple sclerosis**
  1.2 Devic disease/syndrome (neuromyelitis optica)
  1.3 *Acute disseminated encephalomyelitis* (ADEM)
  1.4 Adrenomyeloneuropathy: usually chronic/progressive
2 Other non-infectious inflammatory disorders
  2.1 Post-infectious/post-vaccinal transverse myelitis
  2.2 Primary angiitis of the central nervous system
  2.3 Systemic lupus erythematosis
  2.4 Paraneoplastic myelopathy
    ▪ Some myelopathies associated with breast, lung, lymphomas.
    ▪ Others with anti-Hu antibody associated with dorsal root ganglia degeneration.
  2.5 Sjögren syndrome
  2.6 Mixed connective tissue disease
3 Vascular
  3.1 *Cord infarction*: see Acute paresis/plegia, above.
  3.2 *Spinal dural arteriovenous malformation*
4 Infectious etiologies
  4.1 Viral infections
    4.1.1 **HIV**
    4.1.2 Polio virus
    4.1.3 *Herpes viruses*: herpes simplex, varicella zoster, cytomegalovirus, Epstein-Barr virus

        4.1.4 Human T-cell leukemia virus (types I and II): tropical spastic para-
              paresis

        4.1.5 Group B arboviruses (West Nile virus)

    4.2 Bacterial and mycobacterial infections

        4.2.1 ***Bacterial meningitis, intraparenchymal abscess, epidural abscess***
              (Staphloccocus and/or Streptoccocus species)

        4.2.2 ***Mycobacterium tuberculosis***: including Pott disease

        4.2.3 *Treponemal (syphilis)*

        4.2.4 *Lyme disease (Borrelia burgdorferi)*

    4.3 Parasitic infections

        4.3.1 Schistosomal

Chronic para- or quadriparesis

- Clinically, may present as a mono-, para-, or quadriparesis.
- Associated with upper motor neuron signs and symptoms.
- Motor signs may be weakness or frank paralysis.
- Sensory deficits typically distributed at a spinal level corresponding to the lesion and may affect posterior columns, spinothalamic tracts, or both.

1 **Compressive lesions**

    1.1 **Disc herniation**

    1.2 **Chronic degenerative arthritis and spinal stenosis**

- May be due to osteoarthritis or inflammatory arthritides (rheumatoid, anklyosis spondylitis).
- Sometimes associated with congenital craniocervical or spinal anomalies.
- Patients with spinal stenosis may be more vulnerable to mild cervical trauma.

    1.3 *Neoplasm* (see Chapter 10: Neuro-oncology).

    1.4 *Abscess*

2 Inflammatory/demyelinating lesions

    2.1 **Multiple sclerosis** (see Chapter 7: Infectious, Inflammatory, and Demyelinating Disorders).

    2.2 Chronic inflammatory demyelinating polyneuropathy (see Chapter 8: Peripheral Neurology).

    2.3 Paraneoplastic myelopathy

    2.4 Spinal arachnoiditis

- Associated with chronic infection, repeated spine surgery, intrathecal injections.
- Pain is a primary symptom.

    2.5 Neurosarcoidosis

3 Infectious
    3.1 HIV vacuolar myelopathy
    3.2 Lyme disease
    3.3 Tuberculosis
    3.4 Syphilis
    3.5 Human T-cell lymphotropic virus type 1/2 (HTLV-1/2)
4 Metabolic/toxic
    4.1 Vitamin B_{12} deficiency
    4.2 Nitrous oxide inhalation-induced subacute combined degeneration
    4.3 Post-radiation therapy myelopathy
    4.4 Vitamin E deficiency
5 Hereditary and congenital conditions
    5.1 **Cerebral palsy**: spastic diplegia, hemiplegia, or quadriplegia
    5.2 Arnold-Chiari malformation with or without syringomyelia
    5.3 Hereditary spastic paraplegia
        5.3.1 Pure spastic paraplegia: several types – AD, AR, XL (Xq28, Xq21)
        5.3.2 Complicated spastic paraplegia: many variants, associated with hand amyotrophy, ataxia, myoclonus, choreoathetosis, deafness, dementia, optic atrophy.

Spinal cord tumors (see Chapter 10: Neuro-oncology)

Slowly progressive weakness

Anterior horn cell disease

- Anterior horn cells, named for their location within the spinal cord, are lower motor neurons. The anterior horn cell, with its axon, is referred to as an alpha motor neuron. The axons extend peripherally to innervate a variable number of muscle fibers.
- The most common cause of anterior horn cell disease is degeneration.
- Associated signs include:
  - paralysis or paresis
  - decreased muscle tone
  - muscle atrophy
  - absent or decreased deep tendon reflexes
  - muscle fasciculations and fibrillations
- This differential is distinct from that for 'Combined anterior horn cell and corticospinal tract disease' (see p. 459).

1 **Infantile spinal muscular atrophy (~1:15,000) (Werdnig-Hoffman disease)**
  - (See p. 461, Spinal muscular atrophy)
2 Juvenile spinal muscular atrophy (Kugelburg-Welander disease)
  - (See p. 461, Spinal muscular atrophy)
3 Adult-onset spinal muscular atrophy
  - (See p. 461, Spinal muscular atrophy)
4 *Acute poliomyelitis*
  - Acute illness resembling aseptic meningitis
  - Progression to paralytic disease in as many as 50% of patients
  - Focal asymmetric paralysis, fasciculations, myalgia
5 *Progressive post-poliomyelitis muscular atrophy*
  - Previous infection with the polio virus
  - Extreme fatigue
  - 'Overuse' myalgias
  - Progressive muscle atrophy and weakness
  - Fasciculations

Combined anterior horn cell and corticospinal tract disease

- This syndrome is distinct from pure anterior horn cell disease because 'combined anterior horn cell and corticospinal tract disease' are characterized by a mix of upper and lower motor neuron signs/symptoms.
- Associated signs include:
  - Mixed upper (hyperreflexia, Babinski signs, spasticity) and lower motor neuron (loss of reflexes, fasciculations, atrophy) signs
  - Asymmetric weakness
  - Bulbar signs
  - Absence of sensory or autonomic findings
  - Absence of bowel/bladder incontinence
  - Preservation of ocular movement

1 **Amyotropic lateral sclerosis (ALS) (Lou Gehrig disease)**
(See Chapter 8: Peripheral Neurology)
2 **Cervical spondylosis with myelopathy**
  - Lower motor neuron signs in upper limbs due to nerve root compression.
  - Upper motor neuron signs in lower limbs due to cervical cord compression.
  - Distinction from ALS is presence of painful, stiff neck and upper extremity pain or paresthesias.
3 Syringomyelia
  - Lower motor neuron signs in upper extremities due to ventral horn damage.

- Upper motor neuron signs in lower extremities due to corticospinal tract compression.
- Distinction from ALS is presence of upper extremity pain and loss of pain and temperature in cape-like distribution over shoulders and upper extremities.

4 *Intramedullary spinal cord tumor or hemorrhage*
  - Mixed upper and lower motor neuron signs due to central cord syndrome or anterior cord syndrome.
  - Usually some sensory symptoms in upper extremities.

5 Primary lateral sclerosis
  - Predominance of corticospinal and corticobulbar tract findings.
  - Diagnosis can usually be made once other conditions are excluded.

6 Progressive muscular atrophy (Aran-Duchenne syndrome)
  - Predominance of lower motor neuron signs.
  - Asymmetric muscle atrophy and weakness.
  - Reflexes normal or slightly decreased.

7 Other conditions whose presentation may mimic ALS
  - Important to consider because most are treatable (except Guamanian Parkinson-dementia-ALS complex).
    7.1 Monoclonal gammopathy ALS-like syndrome: anti-MAG antibodies.
    7.2 Multifocal motor neuropathy with conduction block: conduction block on nerve conduction studies.
    7.3 Thyrotoxic state: weakness, fasciculations, hyperactive reflexes
    7.4 Guamanian Parkinson-dementia-ALS complex
    7.5 Late HIV infection
    7.6 Myasthenia gravis: fluctuating proximal weakness, ptosis, or ophthalmoplegia all distinguish from ALS

8 Other disorders with spastic paraparesis
  - Usually lack lower motor neuron findings in upper extremities
  - Usually have additional sensory symptomatology
    8.1 Multiple sclerosis/transverse myelitis
    8.2 Vitamin B_{12} deficiency
    8.3 Tropical spastic paraparesis
    8.4 Adrenoleukodystrophy

9 Pseudosyringomyelia: dissociated pain/temperature loss, weakness.
  - Predominant loss of pain and temperature sensation, preserved vibration and proprioception.
  - Mild weakness, reflexes preserved early on.
    9.1 Amyloid neuropathy: AD
    9.2 Tangier disease: AR

Spinal muscular atrophy (SMA)

- Different types of spinal muscular atrophy are classified by age of onset and clinical course.
- Usually present with hypotonia and muscle weakness with preserved mental status.

SMA	Onset	Survival/ prognosis	Ability to sit	Fasciculations	Serum creatine kinase	Inheritance
Infantile (Werdnig-Hoffman) (type I)	Birth to 6 months	< 4 years	Never	+/-	Normal	AR
Intermediate (type II)	3–18 months	> 4 years / no ambulation	Usually	+/-	Normal	AR
Juvenile (Kugelberg-Welander) (type III)	> 2 years	Adulthood	Always	++	Elevated	AR
Adult-onset (type IV)	> 20 years	50 years + / slow progression	Always	++	Elevated	AR

Chapter 15
Diagnostic Tests

Blood/serum tests   **497**

Other clinical tests   **506**

EEG

Normal or nonpathological EEG

Electroencephalographic rhythms

- The rhythmic EEG activity is due to intrinsic membrane properties of various groups of neurons (summated excitatory and inhibitory postsynaptic potentials, EPSPs and IPSPs), the synaptic connections of these neurons, and thalamocortical inputs that lead to synchronization of this activity.
- There are basically four EEG frequency ranges. No individual band is normal or abnormal by definition. All are interpreted according to the topographic location, age, and conscious state of the patient.

Rhythm	Frequency	Normal	Abnormal
Alpha	8–13 Hz	Posterior dominant rhythm in older children and adults, reactive to eye opening and representing the background activity of the awake state	Diffuse alpha activity in alpha coma May suggest seizure activity in neonates
Beta	>13 Hz	Low-voltage waves that occur predominantly over the anterior and central head regions, normal in sleep in infants and young children	Drug-induced (barbiturates and benzodiazepines) beta activity in frontal regions Breach rhythm over the skull defect
Theta	4–7 Hz	Normal in younger children and during drowsiness, posterior waves of youth may have a theta component	Considered abnormal when theta activity is seen focally, e.g. temporal theta in the elderly and focal theta over a structural lesion
Delta	<4 Hz	Normal in infants and during sleep stages	Delta slowing reflects moderate to severe disturbance of cerebral function Intermittent, polymorphic delta activity with focal lesions
Spikes, sharp waves and spike-and-wave complexes	Duration: • Spike: 25–70 ms • Sharp: 70–200 ms	Vertex waves and frontal sharp transients, positive occipital sharp transients of sleep (POSTs), 14- and 6-Hz positive spikes, and benign epileptiform transients of sleep	Increased likelihood of clinical seizures (both generalized and focal seizures)

Normal electroencephalographic patterns in adults during wakefulness

- Fast frequencies dominate the normal adult waking EEG.
- The posterior dominant rhythm is recorded in the awake state with the eyes closed. Eye opening attenuates the posterior dominant rhythm.
- Increasing age can result in slowing of the background. However, a frequency slower than 8 Hz at any adult age is considered abnormal.

1 Anterior EEG activity
  - Low-voltage fast activity superimposed by eye movement artifacts.

- Rhythmic beta activity may be seen in the frontal and central regions, especially when sedatives are used.
- Drug-induced beta activity includes benzodiazepines and barbiturates.
2 Posterior EEG activity
  - Posterior dominant rhythm during awake state and eyes closed is between 8.5 and 11 Hz. Normally symmetric.
  - Amplitude from the left hemisphere is usually slightly lower than the right.
  - Slowing of the posterior background is common in the elderly, but should not be slower than 8 Hz.

Electroencephalography during drowsiness and sleep

- As the patient progresses from the awake state to drowsiness, the first sign is the attenuation of the posterior dominant rhythm with some spreading anteriorly, associated with background slowing.
- The following patterns are seen during drowsiness and sleep:
  - Background posterior dominant rhythm is lost and replaced by mixed frequencies.
  - Vertex waves: are surface-negative potentials with maximum amplitude at the midline (C3, C4), commonly seen in stage 2 sleep (also stage 1B). They are biphasic waves, which may be followed by a slow wave or spindle and are termed a K complex.
  - Sleep spindles: are rhythmic 11–14 Hz waves lasting 1–2 seconds, most prominent in the central region during stage 2 sleep.
  - Positive occipital sharp transients of sleep (POSTS): are positive potentials, with a maximum at O1 and O2.

Sleep stages	EEG findings
Stage 1: drowsiness	
Stage 1A	• **Attenuation of the posterior dominant rhythm**
Stage 1B	• **Progressive loss of posterior dominant rhythm** • Less than 20% of alpha rhythm in the background • Prominent theta activity
Stage 2: light sleep	• **Sleep spindles** • Vertex waves • Increased theta activity • Appearance of delta activity
Stage 3: slow wave sleep	• **More delta activity seen (20–50% of the record)** • Less vertex waves and sleep spindles

Continued

Sleep stages	EEG findings
Stage 4: slow wave sleep	• **Increasing delta activity, more than 50% of the record** • Fewer vertex waves and sleep spindles
REM sleep: • Roving eye movements • Hypotonia • Irregular respirations	• Low-voltage background of fast frequencies • Sawtooth waves may be seen in the frontal regions and the vertex

REM – rapid eye movement.

Benign electroencephalographic variants and patterns

- There are several benign variants of electroencephalographic activity, including variants of normal rhythms, rhythmic patterns, and patterns with 'epileptiform' morphology.
- It is therefore important for neurologists to recognize these patterns in order to avoid over-interpretation with regard to their significance.

Patterns	Description	Significance
Rhythmic patterns		
Rhythmic mid-temporal theta of drowsiness (psychomotor variant)	Bursts or serial trains of rhythmic theta waves ranging from 5–7 Hz with a flat-topped, sharp-contoured, or notched appearance	Predominant during drowsiness or relaxed wakefulness, usually normal but can be associated with structural lesions
Slow alpha variant	Subharmonic alpha rhythm that has a frequency about half of alpha rhythm (4–5 Hz)	Physiological alpha variant, seen during relaxed wakefulness and is normal
Fast alpha variant	Twice the frequency of the resting alpha rhythm (16–20 Hz), alternating with alpha rhythm	Physiological alpha variant
Midline theta rhythm	A rhythmic train of 5–7 Hz activity (a smooth, sinusoidal, spiky or mu appearance) in the central vertex, tends to wax and wane	Nonspecific variant of theta activity, seen in heterogeneous group of patients, including normal individuals and temporal lobe epilepsy
Frontal arousal rhythm (FAR)	Trains of 7–20 Hz waveforms that occur predominantly in frontal regions in runs up to 20 seconds	Nonspecific pattern of no clinical significance. Occurring in children and tends to disappear when awake

Patterns	Description	Significance
Subclinical rhythmic electrographic theta discharge in adults (SREDA)	Rhythmic theta activity in a widespread distribution with maximum amplitude over the parietal-posterior temporal regions	Seen in patients with diverse clinical complaints and considered to have little or no diagnostic significance
Mu rhythm	A central rhythm of alpha activity, with negative wicket-shaped spikes, blocked by movements of contralateral extremity or even just by thinking of limb movement	Seen in 17–19% of young adults, less common in the elderly or children
Mittens	A partially fused sleep spindle and vertex wave, sleep pattern with an appearance of a mitten with a slow wave bordered by a spike-like components	Normal variant

Patterns with 'epileptiform' morphology

14- and 6-Hz positive bursts	Short trains of arch-shaped waveforms with alternating positive spiky components and a negative, smooth, rounded waveform at a rate of 14 Hz or 6–7 Hz lasting up to 1 second during drowsiness or light sleep	Normal patterns, but have been reported in various clinical symptoms, including headache, vertigo, 'thalamic' epilepsy, etc.
Small sharp spikes (SSS) or benign epileptiform transients of sleep (BETS)	Single monophasic or diphasic spike with an abrupt ascending and a steep descending limb, with aftercoming slow-wave component during drowsiness and light sleep	Seen in ~25% of normal populations
Wicket spikes	Intermittent trains or clusters of monophasic arciform waveforms (6–11 Hz) that look like a Greek mu or wicket, seen mainly during drowsiness and light sleep, predominantly over the temporal regions	Seen in adults older than 30 years (0.9%)
Breach rhythm	Sharply contoured arciform waveforms (6–11 Hz) over the central and temporal regions	Normal variants

Abnormal EEG

Coma patterns on EEG

- Coma refers to a state characterized by a reduction of consciousness to a point where the subject is unable to make meaningful responses to environmental stimuli because of either dysfunction of the reticular activating system or widespread depression of cerebral cortical function.
- Three distinctive patterns of coma are seen on EEG. These patterns help distinguish etiologies and define prognosis.

Coma patterns	Description	Association
Alpha coma	• Generalized, invariable, monorhythmic pattern in the alpha frequency range • No variability or reactivity	• Following cardiopulmonary arrest, usually 2 to 3 days after the anoxic event (60%, most common cause) • Brainstem strokes (30%): 'locked-in syndrome' • Drug overdose (10%)
Beta coma	• Beta frequency activity superimposed on delta slowing	• Drug ingestion, particularly barbiturates and benzodiazepines
Spindle coma	• Resembling a sleep EEG, but the patient cannot be aroused • Spindle activity and V-waves occurring in a continuous or intermittent fashion • Little reactivity to afferent stimulation	• Head trauma • Brainstem lesions • Anoxic-ischemic event

Minimal EEG criteria in suspected brain death

- EEG can be a helpful investigation to confirm brain death, demonstrating electrocerebral silence or inactivity (no EEG activity over 2 µV).
- A number of causes, particularly **DRUG OVERDOSE** and **HYPOTHERMIA** can cause transient or reversible electrocerebral silence. Therefore, these conditions should be considered *and excluded* before the diagnosis of brain death is made.
- It is critically important to adhere to the minimum technical requirements for recording EEG in patients with suspected brain death before interpretation.

1 A minimum of eight scalp electrodes

Montage for determining brain death:

Channel	Recommended montage
1	Fp1-C3
2	C3-O1
3	Fp2-C4
4	C4-O2
5	Fp1-T3
6	T3-O1
7	Fp2-T4
8	T4-O2

2 Interelectrode impedance should be less than 10,000 ohm but more than 100 ohm.
3 Verify the integrity of the recording system.
4 Interelectrode distances of at least 10 cm.
5 A sensitivity of 2 μV/mm for at least 30 minutes of recording.
6 Use of appropriate filtering settings.
7 Use of monitoring techniques.
8 No EEG activity.
9 Performed by a qualified technologist.
10 A repeat EEG should be performed if there is any doubt about the finding of electrocerebral silence.

Spike vs. nonspike potentials on EEG

- Spikes and sharp waves are fast transients. By definition, spikes are usually surface-negative and have a duration of 20–70 ms while sharp waves are also surface-negative but with a longer duration of 70–200 ms. A sharp wave should not be considered abnormal unless it stands out from the background and is reproducible.
- One of the major pitfalls in EEG interpretation is misinterpreting sharply contoured rhythms as sharp waves and spikes. Examples include theta activity that can be pointed and looks like a run of spike-and-wave complexes.

The following features help differentiate true spike from nonspike potentials:

Features	Spike	Nonspike
Background	Standing out from the background	Embedded in the background
Appearance	Stereotyped	Vary in morphology
Duration	20–70 ms	Vary in duration
Electrical potentials	Almost always negative	No consistent pattern
Rising phase	Rising phase is faster than any other component	Rising phase may be slower than falling phase
Following slow wave	Following slow wave	Not followed by a slow wave
Sleep	Activated by sleep	No change with sleep

Modified from: Misulis K.E., Head T.C. *Essentials of Clinical Neurophysiology*, 3rd edition. Butterworth-Heinemann, 2002.

Nonepileptic spike and sharp waves

- Most spikes and sharp waves are abnormal and usually indicate epileptiform activity. However, some normal spike-like potentials are seen and they are not epileptiform in nature.

Nonepileptic spikes	Association
Vertex waves	A surface-negative potential at C3 and C4 during stage 2 sleep
Occipital lambda waves	This usually indicates visual exploration and is blocked by eye closure. It tends to appear when patient is looking at a picture or pattern
14- and 6-Hz positive bursts	A normal variant, but the appearance has been reported in various pathological conditions with no clear association
Wicket spikes	A normal variant during drowsiness and sleep
Benign epileptiform transients of sleep (BETS, or small sharp spikes, SSS)	A normal variant during drowsiness and sleep
Positive occipital sharp transients of sleep (POSTS)	A normal variant with positive potentials at O1 and O2 during sleep

Epileptiform activity

- Epileptiform activity is generated when depolarization of the cortex results in synchronous activation of many neurons.

- The abnormalities in epileptiform activity are the repetitive nature of the discharge and the degree of the synchrony. In fact, synchronous activation of many neurons is required for generation of both normal and abnormal rhythms.

1 **Spike and sharp waves**
   - Epileptiform activities mainly consist of spikes and sharp waves. While epileptiform slow activity and suppression does occur, this is much less common.
   - When the depolarization spreads synchronously to many neurons through associative connections, the summed field potentials are detected on the surface as a spike.
   - Spike waves have a duration of less than 70 ms.
   - Sharp waves have a duration of 70–200 ms.
2 **Paroxysmal depolarization shift (PDS)**
   - PDS comprises extracellular field potentials that are waves of depolarization followed by repolarization, reflecting the foundation of the bursting of spike discharges.

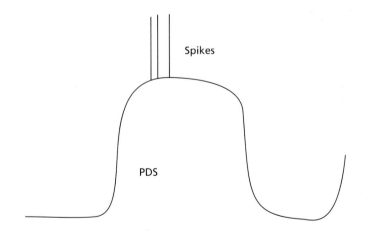

Pathological spikes and sharp waves and clinical correlation

- Focal spikes and sharp waves are usually epileptiform and indicate seizure disorder with a partial onset.
- The location, amplitude, and duration of the spikes as well as the background patterns and clinical history are important to electroencephalographer for accurate interpretation. Different clinical conditions have different predilections of spike morphology and location.

Spike and sharp wave patterns	Clinical correlation
Spikes with triphasic appearance Maximum at C3 and C4 Activated by sleep Otherwise normal background	Benign Rolandic epilepsy
Unilateral or bilateral occipital spikes during light sleep and suppressed by eye opening	Occipital epilepsy
3-per-second spike wave or polyspike-wave complex Activated by hyperventilation	Absence seizure
Midline spikes with prominent negative phase, correlating with simple motor seizure	Simple partial seizures
Temporal or frontal spikes with various patterns associated with focal slowing, correlating with alteration of consciousness	Complex partial seizures
Generalized high-frequency polyspike discharge	Generalized tonic-clonic seizures
Periodic complex of sharp and slow waves, associated with slowing in the frontotemporal area, High-amplitude discharges	Herpes simplex encephalitis
Generalized polyspike discharges, followed by a slow wave with high amplitude in the frontal region	Juvenile myoclonic epilepsy
High-voltage bursts of theta and delta activity with multifocal sharp waves, superimposed by suppression	Hypsarrhythmia seen in infantile spasm
Phantom spikes or 6-per-second spike waves	Frontal predominance: tonic-clonic seizures Occipital predominance: not associated with seizures
Periodic high amplitude bursts of sharp waves with irregular superimposed delta waves between hemispheres with duration of 0.5–2.0 seconds	Subacute sclerosing panencephalitis (SSPE)
Evolving EEG pattern, a periodic pattern with sharp and slow waves or discharges prominent posteriorly, with abnormal low-voltage theta and delta background	Creutzfeldt-Jakob disease (CJD)
Unilateral or bilateral independent sharp and slow-wave complexes at 1–2/second	Periodic lateralized epileptiform discharges (PLEDs)
Bursts of slow waves with superimposed sharp waves, interspersed on periods of relative flattening	Burst suppression
Disorganized background with diffuse slowing and suppression and periodic sharp waves, synchronous between hemispheres, along with clinical history of anoxic injury	Hypoxic-ischemic encephalopathy

Modified from: Misulis K.E., Head T.C. *Essentials of Clinical Neurophysiology*, 3rd edition. Butterworth-Heinemann, 2002.

Periodic patterns on EEG

- The EEG is particularly helpful in patients with impaired consciousness when it shows distinct patterns that help identify the etiology. These patterns include epileptiform activity, periodic patterns, and coma patterns.
- Generalized periodic patterns include triphasic waves, generalized periodic sharp waves, periodic epileptiform discharges, and burst suppression. Focal periodic pattern includes periodic lateralized epileptiform discharges.

Patterns	Description	Associated diagnosis
Triphasic waves	• Broad contoured waveforms with surface negative, positive, and negative peaks that are bilaterally symmetric and synchronous at a rate of 1.5 to 2.5 Hz • Frontal predominance • Typically transient	• Hepatic coma • Metabolic encephalopathies • Degenerative process • Anoxic-ischemic process
Generalized periodic sharp waves	• Widespread, bisynchronous, continuous, periodic, stereotypic sharp waves occurring at the intervals of 0.5 to 1.0 second.	• Creutzfeldt-Jakob disease (CJD) • Metabolic encephalopathies • Drugs, e.g. baclofen, lithium
Generalized periodic epileptiform discharges	• Bisynchronous spike, sharp waves, or spike and wave discharges occurring every 1 to 2 seconds • Often associated with myoclonic jerks	• Status epilepticus • Cardiac arrest
Burst suppression	• Intermittent bursts of spikes, sharp waves, slow waves, or mixed frequency (2 to 7 Hz) activity alternating with periods of electrocerebral silence lasting more than 1 second • Often associated with myoclonic jerks or eye opening/closure	• Severe disturbance of cerebral function from many causes, commonly cardiac arrest • Deep anesthesia • Drug overdose • Hypothermia
Periodic lateralized epileptiform discharges (PLEDs)	• Focal or lateralized epileptiform discharges recurring in a quasiperiodic manner every 1 to 4 seconds • Variable morphology, including spikes, sharp waves, polyphasic sharp and slow complexes	• Acute or subacute disturbance of focal cerebral function • Acute onset of seizures • Focal neurological deficit from an acute vascular event • Herpes simplex encephalitis • Any focal processes

Hypsarrthythmia

- Hypsarrthythmia is the interictal EEG pattern consisting of random high-voltage slow waves mixed with high-voltage multifocal spikes and sharp waves arising from all cortical regions.
- Other variants have been described, including modified hypsarrhythmia and atypical hyparrhythmia.

Hypsarrthythmia is seen in:
1 **Infantile spasms**
   - 66% of patients with infantile spasms demonstrated either hypsarrthymia or modified hypsarrhythmia.
   - The triad of infantile spasms, mental retardation, and hypsarrthythmia is called West syndrome.
2 Metabolic and biochemical diseases
3 Hypoxia-ischemia
4 Others: rare
   - Agenesis of corpus callosum
   - Agyria
   - Hemimegalencephaly
   - Tuberous sclerosis

Prognostic EEG patterns following a hypoxic insult

- The EEG is a very useful investigational tool in determining the prognosis in patients suffering a hypoxic insult.

Below is a summary of EEG features indicating a favorable or poor prognosis.
- Favorable prognosis:
   - Variability
   - Reactivity
   - Varying sleep patterns
   - Increased background frequencies
- Poor prognosis:
   - Invariant pattern
   - No reactivity
   - Monorhythmic pattern
   - Burst suppression
   - Generalized periodic discharges
   - Low-voltage tracing

- Generalized suppression
- Electrocerebral silence

Evoked potentials

Brainstem auditory-evoked potentials (BAEPs)

- Brainstem auditory-evoked potentials test acoustic conduction through the ear, the eighth cranial nerve, into the lower pons, and continuing rostrally in the lateral lemniscus up the brainstem.
- In clinical practice, this is often used to screen hearing in infants. It is also performed in adults for evaluation of possible acoustic neuroma but it is less helpful when evaluating for multiple sclerosis, compared to visual evoked potentials (VEPs). It can also evaluate peripheral and central auditory pathway in sedated and anesthetized patients.
- The waves routinely analyzed in BAEPs testing are I through V. The several succeeding peaks VI–VIII are quite variable and are not used for interpretation.
  - Wave I: the eighth cranial nerve near the brainstem
  - Wave II: near or at the cochlear nucleus at the junction of pons and medulla
  - Wave III: lower pons in the region of superior olive and trapezoid body
  - Wave IV, V: upper pons/lower midbrain in the lateral lemniscus or inferior colliculus

BAEPs findings	Interpretation
Increased I–V interpeak interval	Slow conduction from the eighth nerve to the midbrain, seen in demyelination, ischemia, tumors, and degenerative disorders
Increased wave I latency	Lesion of distal acoustic portion of the eighth nerve
Increased I–III interpeak interval	Lesion of pathway from the proximal eighth nerve into the contralateral lower pons, seen in CP angle tumors (acoustic neuroma), inflammation in the subarachnoid space, or disorders of the pontomedullary junction
Increased III–V interpeak interval	Lesion between lower pons to upper pons or lower midbrain, seen in demyelination or tumors

Continued

BAEPs findings	Interpretation
Absence of wave I, normal wave III and V	Peripheral hearing loss
Absence of wave III, normal wave I and V	Normal study
Absence of wave V, normal wave I and III	Lesion above the lower pons
Absence of all waves	Severe hearing loss

Somatosensory-evoked potentials (SSEPs)

- The somatosensory-evoked potential (SSEP) is the response to electrical stimulation of mixed or cutaneous peripheral nerves.
- SSEPs are usually obtained in the upper extremity with stimulation of the median and ulnar nerves at the wrist, recording at Erb's point in the supraclavicular fossa (N9, afferent volley in plexus), the neck (P14, caudal medial lemniscus), and the scalp (N20, thalamocortical radiations).
- In the lower extremity, the responses are obtained with stimulation of the tibial or peroneal nerves at the ankle, with recording over the lumbar spine (N22, dorsal roots and entry zone), neck (N34, brainstem and thalamus), and scalp (P37, primary sensory cortex).
- Abnormalities seen with SSEPs include slowing of the conduction velocities, decreased amplitude, or loss of the potentials. SSEPs are useful in the evaluation of suspected demyelination or myelopathy. They can also distinguish a central from a peripheral process, and can be helpful in the evalution of plexopathies and root lesions. Other indications include prognostication in patients with coma/brain death.

Median SSEP

Common median SSEP findings	Interpretation
Delayed N9 with normal N9–P14 and P14–N20 intervals	Lesions in the somatosensory nerves at or distal to the brachial plexus
Increased N9–P14 interval with normal P14–N20 interval	Lesions between Erb point and the lower medulla
Increased P14–N20 with normal N9–P14 interval	Lesions between the lower medulla and cerebral cortex
Absent P14, but N9 and N20 are normal, the N9–N20 interval is normal	Lesions between the brachial plexus and the lower medulla

Tibial SSEP

Common tibial SSEP findings	Interpretation
Prolonged N22 with normal N22–P37 interval	Peripheral neuropathy is the most likely. Less likely to be the cauda equina lesion
Normal N22 with prolonged N22–P37 interval	Lesions between the cauda equina and the brain. Median SSEP can be used to localize the lesion further. Normal median SSEP will indicate that the lesion is below the mid-cervical cord. Prolonged median SSEP will indicate that the lesion is above the mid-cervical cord with the possibility of the second lesion below the cervical cord.
Prolonged N22 and prolonged N22–P37 interval	Two lesions affecting both the peripheral and central conductions. The lesion in the cauda equina is also possible.

Visual-evoked potentials (VEPs)

- The visual-evoked potential (VEP) is the potential recorded from the occipital region in response to visual stimuli. It differs from other evoked responses in that the response is long-latency, while it is short-latency in others. VEP is also the only evoked response that is visible without averaging.
- Different types of stimulus are used.
  - Flash is used in patients who cannot cooperate with visual fixation.
  - Full-field pattern reversal is the usual stimulus for VEP, and it is suited for the evaluation of anterior visual pathway.
  - Half-field pattern-reversal stimulation is used for localization of lesions behind the optic chiasm.
- Inspection of normal VEP reveals three identifiable waveforms: N75, P100, and N145. P100 is a positive potential at about 100 ms (the normal limit is up to 117 ms), and is the only one used for VEP interpretation.
- An intact VEP usually suggests continuity of the visual pathways, but it does not fully exclude cortical blindness.

Types of VEP abnormalities	Interpretation
Unilateral prolongation of VEP latency	Slowing of conduction in one optic nerve, for example, optic neuritis in multiple sclerosis
Hemifield prolongation of VEP latency	A conduction defect behind the optic chiasm (sensitivity and specificity are usually not good enough to use this finding to confirm posterior lesions)

Continued

Types of VEP abnormalities	Interpretation
Reduced VEP amplitude	Ischemic and compressive diseases of the eye and optic nerve. Can also be seen in amblyopia and glaucoma
Absent VEPs	• Technical error • Poor visual fixation • Severe optic atrophy

Peripheral electrodiagnostics

Normal electromyographic activity

- Normally, muscle fibers are under neural control and fire only in response to neural activation with little or no spontaneous firing. Therefore, the rate and pattern of firing of muscle fibers in muscle is primarily that of the motor unit potentials under neural control.
- In needle EMG, the recording surface is typically the tip of a small sharp needle inserted through the skin into the muscle under study. The needle electrode should be inserted into the belly of the muscle under study, near the expected region of the motor-end-plate, which is usually the thickest part of the belly muscle.
- Motor unit potential (MUP) is the summation of the potentials of muscle fibers innervated by a single anterior horn cell in the region of the needle electrode.
- Recruitment is the initiation of the firing of additional motor units as the rate of discharge of an active MUP increases.

Normal patterns

Pattern	Procedure	Findings and correlation
Resting activity	Muscle relaxed and needle not moving	No activity
Insertional activity	Movement of the needle in a relaxed muscle, should be close to the end-plate region	Brief volley of action potentials, reflecting spontaneous miniature end-plate potentials (end-plate noise with a typical 'seashell' sound)
Motor unit potentials (MUPs)	Needle is not moved but the patient makes slight contraction	A few motor unit action potentials of short duration, biphasic or triphasic pattern, semirhythmic firing pattern

Pattern	Procedure	Findings and correlation
Recruitment	Patient makes progressive stronger muscle contraction until reaching maximum force	Increase number of functioning movements until the baseline is obscured

Modified from: Misulis K.E., Head T.C. *Essentials of Clinical Neurophysiology*, 3rd edition. Butterworth-Heinemann, 2002.

Abnormal spontaneous activity on EMG

- Spontaneous potentials are defined as any activity that persists beyond the cessation of needle insertion long enough to be recorded.
- There are two normal spontaneous potentials, including end-plate spikes and end-plate noises.
- Abnormal spontaneous potentials can occur with either regular or irregular patterns. These include fibrillations, positive sharp waves, fasciculations, myokymic potentials, complex repetitive discharges, and myotonic potentials.
- The most important feature to distinguish normal from abnormal spontaneous potentials is the initial negative deflection, as almost all pathological spontaneous potentials have positive initial deflection.

	Description	Clinical correlation
Regular pattern		

Fibrillations	• Action potentials of single muscle fibers that are twitching spontaneously in the absence of innervation
	• Rate 0.5–15/second
	• A brief spike or positive wave
	• Resembling 'ticking' or 'tocking' of a clock
	• Develops 1–3 weeks after denervation
		Lower motor neuron diseases
		  • Anterior horn cell diseases
		  • Polyradiculopathies
		  • Plexopathies
		  • Peripheral neuropathies
		Neuromuscular junction disorders
		  • Myasthenia gravis
		  • Botulism
		Muscle disorders
		  • Myositis
		  • Muscular dystrophy
		  • Periodic paralysis
		  • Toxic myopathy
		  • Muscle trauma
		  • Acid maltase deficiency

Continued

	Description	Clinical correlation
Myotonic discharges	• Action potentials of muscle fibers firing spontaneously in a prolonged manner after external excitation • Regular, but vary in frequency between 40 and 100/second, results in 'dive-bomber' sound	Patients with subclinical myotonia • Myotonic dystrophy • Myotonia congenital • Paramyotonia • Hyperkalemic periodic paralysis • Acid maltase deficiency
Complex repetitive discharges (CRD, or pseudomyotonic discharges)	• Action potentials of groups of muscle fibers discharging spontaneously in near synchrony through ephaptic activation of adjacent muscle fibers or split fibers • Abrupt onset and cessation • Frequency ranges 3–40/second • Sound like 'a motor boat that misfires'	Neuropathies • Chronic neuropathies • Chronic radiculopathies • Charcot-Marie-Tooth disease • Spinal muscular atrophy Myopathies • Polymyositis • Muscular dystrophy • Myxedema
Irregular pattern Fasciculations	• Action potentials of a group of muscles fibers innervated by an anterior horn cell that discharge in random fashion • Varying frequency, size, and shape, depending on the character of motor unit • Sounds like 'large raindrops on a roof'	Normal individuals • Fatigue • Cramps Chronic progressive neurogenic disorders • Amyotrophic lateral sclerosis • Peripheral neuropathy Metabolic disorders • Thyrotoxicosis • Tetany
Myokymic discharges	• Spontaneous muscle potentials associated with fine, worm-like quivering of facial myokymia • Bursts of 2 to 10 potentials at 40–60 Hz, at intervals of 0.1 to 10 seconds • Sounds like 'marching soldiers'	Facial muscles • Multiple sclerosis • Brainstem neoplasm • Facial palsy • Polyradiculopathy
Positive sharp waves (PSW)	• Positive sharp potentials with a fast downstroke and slower return to baseline	• Neurogenic lesions with denervation • Inflammatory myopathies

Abnormal insertional activity on EMG

• Insertional activity is the electrical response of muscle membrane to the insertion of the EMG needle.

- In normal individuals, insertional activity disappears as soon as the needle movement stops.
- Abnormal insertional activity can be either increased or decreased. Increased activity suggests the presence of abnormal spontaneous potentials in the muscle. Decreased activity implies fibrosis or fatty replacement of muscle.
- Increased insertional activity alone is not clinically important unless it is associated with fibrillations, positive sharp waves, or myotonic potentials.

1 Increased insertional activity
   - It suggests hyperexcitable muscle membrane.
   - Abnormal spontaneous potentials usually co-exist.
      1.1 Normal variants
         - Short trains of regularly firing positive waves.
         - Short recurrent bursts of irregularly firing potentials, seen commonly in muscular individuals.
      1.2 **Denervated muscles**
      1.3 Myotonic disorders
2 Decreased insertional activity
   - Decreased insertional activity alone is significant despite no other spontaneous activity present.
      2.1 Need to exclude wrong location of the tip of EMG needle
      2.2 **Fibrosis of muscle**
      2.3 **Fatty infiltration of muscle**
      2.4 Periodic paralysis, during attack
      2.5 McArdle disease, during contracture
      2.6 Rippling myopathy, during 'rippling'

Increased jitter

- Single-fiber electromyography (SFEMG) can be used to study the microphysiology of individual muscle fibers and document their physiological constancy.
- Jitter is believed to derive from variation in the time it takes the end-plate potential to reach threshold for action potential to generation at the postsynaptic membrane.
- In neuromuscular junction disorders, there is an increased variation in the time taken to attain an end potential capable of reaching threshold. This will lead to increased jitter.
- Abnormal jitter is an indicator of abnormal neuromuscular transmission.

Increased jitter seen in:

1 Myasthenia gravis (MG)
   - Jitter increases in magnitude, and action potentials may even be blocked.
   - Increased jitter is the most sensitive electrophysiological finding in MG, although not specific.
2 Polyneuropathy (occasionally)

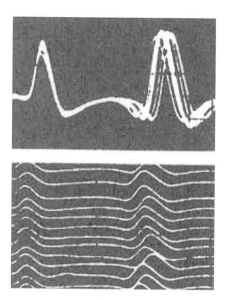

Repetitive nerve stimulation

- Repetitive nerve stimulation is an effective method to fatigue the neuromuscular junction and cause acetylcholine depletion. Slow repetitive stimulation is indicated in patients suspected of MG while rapid stimulation is most useful in patients with suspected presynaptic neuromuscular junction disorders, including Eaton-Lambert syndrome or botulism. Every patient undergoing repetitive stimulation should also complete routine nerve conduction and electromyography.
- In normal subjects, slow (2–3 Hz) repetitive stimulation results in little or no decrement, while a decrement of the compound muscle action potential of 10% or more is characteristic of MG within the appropriate clinical context.
- Although repetitive stimulation is a sensitive test for MG, a variety of other conditions can cause a decremental response. Therefore, decremental response alone from repetitive stimulation test should not be considered diagnostic in patients suspected of MG.

1 **Myasthenia gravis**
  - A decremental response with a slow repetitive stimulation test is reported in approximately 70% of patients with MG.
  - Characteristically, there is a reproducible decrement of more than 10% of the compound muscle action potential (CMAP) with evidence of post-exercise facilitation.
2 Any severe denervating process, amyotrophic lateral sclerosis
3 Myotonic disorders
4 Eaton-Lambert syndrome
  - More typically shows an *incremental response* to rapid repetitive stimulation: indicative of a presynaptic impairment.
  - May show subtle decremental response to slow repetitive stimulation.
5 Congenital myasthenia
6 Botulism
  - Similar to Eaton-Lambert syndrome, shows an *incremental response* to rapid repetitive stimulation: indicative of a presynaptic impairment.
  - May show subtle decremental response to slow repetitive stimulation.
7 Severe myopathy

Nerve conduction studies: types of abnormality

- The most useful information from the analysis of the nerve conduction study is the conduction speed and the amplitude of the waveform. In general, the velocities are greater than 50 m/s in the upper extremity and greater than 40 m/s in the legs.
- While the maximal conduction velocity is the function of the largest nerve fibers that have the most myelin and longest internode length, amplitude reflects the total number of fibers stimulated and the synchronicity of the impulse.
- If the waveform is normal in appearance but low in amplitude, it usually suggests the primary axonal pathology. On the contrary, if the waveform is much broader and has several phases, it points towards demyelination resulting in dispersion and conduction block.

Motor nerve conduction study: types of abnormality

Abnormality	Interpretation
Slow motor nerve conduction velocity	Defect in myelin sheath Could be a result of cool limbs
Increased distal latency	Increased distal latency of the CMAP from the most distal site indicates slowing of conduction in the most distal portion

Continued

Abnormality	Interpretation
Conduction block	Segmental slowing of motor NCV May be related to nerve function or compression
Decreased amplitude or altered waveform of the CMAP	Axonal dropout Damage to myelin can disperse waveform
Relative slowing of motor NCV by comparing segments	Although the value may be normal, it is important to compare for discrepancy between the velocities of segments of the nerve

Sensory nerve conduction study: types of abnormality

Abnormality	Interpretation
Slow conduction (usually with increased distal latency)	Damage to the myelin and the process can be focal, such as entrapment or as part of peripheral neuropathy
Low amplitude	Difficult to interpret alone as the sensory amplitude is normally low. Need to consider the results together with conduction velocity and latency
Absent response	Suggests severe reduction of amplitude. However, it can be due to axonal or demyelinating processes

CMAP – compound muscle action potential, NCV – nerve conduction study.

Electrophysiologic differentiation between axonal and demyelinating neuropathy

- There are two major components in peripheral nerves: axon and myelin, reflecting two types of neuropathy, including axonal and demyelinating neuropathy.
- Differentiation between both types of neuropathy is critically important as it has major influences on differential diagnosis, evaluation, and treatment.
- In axonal neuropathy, the hallmark of abnormalities is the diminution of the amplitude of CMAP in the motor nerve conduction, and of the CNAP in the sensory and mixed nerve conduction in the presence of near-normal NCVs, and of normal shape and duration of the CMAP or CNAP.
- In demyelinating neuropathy, the major findings include conduction block, abnormal temporal dispersion, and marked slowing conduction velocity.

Parameters	Axonal neuropathy	Demyelinating neuropathy
Primary pathology	Axon	Myelin
Motor nerve conduction		
Amplitude	Decreased	Normal or slightly decreased
Duration	Normal	Dispersion
Shape	Normal	Multiphasic
Distal latency	Normal or slightly delayed	Marked delay (>150%)
Conduction velocity	Normal or slightly decreased (>30 m/s)	Marked decrease (<60%, <30 m/s)
Sensory nerve conduction		
Amplitude	Decreased or absent	Can be normal, decreased, or absent
Duration	Normal	Rarely dispersion
Shape	Normal	Rarely multiphasic
Conduction velocity	Normal or slightly decreased	Marked decrease (<60%)
F-wave	Moderate delay (100–150%) or absent	Marked delay (>150%) or absent
H-reflex	Moderate delay (100–150%) or absent	Marked delay (>150%) or absent
Needle EMG		
Fibrillation or positive sharp waves	Common	Absent or occasional
Fasciculation	Absent	Present in chronic form
Biopsy/pathology		
Teasing preparation	Myelin ovoids	Segmental demyelination
Regeneration process	Slow axonal sprouting	Remyelination

CMAP – compound muscle action potential, CNAP – compound nerve action potential.
Modified from: Oh S.J. *Principles of Clinical Electromyography*. Lippincott Williams & Wilkins, Philadelphia, 1998.

Lumbar puncture

- Cerebrospinal fluid can usually be obtained from the lumbar subarachnoid space via lumbar puncture (LP) or spinal tap. Normally, the procedure is carried out at the L3/L4 or L4/L5 interspace with the patient in the lateral decubitus position.
- Because the spinal cord in adults ends at the L1/L2 level, lumbar puncture can be performed below that level without the risk of injury to the spinal cord.
- The most common side-effect associated with lumbar puncture is post-LP headache. The risk is significantly decreased with the use of a small needle. It is controversial if bed rest is necessary after LP in order to prevent post-LP headache.
- The lists below give the common indications and contraindications for LP.

Indications:
- To confirm suspected central nervous system infection.
- To determine if there is hemorrhage within the CNS.
- To determine the chemical and immunologic profile in cases suspected for inflammation or demyelination.
- To obtain opening CSF pressure in cases suspected for pseudotumor cerebri.
- To perform as a diagnostic procedure to determine if patients have shunt-responsive hydrocephalus.
- To obtain cells for cytologic examination, for example, in cases suspected of carcinomatous meningitis.

Contraindications:
- In patients who may have increased intracranial pressure or are suspected of having intracranial space-occupying lesions, especially in the posterior fossa.
- Infection at the site of LP (the needle may introduce organisms into the underlying subarachnoid space).
- Suspicion of epidural abscess at the puncture site.
- Coagulation disorders, for example, thrombocytopenia, hemophilia, vitamin K deficiency, etc.

Routine CSF tests

CSF initial pressure: diagnostic values

- The initial CSF pressure is measured routinely with all diagnostic LPs.
- When dealing with the CSF pressure value, the clinical convention is to express the pressure either in terms of mm CSF or mm H_2O. The pressure level within the right atrium represents the reference zero level in measuring lumbar CSF pressure. The level of CSF pressure is affected greatly by postural influences on central venous pressure, and therefore patients should be positioned so that the cranioverbral axis is horizontal.
- A normal CT or MRI scan cannot exclude the presence of either an elevated or reduced intracranial pressure, especially when not associated with mass lesions.
- A normal lumbar CSF pressure is between 70 and 200 mm H_2O.

Elevated CSF pressure
1 Elevated CSF pressure necessary to establish the diagnosis
  - Pseudotumor cerebri
2 Conditions that are associated with elevated CSF pressure
  - Meningitis
  - Encephalitis

- Hepatic encephalopathy
- Post-anoxic encephalopathy
- Hyponatremia
- Water intoxication

Low CSF pressure
1 Low CSF pressure necessary to establish the diagnosis
- Positional headache with CSF fistula
- Spontaneous intracranial hypotension
2 Other causes of low CSF pressure
- Spinal subarachnoid block in patients with cord, conus or cauda equina syndrome

Intracranial hypotension

- The normal lumbar CSF pressure is between 60 and 200 mm H_2O. Intracranial hypotension is considered when the initial lumbar CSF pressure is below 60 mm H_2O.
- Symptoms of intracranial hypotension include:
  - Positional headache: the most characteristic symptom. Patients experience headache in the erect position, relieved by supine position.
  - Headache can also be precipitated by cough, straining, the Valsalva maneuver, or jugular venous compression.
  - Nausea, vomiting, dizziness.
  - Watery rhinorrhea, salty taste, or fullness in the ear: suggesting the location of CSF leaks.

1 **Technical error**
- Due to incomplete penetration of the subarchnoid space by the needle.
2 **CSF fistulae**
  2.1 **Previous lumbar puncture**
  - The most common cause of CSF fistula.
  - Persistent hole is created from previous LP, resulting in leakage of CSF into the subdural and extradural spaces.
  2.2 Neurosurgical procedures
  2.3 Trauma
  2.4 CSF rhinorrhea: post-traumatic, etc.
  2.5 CSF otorrhea: post-traumatic, etc.
3 Spontaneous intracranial hypotension (Schaltenbrand syndrome)
- This condition refers to the occurrence of the typical postural headache, insidious, subacute in onset, without prior head or spinal injury or lumbar puncture, due to a cryptic CSF leak.

- The condition is self-limited within a few weeks to months.
- It is the diagnosis of exclusion requiring the exclusion of the site of CSF leak.
- In some case reports, the sites of CSF leak were later identified with modern technology.

4 Spinal subarachnoid block
- Causes include tumor, disc, or arachnoiditis.

5 Severe dehydration
- Seen in infants, manifested by sunken fontanelle.

CSF findings in meningoencephalitis and hemorrhage

- The CSF examination is considered essential to establish the diagnosis, the cause, and the choice of treatment in patients with meningoencephalitis.
- In some cases, serial LPs may be needed in order to confirm or exclude certain diagnoses as well as guiding the therapy. Serial LPs are particularly important when the study includes cytologic examination as the positivity increases with repeated examinations.

Diagnosis	Pressure (mm H_2O)	Appearance	White blood cells (per mm³)	Protein (mg/dl)	Glucose (mg/dl)
Normal values	70–200	Clear, colorless	0–5 (0 PMNs, 5 monos)	20–45	60% of serum value
Acute bacterial	Elevated	Cloudy, turbid	100–20000 (mainly PMNs)	100–500	10–40
Acute viral	Normal to mildly elevated	Clear	5–500 (mainly lymphocytes)	Normal to slightly elevated (<100)	Normal except in mumps and HSV, CMV (25% decrease)
Tuberculous	Elevated	Yellowish, fibrin clot on standing	25–100 (mainly lymphocytes, PMNs in early stage)	100–200 (always elevated)	<40
Fungal	Elevated	Opalescent	30–800 (mainly lymphocytes)	50–700 (average 100)	<40
Acute syphilis	Elevated	Opalescent	100–800 (average 500, mainly lymphocytes)	100	Normal (rarely reduced)

Diagnosis	Pressure (mm H$_2$O)	Appearance	White blood cells (per mm^3)	Protein (mg/dl)	Glucose (mg/dl)
Cysticercosis	Elevated	Opalescent	100–200 (mainly mononuclear cells and lymphocytes, also 2–7% of eosinophils)	50–200	Reduced in 20%, others normal
Parameningeal infections (e.g. epidural abscess)	Elevated if spinal block	Clear	0–800, can be normal	>40	Normal
Carcinomatous	Normal or elevated	Clear or opalescent	0–several hundreds (mononuclear cells and malignant cells)	>40	Reduced
Neurosarcoidosis	Normal to low	Clear	0–fewer than 100 (mainly mononuclear cells)	Slightly elevated	Reduced in 50% of cases
Subarachnoid hemorrhage	Elevated	Bloody, xanthochromia	Increased RBCs early, followed by increased WBCs	50–800	Normal or reduced
Traumatic tap	Normal	Bloody but no xanthochromia	RBC:WBC ratio same as peripheral blood (reduced RBCs in successive tubes)	Slightly elevated	Normal

RBC – red blood cell, WBC – white blood cell, PMN – polymorphonuclear cells, monos – mononuclear cells, HSV – herpes simplex virus, CMV – cytomegalovirus.

Cloudy CSF

- The normal appearance of CSF is clear and colorless. In pathological conditions, the CSF may appear cloudy, bloody, purulent, or pigment-tinged. These appearances, if observed carefully with the naked eye, may reveal or suggest an underlying diagnosis.
- The turbidity of CSF can be graded from 0 to 4+.
  0 = crystal clear fluid
  1+ = faintly hazy
  2+ = turbidity, clearly present, but newsprint can be read through the tube
  3+ = newsprint is not easily read through the tube
  4+ = newsprint cannot be seen through the tube
- The Tyndall effect refers to the physical property of suspended particles that scatter ambient light. Normally, spinal fluid appears clear and colorless until there are approximately 400 cells/mm^3. By observing CSF by flicking the tube sample under direct sunlight with the tube viewed against a darker background, the presence of cells in the CSF may be recognized when only 50 cells/mm^3 are present.

CSF appearances	Particles
Bloody CSF	RBCs of at least 6000 cells/mm³
Xanthochromia CSF, pink-tinged	RBCs of between 500–6000 cells/mm³
Hazy, opalescent	Pleocytosis
	RBCs > 400 cells/mm³
	WBCs > 200 cells/mm³
Greenish tinged	Purulent fluid
	Empyema
Oily emulsion	After the intrathecal injection of iophendylate (Pantopaque)
Sudanophilic globules	Fat embolism

RBCs – red blood cells, WBCs – white blood cells.

Elevated CSF glucose

- An increase in CSF glucose is of no diagnostic significance apart from reflecting the presence of hyperglycemia within 4 hours prior to the LP.
- With increasing blood glucose, the CSF glucose is secondarily elevated, but to a lesser degree than in the blood. This observation is clinically important as hyperglycemia may mask the occurrence of relatively low CSF glucose, which is indicative of bacterial meningitis.

Elevated CSF glucose can be seen in:
1 Premature infants and newborns
  - The CSF:blood glucose ratio may be as high as 0.8.
  - The mechanism is still unclear.
2 Hyperglycemia states

Low CSF glucose (hypoglycorrhachia)

- The CSF glucose is derived solely from the plasma and its concentration is dependent upon the blood level as well as the rate of glucose metabolism by the brain.
- The CSF:blood glucose ratio is about 0.6. Therefore, the normal CSF glucose is usually between 45 and 80 mg/dl when a blood glucose is between 70 and 120 mg/dl. Values below 40 mg/dl are considered abnormally low.

1 **Infections of the CNS**
  - Commonly seen in bacterial, tuberculous, and fungal infections, particularly meningitides.
  - The level can be as low as 5 mg/dl in purulent bacterial meningitis, but is usually in the range between 20 and 40 mg/dl.

- Viral infections do not usually cause low CSF glucose except in acute mumps meningoencephalitis, where low CSF glucose can be seen in 25% of cases.
- CSF glucose is not low in neurosyphilis, especially in acute syphilitic meningitis.

2 **Carcinomatous meningitis**
  - Examples include lymphoma, leukemia, metastasis carcinomas, and melanoma.
3 Inflammatory disorder of the CNS
  - Examples include sarcoidosis, vasculitis, and granulomatous infiltrations of the meninges.
4 Subarachnoid hemorrhage
  - The maximal fall of CSF glucose is in between the first and sixth day after hemorrhage, and it depends on the extent of rebleeding.

Elevated CSF protein

- Almost all the proteins normally present in CSF are derived from the serum, with the exception of the beta and gamma trace proteins, tau protein, myelin basic protein, and glial fibrillary acidic protein, which appear to originate from the brain itself.
- An increase in the CSF protein is the single most useful change in the chemical composition of the fluid. However, it serves as a nonspecific indicator of disease.
- Causes of elevated CSF protein vary depending upon the degree of protein elevation in the CSF. While a slight increase in protein content (45–75 mg/dl) is common in many diseases, a very large increase in CSF protein (500–3600 mg/dl) suggests a few certain diagnoses. Therefore, the degree of increased CSF·protein is a useful laboratory value to help confirm or exclude certain neurological disorders.
- When a high CSF protein is obtained, which is unexpected and unexplained, physicians should consider the possibility of myxedema, neurofibroma in the subarachnoid space, and radiculoneuropathy.

1 Mildly increased CSF protein (45–75 mg/dl)
  - A slight increase in CSF protein is relatively common in many diseases. Although it does not suggest any specific disorder, it is characteristic of disorders associated with vasogenic brain edema and increased permeability of the blood-brain barrier.
  - Examples include meningitis, multiple sclerosis, epilepsy, brain tumors, neurosyphilis, and brain trauma
2 Moderately increased CSF protein (75–500 mg/dl)
  - Different pathological processes affecting central and peripheral nervous system can result in moderately high CSF protein.

- Common causes include:
  - 2.1 Infectious causes
    - Bacterial meningitis
    - Tuberculous meningitis (usually >100 mg/dl)
    - Brain abscess
    - Neurosyphilis
  - 2.2 Inflammatory disorders
    - Aseptic meningitis
    - Polyneuritis
  - 2.3 Metabolic disorders
    - Myxedema
    - Uremia
    - Alcoholism
3 Greatly increased CSF protein (>500 mg/dl)
  - The elevated CSF protein of >500 mg/dl is infrequent.
  - When this level is obtained, a few possible diagnoses should be considered:
    - Spinal block due to cord tumors
    - Arachnoiditis
    - Subarachnoid hemorrhage
    - Some cases of purulent meningitis and tuberculous meningitis

Low CSF protein

- Protein level in lumbar CSF between 3 and 20 mg/dl is considered below the normal range.
- The possible mechanism resulting in low CSF protein involves an increased rate of protein removal to the venous system.
- Patients with severe hypoporteinemia or malnutrition do not have low CSF protein.

1 **CSF leaks**
  - CSF extradural leaks occurring following LP can result in mildly low CSF protein in some cases.
  - Usually associated with post-LP headache.
2 **Removal of a large CSF volume**
  - For example, for cytologic study.
3 Pseudotumor cerebri or benign intracranial hypertension
  - About one-third of patients with pseudotumor cerebri have low CSF protein.
4 Acute water intoxication
  - Patients with acute water intoxication may have increased intracranial pressure resulting in low CSF protein.

5 Others
  * Normal young children aged between 6 months and 2 years.
  * Hyperthyroidism, with a return to normal average level after therapy.
  * Leukemias (no clear explanation).

CSF eosinophilia

* Eosinophils are not generally seen in normal fluids, although a single cell can be seen occasionally with a normal total cell count using the cytocentrifuge.
* The most common cause of a prominent CSF eosinophilia (usually 5–10%) is parasitic disease. Inflammatory diseases account for the second most common cause of CSF eosinophilia, although the eosinophilia is usually of a lesser degree (2–4%).

1 **Parasitic diseases**
  * Cysticercosis
  * Trichinosis
  * Toxocara cati
  * Angylostrongylus cantonensis
  * Gnathostoma spinigerum
  * Larva migrans
2 **Inflammatory disorders**
  * Tuberculous meningitis
  * Neurosyphilis
  * Subacute sclerosing panencephalitis
  * Chemical meningitis, for example, following myelography, pneumoencephalography, subarachnoid hemorrhage, intrathecal administration of radioiodinated serum albumin and penicillin
3 Others
  * Tumors, e.g. Hodgkin disease
  * Obstructive hydrocephalus with shunt
  * Allergic reaction to medications, e.g. penicillin

Specialized CSF tests

CSF oligoclonal bands

* The use of a variety of supporting media, including agarose gels and polyacrylamide gels, for the electrophoretic separation provides a visual separation of homogeneous immunoglobulins as bands when stained appropriately.

- Three patterns of bands can be observed in the gamma region: monoclonal, polyclonal, and oligoclonal (a few, 2–5 bands).
- The oligoclonal bands imply that each band represents a homogeneous protein secreted by a single clone of plasma cells. A single oligoclonal band is commonly seen in otherwise normal CSF of normal subjects. However, two or more bands are considered abnormal and their presence usually suggests an immune-mediated process in the CNS.

Oligoclonal bands are commonly seen in the following neurological conditions:
1 **Multiple sclerosis (MS)**
   - Oligoclonal bands are seen in 83–94% of patients with definite MS.
2 Subacute sclerosing panencephalitis (SSPE)
   - Oligoclonal bands are present in 100% of patients with SSPE.
3 CNS infections
   - 50% of patients with bacterial, viral, fungal, or spirochetal CNS infections have oligoclonal bands in the CSF.
4 CNS inflammatory disorders (the percentage of positive CSF oligoclonal bands in these conditions vary).
   - CNS vasculitis
   - Neurosarcoidosis
   - CNS lupus
   - Guillain-Barré syndrome (GBS)
   - Behçet disease

Elevated CSF myelin basic protein

- Myelin basic protein (MBP) is a product of oligodendroglia. It is an antigen in the induction of experimental allergic encephalomyelitis (EAE). When there is damage of the CNS, MBP or its peptides, which represent an important part of the myelin, can appear in the cerebrospinal fluid (CSF), blood, and urine.
- Its concentration in normal CSF is very low, <0.4 mg/dl.
- While it is suggested that elevated CSF MBP may be an indicator for multiple sclerosis, elevated CSF MBP has been found in many other conditions that cause nonspecific myelin breakdown, as listed below, suggesting that it has limited diagnostic usefulness. Therefore, elevated CSF MBP should not be used as a sole criterion in the diagnosis of multiple sclerosis.
- According to McDonald diagnostic criteria for multiple sclerosis, positive CSF defines the presence of oligoclonal bands or a raised IgG index, not by the presence of MBP. CSF MBP cannot serve as a reliable marker of activity in multiple sclerosis.

The list below only includes the common causes of elevated CSF MBP.

1 **Demyelination/multiple sclerosis**
   - Approximately only 20% of MS patients have elevated CSF MBP.
   - Specific correlations have not been established between the CSF IgG level, the presence of oligoclonal bands, the MBP concentration, and the antibody response to MBP.
2 **Stroke**: resulting in very high CSF MBP
3 **Trauma**: resulting in very high CSF MBP
4 Tumors
5 CNS infections
6 Polyneuropathies
7 Dementias
8 Leukodystrophies

CSF 14-3-3 protein

- The 14-3-3 protein is a normal neuronal protein that is released into CSF in association with acute neuronal injury. The 14-3-3 proteins are part of a family of regulatory molecules, located predominantly in the cytoplasm. These proteins are found in large quantities in the cerebral tissue and are involved in several key regulatory processes, including cellular death and apoptosis. Therefore, it is a nonspecific marker for extensive neuronal injury.
- Although it has been suggested that the presence of 14-3-3 protein in CSF is a reliable marker for sporadic Creutzfeldt-Jakob disease (sCJD) and the World Heath Organization and American Academy of Neurology have recommended the use of this test to either confirm or exclude an sCJD diagnosis under appropriate clinical circumstances, more recent studies have found only modestly positive sensitivity in sCJD and reported more false-positive conditions. False-negative results can also occur.
- It is recommended that the CSF 14-3-3 protein test be ordered in patients who have a high degree of clinical suspicion of sCJD. The negative test result does not always rule out the diagnosis of sCJD. The presence of the CSF 14-3-3 protein in an appropriate clinical context reinforces the sCJD clinical diagnosis but may not be able to differentiate sCJD from other causes of rapidly progressive dementia.

Conditions that may result in positive CSF 14-3-3 protein

1 **Sporadic Creutzfeldt-Jakob disease**
   - Sensitivity varies from 53% to 96%, depending on studies.
   - The test is less sensitive in patients with variant CJD, but high specificity means that the detection of CSF 14-3-3 in a patient with suspected vCJD has a high positive predictive value.

- The value of CSF 14-3-3 in GH-related iatrogenic CJD depends on the clinical stage of the disease, being highly sensitive in a later stage.
2 Meningoencephalitis
3 Dementias
   - Multi-infarct dementia
   - Dementia of Alzheimer disease
   - Diffuse Lewy body disease dementia
4 Cerebral neoplasms
5 Various causes of encephalopathy
6 Anoxic brain damage
7 Down syndrome
8 Paraneoplastic syndromes
9 Transverse myelitis

CSF angiotensin-converting enzyme (CSF ACE)

- Angiotensin-converting enzyme (ACE) catalyzes the formation of angiotensin II by cleaving the C-terminal histidylleucine dipeptide from angiotensin I.
- The indications are that ACE is involved in an autonomous renin-angiotensin system of the brain that participates in physiologic processes inside the brain. Since ACE is produced by the epitheloid cells of the sarcoid granulomas, it is implicated as a test for both systemic sarcoidosis and neurosarcoidosis. However, ACE concentration in the CSF can be high and low in various other conditions.
- Elevated levels of serum or CSF ACE are not specific for neurosarcoidosis.

Various neurological conditions are associated with altered levels of CSF ACE.
- Elevated CSF ACE
   - **Neurosarcoidosis** (55%)
   - Systemic sarcoidosis (5%)
   - Guillain-Barré syndrome
   - Bacterial and viral meningitis
   - Brain tumors
   - Behçet disease
- Decreased CSF ACE
   - Alzheimer disease
   - Parkinson disease
   - Progressive supranuclear palsy

Blood/serum tests

Autoantibodies in neurological disorders

- Many autoantibodies are useful in clinical diagnosis of many neurological disorders that may be autoimmune in origin. These include many inflammatory disorders, vasculitides, neuropathies, myopathies, myasthenia gravis, and paraneoplastic syndromes.
- However, the diagnosis of autoimmune disorders should not be made solely on the positivity of the test. False-positive results do occur with many autoantibodies. In addition, the significance of each antibody also depends on the titer level as well as clinical presentations. Most of the time, additional tests are required in conjunction with relevant autoantibodies before a final diagnosis can be made.

Autoantibodies	Suggested clinical diagnosis
Rheumatoid factor	This test is rather nonspecific but sensitive (90%) in rheumatoid arthritis
ANA	Nonspecific (high titer may suggest the presence of autoimmune disorders, >90% of SLE patients have a high ANA titer)
Double-stranded DNA (peripheral pattern)	SLE Active renal diseases
Single-stranded DNA (peripheral pattern)	Sensitive for SLE but nonspecific
Antihistone (homogeneous pattern)	Drug-induced lupus SLE
Anti-Sm (speckled pattern)	Specific for SLE, renal and CNS disorders
Anti-RNP (speckled pattern)	Polymyositis with MCTD SLE Scleroderma Sjögren syndrome
Anti-Jo-1	Polymyositis with interstitial lung disease
Anti-PM-Scl	Polymyositis with scleroderma
Anti-Ro (SSA)	SLE Sjögren syndrome
Anti-La (SSB)	Primary Sjögren syndrome
cANCA	Wegener granulomatosis Microscopic periarteritis

Continued

Autoantibodies	Suggested clinical diagnosis
pANCA	Polyarteritis nodosa Glomerulonephritis
Anti-Scl-70 ANA (nucleolar pattern)	Progressive systemic sclerosis (anti-Scl-70 is specific but insensitive)
Antiphospholipid	SLE Systemic autoimmune disorders
Ach receptor Anti-striated	Myasthenia gravis
VGCC	Lambert-Eaton syndrome
Anti-GM$_1$ ganglioside	Lower motor neuron syndrome that resembles amyotrophic lateral sclerosis
Anti GAD	Stiff man syndrome IDDM Cerebellar ataxias Rarely – epilepsy

ANA – antinuclear antibody, SLE – systemic lupus erythematosus, MCTD – mixed connective tissue disease, cANCA – anti-neutrophilic cytoplasmic antibody, cytoplasmic pattern, pANCA – anti-neutrophilic cytoplasmic antibody, perinuclear pattern, RNP – ribonuclear protein, VGCC – voltage-gated calcium channel, GAD – glutamic acid decarboxylase.

Clinical indications for chromosomal analysis in pediatrics

- Abnormalities in chromosome structure or number are the single most common cause of severe mental retardation, but they still comprise only one-third of total causes.
- Abnormalities of autosomal chromosomes are frequently associated with infantile hypotonia.
- Clinical features that suggest chromosomal aberrations are listed below. These features, *when present in combination with global developmental delay*, should lead the clinician to consider genetic analysis in these patients and/or their families.

1 Head and neck abnormalities
   - Hypertelorism or hypotelorism
   - High nasal bridge
   - Microphthalmia
   - Mongoloid slant (especially in non-Asians)
   - Occipital scalp defect
   - Small mandible
   - Small or fish mouth (hard to open)

- ◆ Small or low-set ear
- ◆ Upward slant of eyes
- ◆ Webbed neck
2 Limb abnormalities
  - ◆ Abnormal dermatoglyphics
  - ◆ Low-set thumb
  - ◆ Overlapping fingers
  - ◆ Polydactyly
  - ◆ Radial hypoplasia
  - ◆ Rocker-bottom feet
3 Genitourinary abnormalities
  - ◆ Ambiguous genitalia
  - ◆ Polycystic kidney

(Ref: Fenichel GM. *Clinical Pediatric Neurology*, 4th edition, 2001. Philadelphia, WB. Saunders.)

Ceruloplasmin

- Ceruloplasmin is an acute phase protein. It is a ferroxidase that has an essential role in iron metabolism and contains greater than 95% of the plasma copper.
- Because ceruloplasmin accounts for 95% of the serum copper, measurement of this value will also be abnormally low in patients with Wilson disease (usually <20 mg/dl, and a level >35 mg/dl almost excludes the diagnosis). On the contrary, the low level of ceruloplasmin can also be seen in the conditions listed below.
- Therefore, the diagnosis of Wilson disease cannot be based solely on the low level of ceruplasmin.
- A separate condition, aceruloplasminemia, is an inherited disorder of iron metabolism caused by the complete lack of ceruloplasmin ferroxidase activity caused by mutations in the ceruloplasmin gene. It is characterized by iron accumulation in the brain as well as visceral organs. Clinically, the disease consists of the triad of adult-onset neurologic disease, retinal degeneration, and diabetes mellitus. The neurological symptoms, which include involuntary movements, ataxia, and dementia, reflect the sites of iron deposition.

The following conditions can cause false-positive low ceruloplasmin:
1 **Hypoproteinemic states**
  - ◆ Nephrotic syndrome
  - ◆ Protein-losing enteropathy

- Malabsorption
- Other causes of malnutrition
2 Others
- Menkes disease

Copper studies: diagnostic values in Wilson disease

- Wilson disease is a rare disorder of copper metabolism that results in an accumulation of copper in the liver and subsequently in other organs, mainly the central nervous system and the kidneys.
- The myriad manifestations of Wilson disease, ranging from psychiatric illness to any types of movement disorders, make its diagnosis dependent on a high index of suspicion. For neurologists, the diagnosis of Wilson disease should be entertained in any patients under 40 years of age with any types of movement disorders, psychiatric symptoms with liver disease, or mood disorders with minor elevations of liver enzymes. If treated promptly, neurological complications may be reversible.
- The measurement of hepatic copper by liver biopsy is considered as a gold standard, and is the most definitive test available for the diagnosis of Wilson disease. Serum ceruloplasmin is a useful screening test in suspected individuals.

Test ordered	Typical result in Wilson disease	False 'negative'	False 'positive'
Serum ceruloplasmin	Decreased (<20 mg/dl)	Normal levels in liver inflammation, pregnancy, estrogen, hyperthyroidism, and myocardial infarction	Low levels in hypoproteinemic states, heterozygotes, and aceruloplasminemia
24-hour urinary copper	>100 μg/day	Incorrect collection, children without liver disease	Cholestasis
Hepatic copper	>250 μg/g dry weight	In patients with active liver disease or with regenerative nodules	Cholestasis
Kayser-Fleischer rings by slit-lamp examination	Present	In up to 60% of patients with hepatic Wilson disease and in most asymptomatic siblings	Primary biliary cirrhosis

Ref: Modified from Ferenci P. Review article: diagnosis and current therapy of Wilson disease. *Aliment Pharmacol Ther* 2004; 19: 157–165.

Marked elevation of serum creatine kinase: neurological causes

- Sustained serum creatine kinase (CK) elevation is often due to myopathies, less commonly with neurogenic disorders.
- CK-MM is the predominant isoenzyme in myopathies. There are many factors involved in the elevation of CK enzyme including:
  - Severity of disease
  - Course of disease
  - Available muscle mass
  - Myofiber necrosis: is the major factor in CK elevation
- Idiopathic hyperCKemia is defined as persistent elevation of serum CK levels of skeletal muscle origin without clinical manifestations of weakness, abnormal neurological examination, EMG, or muscle biopsy. With the advances of genetic tests, it is likely that more patients with this condition will have a defined neuromuscular disease or carrier state of such a disease.

1 **Dystrophinopathies**
  - Associated with the highest recorded CK serum concentration
  - Examples include Duchenne and Becker muscular dystrophy (DMD, BMD)
2 Rhabdomyolysis and myoglobinuria
3 Malignant hyperthermia (only during attack)
4 Neuroleptic malignant syndrome
5 Polymyositis, dermatomyositis
6 Myoshi distal myopathy (dysferlin mutation, AR transmission)

Dystrophin test

- Dystrophin, in normal cells, stabilizes the glycoprotein complex and protects it from degradation. In the absence of dystrophin, the complex becomes unstable.
- Dystrophin can be detected on immunoblots of 100 µg of total muscle protein derived from a small portion of a muscle biopsy by using antidystrophin antibodies.
- If the 427 kDa dystrophin is normal in size and amount, the diagnosis of DMD or BMD can almost be excluded. More than 99% of DMD patients display complete or almost complete absence of dystrophin in skeletal muscle biopsy specimens. Most BMD patients have dystrophin of abnormal molecular weight, which is often low in quantity.
- The test is very specific as patients with other neuromuscular disorders (other than DMD or BMD) have normal dystrophin.
- The quantity of the dystrophin molecule, rather than its size, correlates with the severity of the disease. Therefore, this test can be used to predict the severity of the evolving muscular dystrophy phenotype.

Muscular dystrophy	Dystrophin quantity by Western blot analysis	Dystrophin protein size by Western blot analysis
DMD	0–5%	Normal or abnormal size
Intermediate or severe BMD	5–20%	Normal or abnormal size
Mild or moderate BMD	20–50%	Normal size
	20–100%	Abnormal size

DMD – Duchenne muscular dystrophy, BMD – Becker muscular dystrophy.
Ref: Darras B.T. Muscular dystrophies, In Samuels M.A., Feske S.K. *Office Practice of Neurology*, 2nd edition. 2003, Churchill Livingstone.

Genetic diagnostic tests in autosomal dominant ataxias

- Genetic analysis in patients with autosomal dominant ataxias should be directed according to the frequency of genetic subtypes in the relevant ethnic background and predominant clinical features. For example, in the USA, SCA3 accounts for approximately 20% of cases, while SCA2 and SCA6 each represent 15% of patients with ADCA. About a third of families with ADCA are genetically undefined. On the contrary, DRPLA accounts for approximately 8% of ADCA cases in Japan.
- Because of the huge phenotypic variability of most SCA subtypes, testing for all known genes may be considered in families with rare phenotypes.
- The table below provides as a brief guide for efficient genetic diagnostic tests based on predominant clinical signs. Additional tests should be considered according to the level of clinical suspicion.

Main clinical signs	First line genetic test	Second line genetic test
Pure cerebellar ataxia	SCA6 > SCA5	SCA11, SCA14, SCA15, SCA16, SCA22
Parkinsonism	SCA2, SCA3, SCA12	SCA21
Dystonia	SCA3	
Slow saccades	SCA2	SCA1, SCA3, SCA7, SCA17
Pigmentary retinopathy	SCA7	
Tremor	SCA2, SCA8, SCA12	SCA16, SCA21
Chorea	DRPLA, SCA17	SCA1 (late stage)
Myoclonus	DRPLA	SCA2, SCA19
Dementia	DRPLA, SCA17	SCA2, SCA3, SCA19, SCA21
Psychosis	DRPLA, SCA17	SCA3, FGF14
Peripheral neuropathy	SCA3, SCA4, SCA18, SCA25	SCA1

ADCA – autosomal dominant cerebellar ataxia, SCA – spinocerebellar ataxia, DRPLA – dentatorubral-pallidoluysian atrophy, FGF14 – fibroblast growth factor 14.
Modified from: Schöls L., Bauer P., Schmidt T., Schulte T., Riess O. Autosomal dominant cerebellar ataxias: clinical features, genetics and pathogenesis. *Lancet Neurology* 2004; 3: 291–304.

Serologic tests for Lyme disease

- Culture of B. burgdorferi is difficult and not useful for routine diagnosis of Lyme disease. Therefore, the diagnosis very much depends on the presence of serologic tests in the appropriate clinical setting.
- Screening for Lyme disease is usually performed with ELISA for IgG, although the sensitivity is poor, especially for the first few weeks. Enzyme immunoassay for IgM has been used early in the diseases.
- There is significant cross-reactivity of ELISA tests with other antigens. Therefore, false-positive results do occur with other inflammatory diseases.
- Western blotting is recommended to confirm the diagnosis of Lyme disease with the claimed specificity of 100%.
- Positive serologic tests alone do not indicate that patients have active Lyme infection and it can persist long after successful treatment or exposure.

Timing	Tests	Sensitivity	Specificity
Early Lyme disease	IgM ELISA	40%	94%
	IgM Western blot	32%	**100%**
Lyme disease after a few weeks	IgG ELISA	89%	72%
	IgG Western blot	83%	95%

Ref: Dressler F., Whalen J.A., Reinhardt B.N., Steere A.C. Western blotting in the serodiagnosis of Lyme disease. *J Infect Dis* 1993; 167: 398.

Muscular dystrophy tests

- The muscular dystrophies are progressive, hereditary degenerative diseases of striated muscles. They affect primarily the muscle fibers and leave the spinal motor neurons, muscular nerves, and nerve endings intact.
- The main symptom and sign of muscular dystrophies is weakness, which is usually progressive.
- In the past, the diagnosis of muscular dystrophies was based on myopathic symptoms and signs, CK levels, myopathic changes on EMG, and muscle biopsies, and sometimes a positive family history. Until a few years ago, cloning of defective genes as well as the characterization of protein products have provided a molecular diagnostic tool for accurate diagnosis of this disorder.

Test name	Assays	Phenotypes
Dystrophin test	Dystrophin protein in muscle	Male children exhibiting high serum CK, toe walking, Gower sign, pseudohypertrophy of calf and tongue muscles, and muscle wasting
Duchenne/Becker muscular dystrophy DNA deletion test (males only)	Deletions in dystrophin (65% in DMD, 85% in BMD)	Male children showing high CK, toe walking, Gower sign, pseudohypertrophy of calf and tongue muscles, and muscle wasting
Duchenne/Becker muscular dystrophy DNA carrier test (females only)	Deletions in dystrophin	At-risk female relatives of males with confirmed DMD or BMD diagnosis
Complete myotonic dystrophy evaluation	CTG expansions in DM1 and CCTG expansions in DM2	Adults may present with cataract, myotonia, ptosis, and muscle wasting, while infants may present with severe hypotonia, skeletal deformities, and respiratory insufficiency
DM1 DNA test	CTG expansions in DM1 (> 100 repeats in full mutation)	As above, with a known family history of DM1
DM2 DNA test	CCTG expansions	As above, but without the infantile form, or with a known family history of mutations in DM2
FSHD DNA test	FSHD deletion on chromosome 4q35	Slowly progressive asymmetric wasting of the muscles of face, shoulder, and upper arms
OPMD DNA test	GCG expansions in PABP2, linked to chromosome 14q11	Late-onset weakness and wasting of the facial muscles with ophthalmoplegia and ptosis
LGMD evaluation	Dysferlin (Western blot) FKRP (DNA sequencing)	Face-sparing, proximal > distal progressive myopathy with elevated CK. Age of onset ranges from infancy to late adulthood. May also involve cardiac and respiratory muscles
Dysferlin blood test	Dysferlin protein in blood	Includes LGMD2B, Miyoshi, distal anterior compartment, and scapuloperoneal myopathies. These distinctions are usually identifiable only at disease onset and may appear very similar and as described above, as the disease progresses
FKRP DNA sequencing test	FKRP DNA sequencing	Includes a severe form termed MDC1C and a milder form termed LGMD2I. MDC1C may cause loss of ambulation by teenage years, while LGMD2I is relatively benign

DMD – Duchenne muscular dystrophy, BMD – Becker muscular dystrophy, DM – myotonic dystrophy, FSHD – facioscapulohumeral muscular dystrophy, OPMD – oculopharyngeal muscular dystrophy, PABP-2 – poly-A binding protein 2, LGMD – limb-girdle muscular dystrophies, FKRP – fukutin-related protein gene, MDC1C – congenital muscular dystrophy 1C.
Ref: Athena diagnostic, Inc. Worcester, MA, USA.

Serological tests for neurosyphilis

- In immunocompetent patients, the clinical manifestations of neurosyphilis include:
  1 Asymptomatic neurosyphilis
  2 Meningitis
  3 Meningovascular syphilis
  4 Dementia paralytica
  5 Tabes dorsalis
- The diagnosis of neurosyphilis depends on the clinical manifestations as above, along with CSF findings. CSF abnormalities usually consist of mild mononuclear pleocytosis, mild protein elevation, and normal glucose and a positive CSF VDRL.
- It is important to be aware that a nonreactive CSF VDRL does not rule out neurosyphilis.
- After successful treatment, we expect that the serum VDRL titer should decrease, but that the serum FTA-ABS and MHA-TP should remain reactive for life.

1 Nonspecific nontreponemal globulin complex
  - The tests depend upon the combination of reagin in the patient's serum with an antigen composed of a suspension of cardiolipin activated by the addition of cholesterol and lecithin.
    1.1 Venereal Disease Research Laboratory (VDRL)
      - The presence of a positive VDRL in CSF implies that there is evidence of either asymptomatic or symptomatic neurosyphilis. The exception is that a positive CSF VDRL may be observed in purulent meningitis, which allows serum regain across the blood-brain barrier in sufficient concentration.
      - **The CSF-VDRL is nonreactive in 30–57% of patients with neurosyphilis. Therefore, a nonreactive result does not exclude the diagnosis.**
    1.2 Rapid plasma regain (RPR)
      - Now widely used for screening as it is more sensitive than VDRL.
      - Not suitable for CSF analysis.
2 Specific treponemal antibody tests
    2.1 Fluorescent treponemal antibody absorption (FTA-ABS)
    2.2 Microhemagglutination assay for treponemal antibody (MHA-TP)
  - There is little rationale to perform FTA-ABS or MHA-TP on the CSF because both tests depend upon the presence of circulating IgG from the serum. Therefore, the antibody present in CSF only represents a diluted serum sample.

Other clinical tests

Autonomic dysfunction: clinical tests

- Different clinical tests have been utilized to assess patients with autonomic dysfunction. The tests mainly evaluate cardiovascular and thermoregulatory functions.
- In cardiovascular circuits, baroreceptor dysfunction may produce severe hypertension, arterial pressure fluctuations, or syncope. Lesions of the cardiovascular regulatory centers, descending vasomotor pathways, or peripheral sympathetic fibers produce orthostatic hypotension.
- For thermoregulatory function, sympathetic denervation may produce warm, dry skin, while sympathetic overactivity can cause coldness and sweating. Diffuse sudomotor failure may cause heat intolerance.

Tests	Central sympathetic dysfunction	Peripheral sympathetic dysfunction	Vagal dysfunction
Head tilt test: • Blood pressure	Orthostatic hypotension	Orthostatic hypotension	Variable
Head tilt test: • Heart rate	No increase	No increase	No increase
Heart rate fluctuations during deep breathing or respiratory sinus arrhythmia	Presence	Presence	Absent
Valsalva maneuver (voluntary expiration against resistance)	Abnormal	Abnormal	Abnormal
Thermoregulatory sweat test (measuring sudomotor response to increased body temperature)	Abnormal	Abnormal	Normal
Acetylcholine sudomotor reflex test (stimulating sympathetic sudomotor receptors by application of acetylcholine)	Normal	Abnormal	Normal

Modified from: Benarroch E.E., Wastmoreland B.F., Daube J.R., Reagan T.J., Sandok B.A. *Medical Neurosciences*.1999, Philadelphia, Lippincott Williams & Wilkins.

Tensilon or edrophonium test

- Tensilon or edrophonium hydrochloride is a short-acting acetylcholinesterase inhibitor.

- When performing a tensilon test, a double-blind study is preferable, and it is most useful when there is an obvious objective clinical parameter to monitor the improvement, for example, the degree of ptosis and extraocular muscle weakness.
- Although tensilon is considered to be a safe test, care must be exercised in all patients, particularly the elderly. Bradycardia, hypotension, tearing, flushing, gastrointestinal cramps are common adverse effects and they are transient. Atropine should be available to counteract side-effects if needed.
- Although the improvement in strength after intravenous injection of edrophonium is the hallmark of postsynaptic neuromuscular transmission disorders, particularly myasthenia gravis, positive results have been reported in many other conditions. False-negative tests are relatively common and repeated tests are of value.

The following conditions may have a positive response to the edrophonium test:
1 **Myasthenia gravis**
   - The sensitivity is estimated to be 86% in ocular and 95% in generalized MG. The specificity is much more difficult to estimate but is likely to be higher in generalized disease.
2 Other disorders of neuromuscular transmission
   - Eaton-Lambert syndrome
   - Botulism
   - Congenital myasthenia
   - Snake envenomation
3 Motor neuron disease
4 Others
   - Guillain-Barré syndrome
   - Brainstem gliomas
   - Multiple sclerosis
   - Pituitary tumors
   - Compressive aneurysm

Urodynamic findings on neurogenic bladder

- Cystometry is an investigation that should be considered in the work-up of patients with incontinence or voiding difficulties resulting from neurologic causes. It provides information about the pressure-volume relationship on filling (bladder compliance), bladder capacity, volume at first sensation and at urge to void, voiding pressure, and the presence of uninhibited detrusor contractions.

- A micturition cystourethrogram (MCUG) is often combined with cystometry. It can visualize the position, opening of the bladder neck, sphincter dyssynergia as well as ureteric reflux.
- In a normal adult, the bladder can usually be filled with 500 ml of fluid without the pressure rising to more than 10 cm of water.

Features	Spastic bladder	Atonic (flaccid bladder)	Detrusor sphincter dyssynergia (often occurs with spastic bladder, DSD)
Urodynamic findings			
Bladder capacity	Decreased	Increased	Fluctuating capacity
Bladder compliance	Reduced	Increased	Fluctuating flow rate
Intravesical pressure	Increased	Decreased	
Symptoms and signs			
Incontinence	Yes	Yes	
Retention	No or late if combined with DSD	Yes	
Perianal sensation	Yes or diminished	No	
Anal or bulbocavernosus reflex	Yes	No	
Disease examples	Multiple sclerosis Trauma	Diabetes mellitus Radiculopathy Disc prolapse Pelvic injury	

Appendix A
Clinical Pearls

Medications

Emergency neurological medications

Status epilepticus

- Much current evidence supports a conservative definition of status epilepticus to prevent neuronal injury. The condition of status is characterized as a generalized tonic-clonic seizure lasting >5 minutes or multiple GTC seizures in a 24-hour period in which the patient does not return to baseline during the interictal period.
- Ensure ABCs, provide oxygen, airway protection, chem 7 panel, AED levels, drug (tox) screen.
- Always provide cardiac and blood pressure monitoring during drug loading. Hypotension is commonly seen with many of the drugs listed below.

Medication	Dose	Rate	Comments
Lorazepam	0.1 mg/kg	2 mg/min	Slower onset than diazepam, but prevents rebound seizure from volume redistribution which may occur with diazepam
Diazepam	0.4 mg/kg	IV push, max 30 mg	Initiate definitive therapy after IV load as volume redistribution out of CNS may lead to rebound seizures
Diazepam rectal gel	0.5 mg/kg	Per rectum	Especially useful for at home administration in pediatric population
Phenytoin	20 mg/kg	50 mg/min	Refer to phenytoin pearls for additional information. Do not administer with glucose solution as it will precipitate
Fosphenytoin	20 mg/kg	150 mg/min	Order as phenytoin equivalent. Much less toxicity than phenytoin
Phenobarbital	10–20 mg/kg	100 mg/min	Monitor respiratory depression, especially if preceded by benzodiazepines
Pentobarbital	5–20 mg/kg IV load over 1 hour	1–4 mg/kg/hr IV drip	May be utilized to induce coma in refractory cases. Titrate for burst suppression on EEG telemetry
Propofol	2 mg/kg IV push	2–10 mg/kg/hr IV drip	Titrate drip for burst suppression on EEG telemetry

Medication	Dose	Rate	Comments
Midazolam	0.1–0.3 mg/kg IV push	0.05–0.4 mg/kg/hr IV drip	Rapid action, short half-life, monitor for respiratory depression
Thiamine	100 mg	IV push	Always administer when there is suspicion of chronic ethanol use. Give prior to glucose
Glucose 50%	50 ml	IV push	Always give thiamine first if there is any suspicion of malnutrition or ethanol abuse. Give emergently in setting of hypoglycemia. Never co-administer with phenytoin

Cerebral edema

- Maintain ABCs.
- Use non-pharmacologic methods, including hyperventilation acutely as well as elevating head of bed.
- Ensure iso-/hyperosmolality with 3% NaCl (Na^+ >135, <150).
- Manage in consultation with neurosurgery.

Medication	Dose	Rate	Maintenance	Comments
Dexamethasone	10 mg	IV push	4 mg IV q6°	For edema associated with tumor or abscess
Mannitol	1.5 g/kg	Over 30 minutes	50–300 mg/kg IV q6°	Half-life ~100 minutes, osmotic effect in ~15 minutes, reduction in elevated ICP effect ~3–8 hours, monitor for electrolyte abnormalities, volume overload, and pulmonary edema

Acute stroke

- Maintain ABCs.
- Must establish symptom onset within 180 minutes of anticipated administration.
- Must rule out evidence for intracranial or subarachnoid hemorrhage.
- Absolute contraindications include: active bleeding, stroke, or intracranial/spinal surgery in past two months, intracranial neoplasm, aortic dissection, intracranial AVM or aneurysm, and seizure at stroke onset.

- Relative contraindications include: recent puncture of non-compressible vessel, surgery, or organ biopsy in past 10 days, serious GI bleed in last 3 months, serious trauma or CPR in past 10 days, diabetic proliferative retinopathy, anticoagulation, platelets <100,000, severe liver or renal disease, uncontrolled hypertension (SBP >185 or DBP >110) despite conservative control measures (topical NTG or labetolol up to 20 mg IV), bacterial endocarditis, 10 days postpartum period, or active menstruation.
- Tissue plasminogen activator (tPA):
  - Action: converts plasminogen to plasmin which degrades fibrin clots.
  - Half-life: 5–8 minutes, prolonged in liver failure.
  - Dosing: 0.9 mg/kg to a maximum of 90 mg. 10% total dose IV bolus over 1 minute, remaining 90% over 1 hour.
  - Follow-up: ICU monitoring, maintain blood pressure <185/110, no anticoagulant or antiplatelet therapy for 24 hours.
  - Reversal: in setting of hemorrhage, administer fresh frozen plasma and cryoprecipitate.

Spinal cord pathology

- Initiate therapy immediately upon suspicion of trauma or lesion.
- Obtain neurosurgical consultation.
- Immobilize patient in setting of possible traumatic injury.

Medication	Bolus dose	Bolus rate	Maintenance/rate
Spinal cord mass			
Dexamethasone	10 mg	IV push	4 mg IV q6°
Spinal cord trauma			
Methylprednisolone	30 mg/kg	IV push	5.4 mg/kg/hr for 24 hours

Drug overdose

- Commonly encountered drug overdoses in neurology include opiates and benzodiazepines.
- Pharmaceutical effects of these overdoses can be reversed, though typically only transiently. Reversal is often utilized for diagnostic purposes.
- Because reversal is often transient, primary management is supportive, including cardiovascular monitoring and respiratory support.

Medication	Dose	Max	Comments
Opiate overdose			
Naloxone	0.4–2 mg IV q2 min	10 mg	Monitor for hypertension, tachycardia, agitation, seizure
Benzodiazepine overdose			
Flumazenil	0.2mg IV over 30 s Repeat 0.5 mg IV over 30 s q1 min	3 mg	Monitor for withdrawal: including agitation, seizures, myoclonus. Sedation reversal may precede reversal of respiratory depression.

Malignant hyperthermia

- Autosomal dominantly inherited condition predisposing individuals to fever, rhabdomyolysis, muscle rigidity, and metabolic acidosis following exposure to inhaled anesthetics and succinyl choline.
- Co-treatment with antipyretics or external cooling, oxygen, and correction of acidosis.

Medication	Dose	Max	Maintenance	Comments
Dantrolene	1–2 mg/kg IV push Repeat as needed	10 mg/kg	1–4 mg/kg po qid for 3 days	Stop offending anesthetic

Anticoagulation

- Although controlled clinical trials do not support the use of anticoagulation in acute stroke therapy, most neurologists agree that it is appropriate to use them in the setting of stroke progression believed to be the result of clot propagation, in suspected/confirmed basilar artery stenosis/occlusion, suspected critical carotid stenosis, and ongoing cardioembolism.
- Appropriate anticoagulants in the setting of acute stroke include heparin, enoxaparin, and dalteparin.
- Long-term anticoagulation should be effected with warfarin. Refer to warfarin dosing guide (See pp. 517–18).
- Goal PTT is 45–65 seconds.
- PTT should be checked q4 hours after any dosing change.
- PTT should be checked q12 hours in all patients.
- Check CBC and platelets qd on all patients receiving anticoagulation.
- Provide all patients with GI prophylaxis (H2 blocker or proton pump inhibitor).

Medication	Circumstance	Dose/rate	Comments
Heparin	Bolus	50 U/kg (max 8000 U) IV push	Stroke progression or basilar stenosis only
	Initial infusion	15 U/kg/hr (max 2000 U/hr)	
	PTT <35 s	Increase by 3 U/kg/hr	
	PTT 35–44 s	Increase by 2 U/kg/hr	
	PTT 45–65 s	No change	
	PTT 66–90 s	Decrease by 2 U/kg/hr	
	PTT >90 s	Hold for 1 hr, then restart at rate decreased by 3 U/kg/hr	
Enoxaparin	Maintenance	1 mg/kg sq bid	
Dalteparin	Maintenance	120 U/kg sq bid	

Phenytoin pearls

- Despite the availability of many newer anticonvulsants, phenytoin remains one of the most commonly prescribed epilepsy medications. Useful features include: once-a-day dosing, easy level monitoring, prescriber familiarity, patient tolerance, good efficacy, many years of user data, easy loading both PO and IV.
- Due to its high protein binding (~90%), it is particularly useful in dialysis patients.
- It is prescribed for multiple seizure types, though usually for secondarily generalized seizures. It is contraindicated in absence seizures.
- Toxicity is heralded by nausea, emesis, diplopia, ataxia, slurred speech, and nystagmus.
- Excessively supratherapeutic levels may trigger seizures.
- When loading IV, strongly consider using fosphenytoin (ordered as phenytoin equivalents) as there is significantly lowered morbidity despite the higher cost.
- Remember that true therapeutic levels are those in which the patient is seizure free in the absence of toxic side-effects.
- Liver transaminases should be periodically monitored, especially after initial dosing.
- Women of child-bearing age should always be co-treated with folate.
- Long-term side-effects may include coarsening of facial features, hirsutism, and gingival hyperplasia.
- Phenytoin is metabolized via the cytochrome P450 oxidase system (CYP2C9 and CYP2C19 isoforms in particular). The metabolism is non-linear because the system is saturable. Therefore, small increases in phenytoin dosing may result in marked elevation of plasma levels. Saturation points are different for every individual, therefore care should be taken when increasing dosing above 5 mg/kg.

- Phenytoin acts as a sodium channel inhibitor.
- Due to saturable GI absorption, doses greater than 400 mg should be divided.

Typical serum therapeutic levels
- Total serum levels: 10–20 µg/ml
- Free serum levels: 1–2 µg/ml

Serum level correction for low albumin

$$\text{adjusted concentration} = \frac{\text{measured concentration}}{[(0.2 \times \text{albumin}) + 0.1]}$$

Serum level correction for patients with renal failure ($Cl_{CR} < 10$ ml/min)

$$\text{adjusted concentration} = \frac{\text{measured concentration}}{[(0.1 \times \text{albumin}) + 0.1]}$$

Estimated creatinine clearance in ml/min/70 kg

- $$\text{males} = \frac{[140 - \text{age (in years)}]}{\text{serum creatinine (in mg/dl)}}$$

- females = (male value) $\times 0.85$

Loading phenytoin

Intravenous
- 10–20 mg/kg at <50 mg/minute
- Monitor vital signs during load, especially blood pressure.
- May check levels from IV load approximately 2 hours after completion of dosing.

Oral
- 20 mg/kg in 3–4 divided doses given 2 hours apart.

Adjusting doses for sub-optimal serum levels

Intravenous
Dose (in mg/kg) = $0.7 \times (\text{plasma } C_{desired} - C_{observed})$

Oral

Dose (in mg/kg) = IV dose (in mg/kg) + 10%

Phenytoin (PHT): drug interactions

- Phenytoin has many drug interactions which should be carefully considered and may make its use undesirable.
- In general, phenytoin induces the CYP1A2, 2C, and 3A4 isoforms of the P450 oxidase system. In contrast, it inhibits the CYP2C9 isoform.
- A few important interactions are listed below.

Drugs which may increase PHT levels
- amiodarone
- diazepam
- disulfiram
- H_2-blockers
- isoniazid
- methylphenidate
- pheothiazines
- sulfonamides
- tobutamine
- trazadone

Drugs which may decrease PHT levels
- carbamazepine
- reserpine
- sucralfate
- Ca^{2+}-based antacids

Drugs with lowered efficacy on PHT
- corticosteroids
- oral contraceptives
- warfarin
- doxycycline
- furosemide
- estrogens
- rifampin
- theophylline
- vitamin D

Warfarin dosing and indications

Indications and goal INR

Indication	Goal INR
Atrial fibrillation	2–3
Tissue heart valves	2–3
Mechanical heart valves	2.5–3.5
Antiphospholipid antibody syndrome	3–4
Prevention/recurrent systemic embolism	2–3
DVT treatment	2–3
PE treatment	2–3

Dosing

Weight	Day 1	Day 2	Day 3	Day 4+
Loading method				
<50 kg or age >85 years	5 mg	5 mg	5 mg	2.5 mg (adjust PRN)
50–75 kg	7.5 mg	7.5 mg	5 mg	2.5 mg (adjust PRN)
75–100 kg	10 mg	10 mg	7.5 mg	2.5 mg (adjust PRN)
>100 kg	12.5 mg	12.5 mg	7.5 mg	2.5 mg (adjust PRN)
Nonloading method				
<50 kg or age >85 years	2 mg/day			Check INR in 5 days and adjust PRN
50–100 kg	2.5 mg/day			Check INR in 5 days and adjust PRN
>100 kg	4 mg/day			Check INR in 5 days and adjust PRN

Adjustment of dosing for goal INR of 2–3

INR	Adjustment	RECHECK INR
1.1–1.4	Increase total weekly dose 10–20%	1 week
1.5–1.9	Increase total weekly dose 5–10%	2 weeks
2–3	No change	4 weeks
3.1–3.9	Decrease total weekly dose 5–10%	2 weeks
4–5	Decrease total weekly dose 10–20%	1 week
>5	Stop warfarin until INR <3 then restart at 50% previous total weekly dose	Daily

Adjustment for dosing with supratherapeutic INR

- These serve as guidelines only, patient-specific plans should be developed based on overall clinical situation and inpatient/outpatient/fall-risk status.
- Use of subcutaneous vitamin K may cause warfarin resistance for up to a week.

INR	Patient condition	Adjustment
Above goal but <6	No bleeding, rapid reversal not required for specific intervention	Hold dosing until INR is in therapeutic range then reinitiate therapy at lower dose
6–10	No bleeding or rapid reversal is required for specific intervention	Administer 1 mg vitamin K sq. Reassess in 24 hours. May administer additional 0.5 mg if remains elevated
>10	No bleeding	Administer 3 mg vitamin K sq. Reassess in 6 hours. Repeat PRN
>20	Serious bleeding	Administer 10 mg vitamin K sq with fresh frozen plasma as needed. Reassess in 6 hours. Repeat PRN
>20	Life-threatening bleeding	Administer 10 mg vitamin K sq along with sq prothrombin complex concentrate. Reassess in 6 hours. Repeat PRN

Prognostication

Predicting outcome in hypoxic-ischemic coma

- The following algorithm is provided to assist in predicting long-term outcomes in comatose patients surviving hypoxic-ischemic insult.
- The actual outcomes should not be applied in absolute terms to any particular patient, as these are based on cohort series analyses.
- The statistics should only be used as guidelines as each patient must be evaluated as an individual case.
- Prior to evaluation, great care should be taken to ensure that:
  1 all toxic, infectious, metabolic, and medical comorbidities have been maximally managed,
  2 the patient is cleared of all sedating medications, and
  3 core body temperature is >35°C.
- Severe disability implies complete dependence for all ADLs, moderate disability implies some, though not complete, functional independence.

Initial exam

	Best 1 year recovery		
	Veg. state	Sev. disab.	Mod. disab.
Any two reactive? corneal, pupil, oculovestibular			
no	97%	2%	1%
yes → verbal: moans?			
yes	46%	13%	41%
no → motor: withdrawal?			
yes	58%	19%	23%
no → motor: extensor or flexor?			
yes	69%	14%	17%
no	80%	8%	12%

Exam @ 1 day

	Best 1 year recovery		
	Veg. state	Sev. disab.	Mod. disab.
Any three reactive? corneal, pupil, oculovestibular, motor			
no	98%	0%	2%
yes → verbal: at least inappropriate words?			
yes	0%	33%	67%
no → motor: at least withdrawal?			
yes	42%	21%	37%
no → any 1 present? oculoceph.: nl, oculovestib.: nl, spont. eye movt: nl, motor: ext. or flex.			
yes	76%	13%	11%
no	84%	11%	4%

Exam @ 3 days

	Best 1 year recovery		
	Veg. state	Sev. disab.	Mod. disab.
both reactive? corneal, motor			
no	96%	4%	0%
yes → verbal: at least inappropriate words			
yes	0%	26%	74%
no → motor: at least withdrawal?			
yes	40%	27%	33%
no	76%	16%	8%

Exam @ 7 days

	Best 1 year recovery		
	Veg. state	Sev. disab.	Mod. disab.
eye opening; at least to pain			
no	92%	8%	0%
yes → motor: at least localizing			
yes	1%	24%	75%
no	63%	28%	10%

Ref: Levy, *et al.*, *Ann Intern Med*, 1981; 94: 293–301

Predicting risk of stroke during coronary artery bypass surgery

- The following chart is provided to assist in assessing risk of stroke in patients with comorbidities undergoing coronary artery bypass surgery.
- The risks should not be applied in absolute terms to any particular patient, as they are based on cohort series analyses.
- The statistics should only be used as guidelines as outcomes may vary widely based on patients overall preoperative health, precise type and complexity of surgery, surgeons, and institutions.
- Risk of CNS injury (%) is determined on the y-axis after generating the cumulative stroke risk index (x-axis) by adding the age multiple to any additional applicable comorbidities.

Preoperative stroke risk for CABG surgery

Risk factor	Score
Age multiple	(age − 25) × 1.43
Unstable angina	14
Diabetes mellitus	17
Neurological disease	18
Prior CABG	15
Vascular disease	18
Pulmonary disease	15

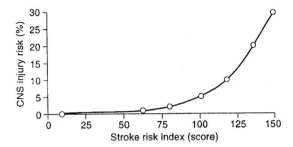

Definitions

- Diabetes mellitus: history of type I or II or preoperative insulin requirements.
- Vascular disease: PVD, carotid disease, claudication, or prior vascular surgery.
- Pulmonary disease: emphysema, chronic bronchitis, asthma, restrictive lung disease.
- Neurological disease: previous stroke or TIA.

Reference: Newman, *et al. Circ*, 1996; 94: 1174–80; Roach, *et al.*, *NEJM*, 1996; 335: 1857–1863.

Appendix B
Abbreviations

ACA anterior cerebral artery

ACoA anterior communicating artery

ACTH adrenocorticotrophic hormone

AlzD Alzheimer disease

AD autosomal dominant

ADL activity of daily living

AED antiepileptic drug

ALS amyotrophic lateral sclerosis

ALT alanine aminotransferase

Anti-MAG anti-myelin-associated glycoprotein

ASD atrial septal defect

AST aspartate aminotransferase

CABG coronary artery bypass graft

CBC complete blood count

CMT charcot-Marie-Tooth disease

CMV cytomegalovirus

CO carbon monoxide

CPK creatinine phosphokinase

CPR cardiopulmonary resuscitation

CaT capillary telangiectasia

CT computed tomography

DM diabetes mellitus

DSM diagnostic and statistical manual of mental disorders

DVT deep vein thrombosis

ESR erythrocyte sedimentation rate

FDG fluorodeoxyglucose

FLAIR fluid-attenuated inversion recovery

FSH follicle stimulating hormone

GH growth hormone

GRE gradient-recalled echo

GTC generalized tonic clonic

HTN hypertension

ICA   internal carotid artery
IDDM   insulin dependent diabetes mellitus
IHS   international headache society
INR   international normalized ratio
LH   luteinizing hormone
LMN   lower motor neuron
MCA   middle cerebral artery
MRA   magnetic resonance angiography
MRI   magnetic resonance imaging
MSG   monosodium glutamate
NM   neuromuscular
NOS   not otherwise specified
NREM   non-rapid eye movement
NTG   nitroglycerine
PCR   polymerase chain reaction
PE   pulmonary embolism
PMN   polymorphonuclear
PNET   primitive neuroectodermal tumor
PNS   peripheral nervous system
PO   per oral
PRN   when needed
PT   prothrombin time
PVD   peripheral vascular disease
REM   rapid eye movement
RPR   rapid plasma regain
SCA   spinocerebellar ataxia
SuCA   superior cerebellar artery
SE   spin echo
SIADH   syndrome of inappropriate antidiuretic hormone secretion
SSRI   selective serotonin reuptake inhibitor
STD   sexually transmitted disease
TIA   transient ischemic attack
TSH   thyroxine stimulating hormone
UMN   upper motor neuron
VEP   visual evoked potential
VF   visual field
Vim   ventral intermediate nucleus
VP   ventriculo-peritoneal
VSD   ventricular septal defect

Index